THE NATIVE AMERICAN HERBALIST'S BIBLE

6 in 1. The Complete Native American Herbalist Remedies Encyclopedia. Ancient Traditions and Practices to Naturally Improve Your Wellness

TATANKA DAVIS

First Printing Edition, 2021

Printed in the United Stated of America

Available from Amazon.com and Other Retail Outlets

TABLE OF CONTENTS

NATIVE AMERICAN HERBALISM ENCYCLOPEDIA

A Complete Medical Handbook of Native American Herbs

Taahira Maskwa

INTRODUCTION

Native American cultures across the United States are notable for their wide variety and diversity of lifestyles, regalia, art forms, and beliefs. The culture of indigenous North America is usually defined by the concept of the Pre-Columbian culture area, namely a geographical region where shared cultural traits occur. The northwest culture area, for example, shared common traits such as salmon fishing, woodworking, large villages or towns, and a hierarchical social structure. Though cultural features, language, clothing, and customs vary enormously from one tribe to another, certain elements are encountered frequently and shared by many tribes. Early European American scholars described the Native Americans as having a society dominated by clans.

Native American Cultures

Many thousands of years before Christopher Columbus' ships landed in the Bahamas, a different group of people discovered America: the nomadic ancestors of modern Native Americans who hiked over a "land bridge" from Asia to what is now Alaska more than 12,000 years ago. In fact, by the time European adventurers arrived in the 15th century A.D., scholars estimate that more than 50 million people were already living in the Americas. Of these, some 10 million lived in the area that would become the United States. As time passed, these migrants and their descendants pushed south and east, adapting as they went. To keep track of these diverse groups, anthropologists and geographers have divided them into "culture areas," or rough groupings of contiguous peoples who shared similar habitats and characteristics. Most scholars break North America excluding present-day Mexico into separate cultural areas: the Arctic, the Subarctic, the Northeast, the Southeast, the Plains, the Southwest, the Great Basin, California, the Northwest Coast, and the Plateau.

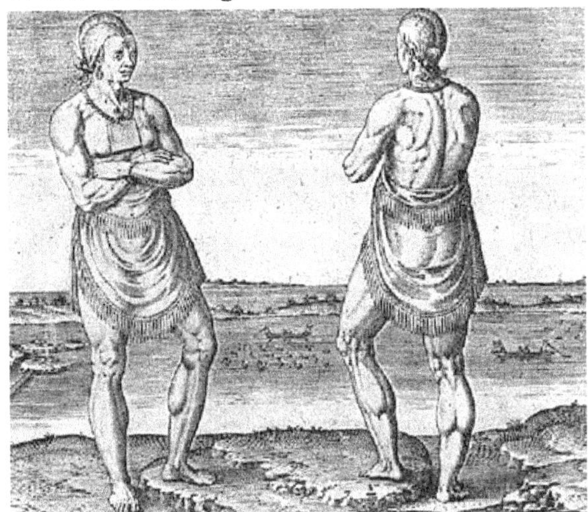

1. The Arctic

The Arctic culture area, a cold, flat, treeless region (actually a frozen desert) near the Arctic Circle in present-day Alaska, Canada, and Greenland, was home to the Inuit and the Aleut. Both groups spoke, and continue to speak, dialects descended from what scholars call the Eskimo-Aleut language family. Because it is such an inhospitable landscape, the Arctic's population was comparatively small and scattered. Some of its peoples, especially the Inuit in the northern part of the region, were nomads, following seals, polar bears, and other game as they migrated across the tundra. In the southern part of the region, the Aleut were a bit more settled, living in small fishing villages along the shore.

The Inuit and Aleut had a great deal in common. Many lived in dome-shaped houses made of sod or timber (or, in the North, ice blocks). They used seal and otter skins to make warm, weatherproof clothing, aerodynamic dogsleds, and long, open fishing boats (kayaks in Inuit; baidarkas in Aleut). By the time the United States purchased Alaska in 1867, decades of oppression and exposure to European diseases had taken their toll: The native population had dropped to just 2,500; the descendants of these survivors still make their home in the area today.

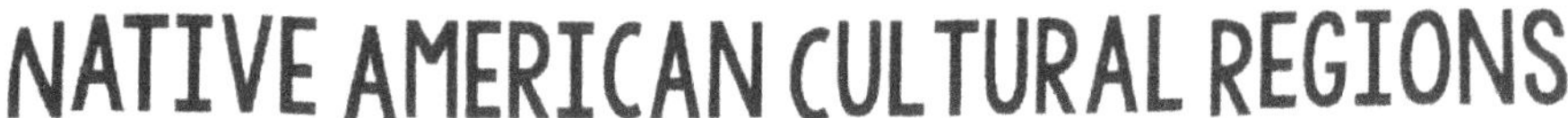

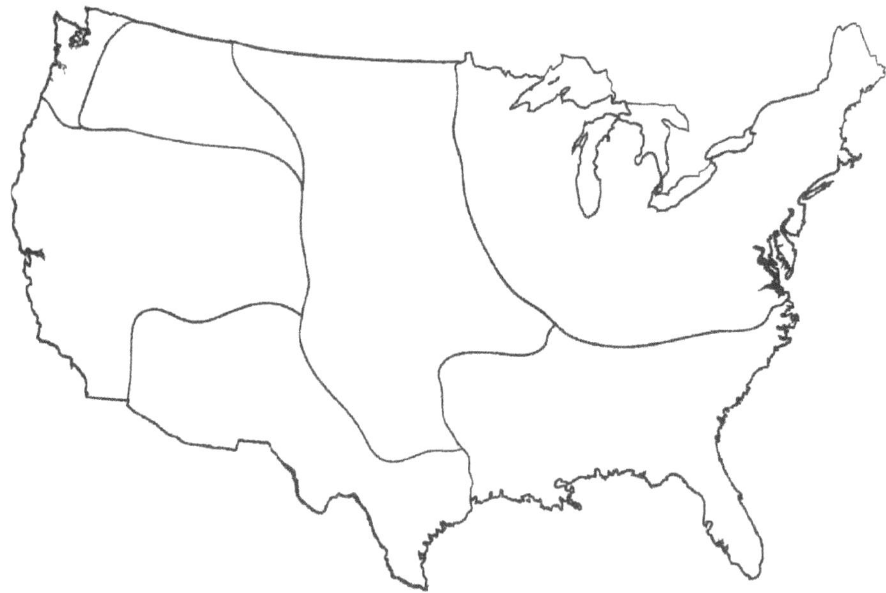

2. The Subarctic

The Subarctic culture area, mostly composed of swampy, piney forests (taiga) and waterlogged tundra, stretched across much of inland Alaska and Canada. Scholars have divided the region's people into two language groups: the Athabaskan speakers at its western end, among them the Tsattine (Beaver), Gwich'in (or Kuchin) and the Deg Xinag (formerly and pejoratively known as the Ingalik), and the Algonquian speakers at its eastern end, including the Cree, the Ojibwa, and the Naskapi. In the Subarctic, travel was difficult toboggans, snowshoes and lightweight canoes were the primary means of transportation and the population was sparse. In general, the peoples of the Subarctic did not form large permanent settlements; instead, small family groups stuck together as they traipsed after herds of caribou. They lived in small, easy-to-move tents and lean-tos, and when it grew too cold to hunt they hunkered into underground dugouts.

3. The Northeast

The Northeast culture area, one of the first to have sustained contact with Europeans, stretched from present-day Canada's Atlantic coast to North Carolina and inland to the Mississippi River valley. Its inhabitants were members of two main groups: Iroquoian speakers (these included the Cayuga, Oneida, Erie, Onondaga, Seneca, and Tuscarora), most of whom lived along inland rivers and lakes in fortified, politically stable villages, and the more numerous Algonquian speakers (these included the Pequot, Fox, Shawnee, Wampanoag, Delaware, and Menominee) who lived in small farming and fishing villages along the ocean. There, they grew crops like corn, beans, and vegetables.

Life in the Northeast culture area was already fraught with conflict the Iroquoian groups tended to be rather aggressive and warlike, and bands and villages outside of their allied confederacies were never safe from their raids and it grew more complicated when European colonizers arrived. Colonial wars repeatedly forced the region's natives to take sides, pitting the Iroquois groups against their Algonquian neighbors. Meanwhile, as white settlement pressed westward, it eventually displaced both sets of indigenous people from their lands.

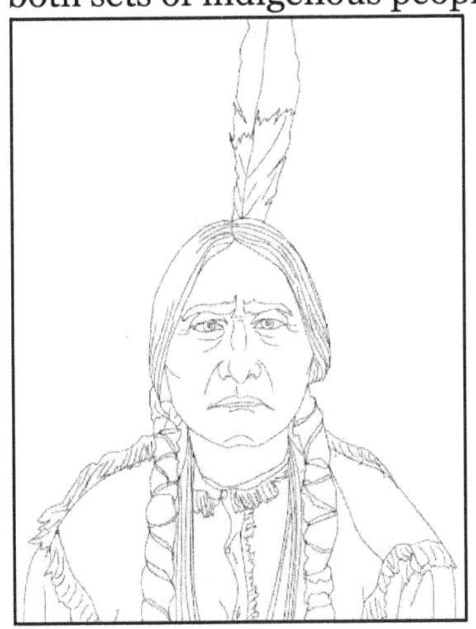

4. The Southeast

The Southeast culture area, north of the Gulf of Mexico and south of the Northeast, was a humid, fertile agricultural region. Many of its natives were expert farmers they grew staple crops like maize, beans, squash, tobacco, and sunflower who organized their lives around small ceremonial and market villages known as hamlets. Perhaps the most familiar of the Southeastern indigenous peoples are the Cherokee, Chickasaw, Choctaw, Creek, and Seminole sometimes called the Five Civilized Tribes, some of whom spoke a variant of the Muskogean language.

By the time the U.S. had won its independence from Britain, the Southeast culture area had already lost many of its native people to disease and displacement. In 1830, the federal Indian Removal Act compelled the relocation of what remained of the Five Civilized Tribes so that white settlers could have their land. Between 1830 and 1838, federal officials forced nearly 100,000 Indians out of the southern states and into "Indian Territory" (later Oklahoma) west of the Mississippi. The Cherokee called this frequently deadly trek the Trail of Tears.

5. The Plains

The Plains culture area comprises the vast prairie region between the Mississippi River and the Rocky Mountains, from present-day Canada to the Gulf of Mexico. Before the arrival of European traders and explorers, its inhabitant's speakers of Siouan, Algonquian, Caddoan, Uto-Aztecan, and Athabaskan languages were relatively settled hunters and farmers. After European contact, and especially after Spanish colonists brought horses to the region in the 18th century, the peoples of the Great Plains became much more nomadic. Groups like the Crow, Blackfeet, Cheyenne, Comanche, and Arapaho used horses to pursue great herds of buffalo across the prairie. The most common dwelling for these hunters was the cone-shaped teepee, a bison-skin tent that could be folded up and carried anywhere. Plains Indians are also known for their elaborately feathered war bonnets.

As white traders and settlers moved west across the Plains region, they brought many damaging things with them: commercial goods, like knives and kettles, which native people came to depend on; guns; and disease. By the end of the 19th century, white sport hunters had nearly exterminated the area's buffalo herds. With settlers encroaching on their lands and no way to make money, the Plains natives were forced onto government reservations.

6. The Southwest

The peoples of the Southwest culture area, a huge desert region in present-day Arizona and New Mexico (along with parts of Colorado, Utah, Texas, and Mexico) developed two distinct ways of life. Sedentary farmers such as the Hopi, the Zuni, the Yaqui, and the Yuma grew crops like corn, beans, and squash. Many lived in permanent settlements, known as pueblos, built of stone and adobe. These pueblos featured great multistory dwellings that resembled apartment houses. At their centers, many of these villages also had large ceremonial pit houses or kivas.

Other Southwestern peoples, such as the Navajo and the Apache, were more nomadic. They survived by hunting, gathering, and raiding their more established neighbors for their crops. Because these groups were always on the move, their homes were much less permanent than the pueblos. For instance, the Navajo fashioned their iconic eastward-facing round houses, known as hogans, out of materials like mud and bark.

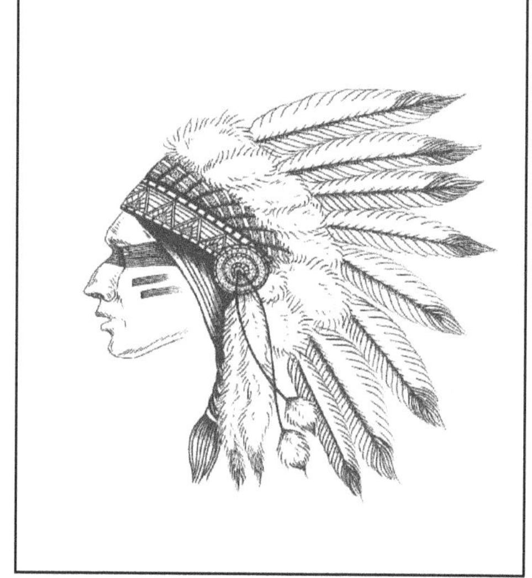

By the time the southwestern territories became a part of the United States after the Mexican War, many of the region's native people had already been exterminated. (Spanish colonists and missionaries had enslaved many of the Pueblo Indians, for example, working them to death on vast Spanish ranches known as encomiendas.) During the second half of the 19th century, the federal government resettled most of the region's remaining natives onto reservations.

7. The Great Basin

The Great Basin culture area, an expansive bowl formed by the Rocky Mountains to the east, the Sierra Nevadas to the west, the Columbia Plateau to the north, and the Colorado Plateau to the south, was a barren wasteland of deserts, salt flats, and brackish lakes. Its people, most of whom spoke Shoshonean or Uto-Aztecan dialects (the Bannock, Paiute, and Ute, for example), foraged for roots, seeds, and nuts and hunted snakes, lizards, and small mammals. Because they were always on the move, they lived in compact, easy-to-build wikiups made of willow poles or saplings, leaves, and brush. Their settlements and social groups were impermanent, and communal leadership (what little there was) was informal.

After European contact, some Great Basin groups got horses and formed equestrian hunting and raiding bands that were similar to the ones we associate with the Great Plains natives. After white prospectors discovered gold and silver in the region in the mid-19th century, most of the Great Basin's people lost their land and, frequently, their lives.

8. California

Before European contact, the temperate, hospitable California culture area had more people an estimated 300,000 in the mid-16th century than any other. It was also more diverse: Its estimated 100 different tribes and groups spoke more than 200 dialects. (These languages derived from the Penutian (the Maidu, Miwok, and Yokuts), the Hokan (the Chumash, Pomo, Salinas, and Shasta), the Uto-Aztecan (the Tubabulabal, Serrano and Kinatemuk; also, many of the "Mission Indians" who had been driven out of the Southwest by Spanish colonization spoke Uto-Aztecan dialects) and Athapaskan (the Hupa, among others). As one scholar has pointed out, California's linguistic landscape was more complex than that of Europe.

Despite this great diversity, many native Californians lived very similar lives. They did not practice much agriculture. Instead, they organized themselves into small, family-based bands of hunter-gatherers known as tribelets. Inter-tribelet relationships, based on well-established systems of trade and common rights, were generally peaceful.

Spanish explorers infiltrated the California region in the middle of the 16th century. In 1769, the cleric Junipero Serra established a mission at San Diego, inaugurating a particularly brutal period in which forced labor, disease, and assimilation nearly exterminated the culture area's native population.

9. The Northwest Coast

The Northwest Coast culture area, along the Pacific coast from British Columbia to the top of Northern California, has a mild climate and an abundance of natural resources. In particular, the ocean and the region's rivers provided almost everything its people needed salmon, especially, but also whales, sea otters, seals and fish, and shellfish of all kinds. As a result, unlike many other hunter-gatherers who struggled to eke out a living and were forced to follow animal herds from place to place, the Indians of the Pacific Northwest were secure enough to build permanent villages that housed hundreds of people apiece. Those villages operated according to a rigidly stratified social structure, more sophisticated than any outside of Mexico and Central America.

CHAPTER 1 : NATIVE AMERICAN MEDICINE AND MODERN USES

Native American medicine refers to the combined health practices of over 500 nations. The specific practices varied among tribes but all are based on the basic principle that man is part of nature and health is a matter of balance. The natural world drives when it's interrelationships are honored, nurtured, and kept in harmony. The natural world cannot be seen by the eye and is not involved in technology, but is experienced directly and intuitively. Just as one cannot measure the inner life of a human being, nature has compelling forces that need to be integrated for balance. Native medicine is 40,000 years old. Documentation has only now begun and has been limited to observations therefore is incomplete. Native medicine honors all creation and is not just an academic body of knowledge or technique. Native American elders usually do not share their knowledge for fear of exploitation. Native American medicine addresses the balance in the inner life and overt behavior. The body, mind, spirit, emotions, social group, and lifestyle are all taken into account. A patient's choice and preferences are always honored to create harmony.

Each Native American healer has their approach and can include bodywork, bone setting, midwifery, naturopathy, hydrotherapy, and botanical and nutritional medicine. Ceremonial and ritual medicine are also included. Much of this has been lost as this undocumented living tradition has only survived through living practitioners. More Native Americans have become interested in preserving their culture and through this effort Native, American medicine is as fluid today as ever.

Treatment Approaches - Different Types Of Treatments

Native American medicine is a complete system that balances every sphere of one's life from their inner world to lifestyle and social connections. Native medicine believes the roots of any imbalance are in the spiritual world. The spiritual interventions are critical to the process of any treatment plan.

Treatment approaches are always specifically and uniquely designed for the patient including fees and prices. They include the process of negotiating a fee as part of the healing process. The healing Elder has the most healing power and when treatment fails the elder practitioner loses the reputation as a powerful healer. The client in need of healing makes an offer to the medical practitioner and waits to see if it is accepted. They never negotiate face-to-face. The client leaves the offering outside the healer's door and if it is still there in the morning it has not been accepted and one can go elsewhere. Once they both agree, treatment may begin with the behavioral prescription, for example, a commitment, a selfless act, making amends, or climbing a sacred mountain. Techniques include self-inquiry and discovery to identify whether a lifestyle modification, herbs, prayer, massage, a sweat lodge ceremony, or a vision quest are necessary. GNC has been researching Indian herbs for a long time and has created some well-known supplements. You can try some with GNC coupons.

Training

Native American healers train their students through apprenticeships. Many years of testing a student's intention and commitment are essential for preparation. An apprentice learns patience, respect, and receives knowledge. Native medicine continues to be an oral tradition and cannot be learned in an academic setting. Only through experience can students learn the skills necessary and only when the student is ready does the elder teacher allow them to begin the practice of medicine.

Short Summary Of Native American Medicine

Many aspects of Native American healing have been kept secret and are not written down. The traditions are passed down by word of mouth from elders, from the spirits in vision quests, and through initiation. It is believed that sharing healing knowledge too readily or casually will weaken the spiritual power of the medicine.

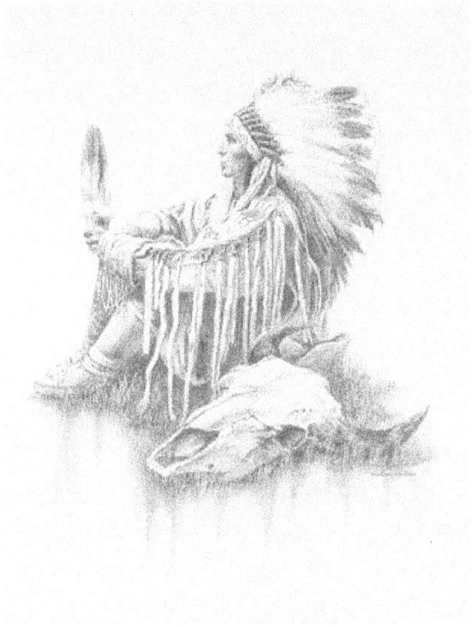

There are, however, many Native American healers who recognize that writing down their healing practices is a way to preserve these traditions for future generations. Many also believe that sharing their healing ways and values may help all people to come into a healthier balance with nature and all forms of life.

Benefits

Native American medicine can benefit anyone who sincerely wishes to live a life of wholeness and balance. These benefits may be physical, emotional, or spiritual. There is, however, the understanding that "the diseases of civilization," or white man's diseases, often need white man's medicine. In those cases, Native American medicine can be an important part of an integrative approach to healing. For example, the most successful programs for treating alcohol addiction in Native communities have combined Western approaches to psychological counseling, social work, and traditional Native American healing practices.

Such inherited conditions as birth defects or retardation are not easily treatable with Native American medicine. Native healers also believe that some illnesses are the result of a patient's behavior. Sometimes they will not treat a person because they do not want to interfere with the life lessons the patient needs to learn. Other illnesses are not treated because they are "callings" or initiation diseases. Native healer Medicine Grizzly Bear Lake explains, "The calling comes in the form of a dream, accident, sickness, injury, disease, near-death experience, or even actual death."

Description

Native American medicine is based upon a spiritual view of life. A healthy person is someone who has a sense of purpose and follows the guidance of the Great Spirit. This guidance is written upon the heart of every person. To be healthy, a person must be committed to a path of beauty, harmony, and balance. Gratitude, respect, and generosity are also considered to be essential for a healthy life.

Ken Cohen writes, "Health means restoring the body, mind, and spirit to balance and wholeness: the balance of life energy in the body; the balance of ethical, reasonable, and just behavior; balanced relations within family and community; and harmonious relationships with nature."

Theories of disease causation and even the names of diseases vary from tribe to tribe. Diseases may be thought to have internal or external causes or sometimes both. According to Cherokee medicine man Rolling Thunder, negative thinking is the most important internal cause of disease. Negative thinking includes not only negative thoughts about oneself but also feelings of shame, blame, low self-esteem, greed, despair, worry, depression, anger, jealousy, and self-centeredness. Johnny Moses, a Nootka healer, says "No evil sorcerer can do as much harm to you as you can do to yourself."

Diseases have external causes too. "Germs are also spirits," according to Shabari Bird of the Lakota Nation. A person is particularly susceptible to harmful germs if they live an imbalanced life, have a weak constitution, engage in negative thinking, or are under a lot of stress. Other people or spirits may also be responsible for an illness. Another external source of the disease is environmental poisons. These poisons include alcohol, impure air, water, and some types of food.

Native American healers believe that disease can also be caused by physical, emotional, or spiritual trauma. These traumas can lead to mental and emotional distress, loss of soul, or loss of spiritual power. In these cases, the healer must use ritual and other ways to physically return the soul and power to the patient. Some diseases are caused when people break the "rules for living." These rules may include ways of showing respect for animals, people, places, ritual objects, events, or spirits.

Native American healers have several different techniques for diagnosing an illness. These may include a discussion of one's symptoms, personal and family history, observation of non-verbal cues like posture or tone of voice, and medical divination. More important than the particular technique is the healer's intuition, sensitivity, and spiritual power.

There is no typical Native American healing session. Methods of healing include prayer, chanting, music, smudging (burning sage or aromatic woods), herbs, laying-on of hands, massage, counseling, imagery, fasting, harmonizing with nature, dreaming, sweat lodges, taking hallucinogens (e.g., peyote), developing inner silence, going on a shamanic journey, and ceremony. Family and community are also important in many healing sessions. Sometimes healing happens quickly. Sometimes a long period is needed for healing. The intensity of the therapy is considered to be more important than the length of time required. Even if the healing happens quickly, however, a lifestyle change is usually required to make the healing last.

A medicine bundle may also be used in Native American healing. The medicine bundle is a bag made of leather or an animal pelt in which the healer carries an assortment of ritual objects, charms, herbs, stones, and other healing paraphernalia. The bundle is a concrete token of the medicine power that the spirits have given the healer, either for healing in general or for healing a particular illness. The bundles vary according to the clan, tribe, and individual.

Native American medicine is not covered by insurance unless perhaps the practitioner is a licensed health care provider. Most Native healers do not charge a set fee for their services. Healing is considered to be "a gift from the Great Spirit." Gifts to the healer are welcomed, however. The offering of a gift "ensures the success of treatment because healing spirits appreciate the generosity." Gifts may include groceries, cloth, money, or another personal expression of respect and appreciation. Frequently the only gift that is required is a pouch of tobacco.

Preparations

The medicine person tells the patient what preparations are necessary before the healing ceremony.

Precautions

A medicine person is essential to ensure safe healing through Native American medicine. People with hypertension should watch themselves during a sweat lodge ceremony for a possible increase in blood pressure. People with asthma may have difficulty when sage or cedar is used in a ceremony. Claustrophobic people may find the close, hot, dark environment of a sweat lodge overwhelming.

Side Effects

Some herbs may cause vomiting, nausea, or diarrhea. From the Native American point of view, these reactions are usually welcomed and considered a form of purging or cleansing of the physical body.

Research & General Acceptance

There has been no formal scientific research conducted on Native American healing practices. Medicine people do not write down their practices out of fear that they might be misused by people who are not trained in their sacred ways. The most prominent users of this form of medicine are Native Americans or others who want a spiritually-based approach to medicine.

Training & Certification

Native American medicine has been passed down by word of mouth for thousands of years. Healing power can come from one's ancestors, another healer, or through training and initiation. Generally, healers train under one primary mentor. Today, however, with the ease of long-distance travel and communication, many healers have several mentors. Training as a medicine person is a long process that requires strength, sacrifice, and patience. Denet Tsosie, a Navajo medicine man, said that it took him six years to learn one of the chants.

Native American Herbal Medicine And Modern Health Supplements

Herbals And Herbalists

For most of human history, people have relied on herbalism for at least some of their medicinal needs, and this remains true for more than half of the world's population in the twenty-first century. Much of our modern pharmacopeia also has its roots in the historical knowledge of medicinal plants.

What Are Herbs, Herbals, And Herbalists?

To botanists, herbs are plants that die back to the ground after flowering, but more generally, herbs are thought of as plants with medicinal, culinary (especially seasoning), or aromatic uses. Traditional herbals are compilations of information about medicinal plants, typically including plant names, descriptions, and illustrations, and information on medicinal uses. Herbals have been written for thousands of years and form an important historical record and scientific resource. Many plant medicines listed in older herbals are still used in some form, but some herbals, especially earlier ones, also contain much inaccurate information and plant lore.

Herbalists follow a long tradition of using plants and plant-based medicines for healing purposes. Some gather medicinal plants locally, while others use both local and foreign plant material. Some rely on age-old knowledge and lore, while others also consult the findings of new research.

Herbal Medicine Today

Today, traditional herbalist healers continue to use the knowledge passed down for generations. Some ethnobotanists are studying with traditional healers to save such knowledge before it disappears. Due to a growing interest in alternative medicine, herbalism is also attracting new practitioners, and herbal research is constantly underway. Critics note that dosages can be difficult to control, even among plants of the same species, and side effects can be unpredictable.

Several essential modern drugs are derived from plants and scientists generally agree that only a fraction of the world's plants have been studied for their medicinal potential. However, threats to the environment, particularly in tropical forests where the highest numbers of species (many still unknown to science) reside, may reduce the possibility of identifying new plant-derived drugs.

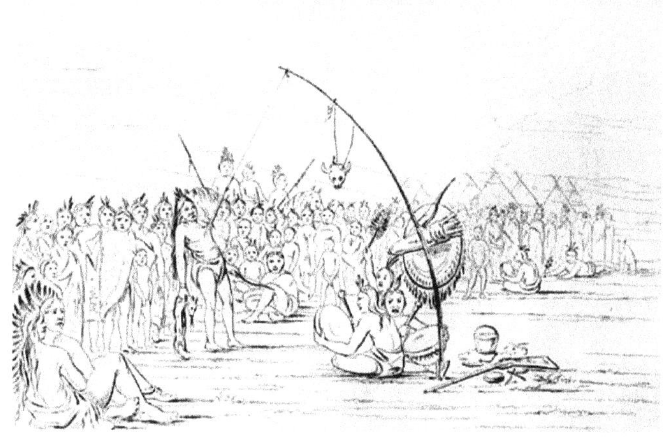

How Plant Pharmaceuticals Are Discovered

The search for new pharmaceuticals from plants is possible using several distinct strategies. Random collecting of plants by field gathering is the simplest but least efficient way. The chances are much greater than new compounds of medicinal value will be discovered if there is some degree of selectivity employed by collecting those plants that a botanist knows are related to others already having useful or abundant classes of secondary metabolites. Even more relevant is to collect plants already targeted for specific medicinal purposes, possibly among indigenous or ethnic peoples who use traditional, plant-derived medicines often with great success to provide for their well-being. Such data are part of ethnobotany when researchers often obtain detailed information on the plants people use to treat illnesses, such as the species, specific disease being treated, plant part preferred, and how that part is prepared and used for treatment. This strategy can provide rapid access to plants already identified by traditional practitioners as having value for curing diseases, and this shortcut often sets the researcher rapidly on the road to the discovery of new drugs.

Taking the ethnobotanical approach, a specific part of the targeted ethnomedicinal plant is extracted, usually in a solvent like ethanol, and then studied in directed assays or tests to determine its value using, for instance, tissue-cultured cells impregnated with the organism known to cause the disease. For example, to assay for malaria the procedure could involve culturing red blood cells infected with the malarial-causing protozoan Plasmodium falciparum, placing a few drops of extract into the culture, and examining after a few days what effect, if any, the addition of the extract had on the protozoa. One final step in this process leading to the discovery of a new drug is to establish the mechanism of action of the compound, reactions in the body, and side effects or toxicity of taking it. The whole process from field discovery to a new pharmaceutical takes up to ten years and requires a multidisciplinary-interactive approach involving ethnobotanists, natural products chemists, pharmacognosists (those who study the biochemistry of natural products), and cell and molecular biologists.

CHAPTER 2 : MEDICINAL PLANTS

Plants can not run away from their enemies nor get rid of troublesome pests as humans or other animals do, so what have they evolved to protect themselves? Whatever this protection is it must be successful, for the diversity and richness of green plants is extraordinary, and their dominance in most ecosystems of the world is unquestioned. Plant successes are closely intertwined with the evolution and production of highly diverse compounds known as secondary metabolites, compounds that are not essential for growth and reproduction, but rather, through interaction with their environment, enhance plant prospects of survival. These metabolites are therefore planted agents for chemical warfare, allowing plants to ward off microorganisms, insects, and other animals acting as predators and pathogens. Such compounds may also be valuable to humans for the same purposes, and therefore may be used as medicines.

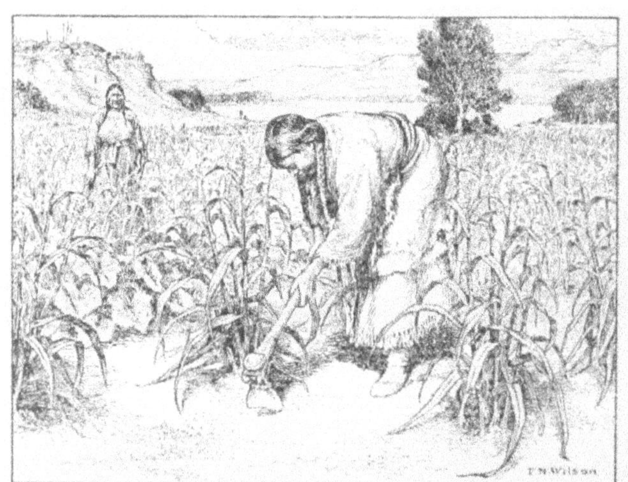

What Characterizes Medicinal Plants

There are twenty thousand known secondary plant metabolites, all exhibiting a remarkable array of organic compounds that provide a selective advantage to the producer, which outweighs their cost of production. Humans benefit from their production by using many of them for medicinal purposes to fight infections and diseases. An estimated two-fifths of all modern pharmaceutical products in the United States contain one or more naturally derived ingredients, the majority of which are secondary metabolites, such as alkaloids, glycosides, terpenes, steroids, and other classes grouped according to their physiological activity in humans or chemical structure.

To illustrate the breadth of human reliance on medicinal plants, the accompanying table provides a list of the most significant plants, their uses in modern medicine, and the major secondary metabolites responsible for their activities. This list grows annually as new plants are found with desired activities and remedies to become pharmaceuticals for use in medicine.

Wildcrafting

Wildcrafting is the practice of foraging for useful plants from their natural, wild habitat for edible or medicinal purposes. It applies to uncultivated plants wherever they may be found, and is not necessarily limited to wilderness areas. Ethical considerations are often involved, such as protecting endangered species, the potential for depletion of commonly held resources, and in the context of private property, preventing theft of valuable plants, for example, ginseng.

Tips For Wildcrafting Medicinal Herbs

Here are 10 tips for wildcrafting medicinal herbs that will help you on your plant foraging journey.

1. Get A Few Good Plant Identification Books For Your Area.

You will want to invest in 2 or 3 good plant identification books to help you. It's especially helpful to find books that are geared towards medicinal and edible plants, and even better if you can find one specifically for your region. Try to go on a few plant walks with a local expert before venturing out on your own, and be 100% sure of your plant identification before harvesting, as there are some toxic lookalikes.

2. Be Prepared.

Before you leave, put together a backpack or bag with your plant books, water, a snack or two, extra clothing, and even a small first aid kit (make a Hiking First Aid Kit). You will also want to bring a pocket knife and scissors and/or small pruners for collecting. If you think you might be collecting some roots, a small gardener's trowel is also handy. Small baggies of some sort for your collections are helpful as well.

3. Get Outside!

This is the best part about wildcrafting, it gets you outside, exercising in nature, all with a purpose. It doesn't matter if you go for a long hike in the woods or a stroll in your neighborhood, medicinal plants grow everywhere. You just have to get outside and start looking!

4. Walk Slowly.

As a longtime hiker, this one was hard for me to start doing. I like to walk fast and get in some good mileage, but when your goal is to collect wild plants, you need to take it slow so that you have the chance to notice your surroundings. If you're like me and you have a hard time with slowing down, maybe take a child or an elderly person with you. They naturally walk slow and force you to move at a different pace, plus I'm sure they would love the adventure!

5. Keep Your Eyes Peeled.

As you're walking slowly, look down. Scan the trail, path, or sidewalk that you're walking on. Look in all directions, and sometimes even behind you. Look up. Stop from time to time just to take in your surroundings. Pick out plants and practice looking them up in your identification books. Just keep looking!

6. Look In Uncommon (And Common) Places.

When you're on the trail, try going off trail for a bit. Be gentle when doing this, as you don't want to disturb the natural habitat. Beyond the woods, however, there are many places to wildcraft.

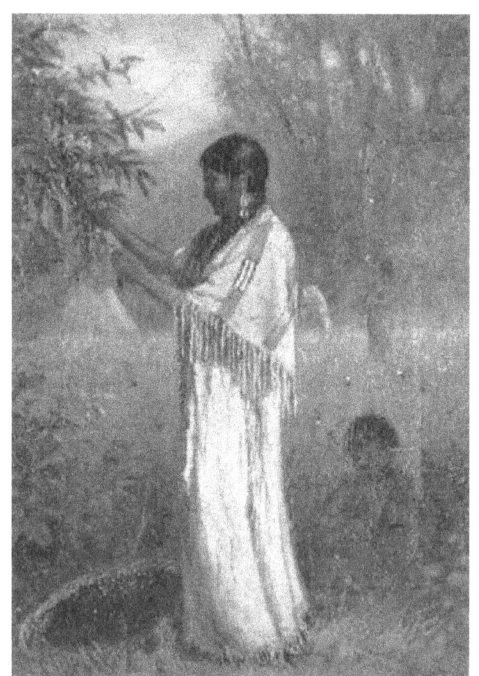

Sidewalks and quiet gravel road edges are good places to look, as are open fields and empty lots. Make sure to get permission first for anything that is private property, and steer clear of busy roadsides to avoid runoff and pesticide contaminants. Also avoid areas that are close to industrial and construction sites, under power lines, or near commercial farms that could be using pesticides and have a toxic runoff. Many local places like parks, green spaces, and school grounds can also be good; just be sure to check that collecting wild plants is allowed before you start. Wherever you collect, be sure that the plants aren't being sprayed with pesticides and are not growing on polluted land, and always check if foraging is allowed. You might even want to look in your backyard!

7. Don't Set Out To Find A Specific Plant.

Unless you know without a doubt that a specific plant grows in a specific place, you don't want to set yourself up for failure by thinking that you're going to go out and collect a whole bunch of a certain plant. Half of the fun is the adventure and not knowing what you're going to find. Often, I will find several plant varieties, but on rare occasions, I won't find any. That's just how it goes sometimes.

8. Don't Overlook Common Plants.

There are so many medicinal plants that we have all grown up with that are easily identifiable. Dandelion, red clover, plantain, yarrow, mullein, rosehips, and elderberry are just a few. Learn about common plants like these first, then move on to more uncommon or harder to find plants.

9. Be Mindful Of Plants That Are Rare Or Endangered.

Research which medicinal plants are rare or endangered, and do not take any of those. Overharvesting can be devastating for many threatened plant species. Some examples of medicinal plants that are at-risk are slippery elm, American ginseng, black cohosh, and goldenseal.

10. Leave More Than You Take.

Finally, even for abundant plants, do not take them all. If you want these wonderful medicinal plants to keep on giving us their wonderful benefits, we have to leave some for future years. So always leave more than you take (a general rule is to harvest just 5-10% of a population), and better yet, plant a seed of the same variety whenever you remove a plant.

Wildcrafting is an endeavor that every herbalist should try. These 10 tips for wildcrafting medicinal herbs should give you a good head start. The most important part is to just start looking, soon you'll be surprised by how many plants you can identify!

Growing And Propagation

Medicinal plants can be cultivated by two methods (applicable to non-medicinal plants): Sexual and Asexual method

1. Sexual Method (Seed Propagation):

In this method, the plants are raised from seeds. Such plants are known as seedlings. Seeds are sown in the fields by methods like broadcast, dibbling, or placing them in drills or holes. The seeds must be of good quality, capable of high germination rate, and free from diseases.

Advantages:

- Seedlings are comparatively much cheaper and easy to raise.
- Seedlings are long-lived, bear more heavy fruits, and plants obtained are more sturdy.
- In those plants where other methods of cultivation cannot be utilized, seed propagation becomes the only method of choice.
- There are chances of production of some chance-seedlings of very high superiority which may be of great importance e.g., orange, papaya, etc.

Disadvantages:

- The seedlings obtained from this method require more time to bear and are not uniform in their growth and yielding capacity as compared to other methods like grafting.
- Also, the cost involved in harvesting and protection from pests is more.

2. Asexual Methods (Vegetative Propagation):

In this method, any of the vegetative parts of the plant like root or stem is provided such an environment that it develops into a new plant. The environment is provided by setting various parts of the plant in well-prepared soil.

1. Bulbs: A bulb is originally and structurally a bud, which possesses the capability of perennation. It consists of a very short stem ending in an apical meristem and enclosed by closely set leaves, which are thick and fleshy, being stored with reserves of food. Each of the leaves has of course its axillary bud.

After flowering, the foliage leaves persist for a time, forming food materials, which are now stored in one or more of the axillary buds. The axillary buds thus used as storehouses become the bulbs of the new generation. Whenever more than one new bulb is formed from an old one, there has been vegetative reproduction as well as perennation e.g., Squill, garlic.

2. Corms: In a corm, the storage organ is swollen base of the stem and this is wrapped in thin scale-leaves, each of which, of course, has an axillary bud e.g. colchicum, saffron.

3. Tubers: It is a swelling on an underground stem branch. The stem grows axillary buds formed low down on the aerial stem and push through the soil, swelling at their ends to form the tubers e.g., jalap, aconite, potato.

4. Rhizomes: In underground stems, the older parts of the rhizome die off. The buds borne on the detached younger portions thus become separate new plants e.g., ginger, turmeric.

5. Runners: The stem grows along the ground (horizontally over the surface of the soil), and produces roots and erect flowering shoots from lateral buds at many of its nodes. The growth of the creeping stem is continued by the terminal bud. Some of the older internodes die, and the detached rooted and shoot bearing parts become independent plants e.g., peppermint, strawberry.

6. Suckers: A shoot arising from a root of a woody plant e.g., mint, pineapple, banana.

7. Offsets: These originate from the axil of the leaf as short thick horizontal branches and are also characterized by the presence of rosette types of leaves and a cluster of roots at their bottom e.g., aloe, valerian.

8. Stolons: A creeping stem that roots at nodes e.g., arrow-root, licorice.

9. Cutting: A clear cut is made preferably below the node and the lower leaves are removed. It is then placed in a suitable medium and provided with suitable conditions of the moist atmosphere, temperature which favoring the development of roots e.g., mint, vanilla.

10. Layering: A layer is a branch or a shoot that is induced to develop roots before it is completely severed from the parent plant. It is done by a cut or ligature and embedding the part so treated in the soil e.g., cascara.

11. Grafting And Budding: Grafting is a process in which two cut surfaces of different but closely related plants are placed to unite and grow together. The rooted portion is called the stock and the cut-off is the scion or graft e.g., female scion of Myristica fragrans on the male stock to increase the fruit-bearing proportion.

12. Aseptic Methods Of Propagation: In this method, the plants are developed in an artificial medium under aseptic conditions from very fine pieces of plants like single cells, callus, seeds, embryos, root tips, shoot tips, pollen grains, etc. They are provided with nutritional and hormonal requirements.

Advantages (Asexual Method):

- There is no variation between the plant grown and the plant from which it is grown. As such, the plants are uniform in growth and yielding capacity.
- Seedless varieties of fruits can only be propagated vegetatively e.g., pomegranates, grapes, lemon.
- Plants start bearing earlier as compared to seedlings.
- Budding or grafting encourages disease-resistant varieties of plants.

Disadvantages:

- In comparison to seedling trees, these are not vigorous in growth and are not long-lived.
- No new varieties can be evolved by this method.

Collecting, Drying, And Storing Medicinal Plants

Drying Herbs

After you harvest your herbs, the next step is to preserve them in a way that prolongs their potency for future use. This allows us to have access to these medicinal herbs all year long. Drying (dehydrating) your herbs can be done in one of two easy ways at home.

Herbs dry best in warm, shaded, well-ventilated areas. It is not recommended to dry them in the sun; the intense heat and rays of the sun can quickly degrade the plant's medicinal constituents. Instead, I prefer to create small bundles of herbs that I hold together with a rubber band placed at the end of the stems. I then hang them upside down on a string in my kitchen window until they are dried completely. For each herb, the drying time will be different so check them daily. You may also choose to lay your herbs flat on a screen or oven rack placed on the counter. This way allows air to flow freely through the plant while they dry but it does take up valuable counter space for several days to a week.

If you have a food dehydrator, you can complete the drying process very quickly. You just set your dehydrator and be on your way.

If you are choosing to dry roots of herbs, I recommend that you clean and chop your roots while they are fresh, before drying. Once a root dries it may become so dense and tough that cutting it into small pieces could take an act of God. Doing some shopping ahead of time will save you a great deal of heartache.

Garbling Your Dried Herbs

Once you have completed the drying process, it is time to garble your herbs. Garbling is the process of separating the leaves, flowers, and stem portions and discarding the unwanted parts. Each medicinal herb has its medicinal part so be sure to research which part you are wanting from your chosen herb.

Storing Your Herbs

Once you have completed your drying and garbling it is time to store your herbs. For best preservation, you want to keep your herbs in airtight containers and away from excess heat and sunlight. I prefer to store my herbs in large mason jars with a tight-fitting lid and then placed them in a cupboard. If you have open shelves in your kitchen that do not receive direct sunlight then your jars of herbs would be a beautiful addition to your décor.

Herbs should maintain their potency in your mason jars for up to two years as long as they were dried properly. It would be wise to check them periodically to be certain there is no mold growth; A few ways to determine if your herbs are still good is to observe any changes in their color and aroma. If you find that they just don't look or smell right, then it is time to toss them.

6 Tips For Storing Dried Herbs

When putting together an herbal apothecary, dried herbs take center stage. Dried herbs are the first ingredient in so many different herbal preparations like herbal teas, infused oils, and tinctures. As one starts amassing a collection of dried herbs, it becomes increasingly important to be sure that you are storing dried herbs properly to ensure the highest level of potency.

The main culprits to the degradation of dried herbs are moisture, oxygen, sunlight, heat, and time. Different types of herbs also have different storage lives. Dried flowers and leaves will lose their potency faster than roots and seeds, for example. Keeping track of when the herbs were acquired is also important to have the highest quality herbs for your preparations. These 6 tips for storing dried herbs will greatly help you to increase their shelf life, keeping them fresh for as long as possible.

1. Whole Herbs Last Longer

The first thing to consider is that herbs in their whole form last longer. If you can store the whole herb and then grind them as needed, you will get a much fresher and stronger product. A good rule of thumb is to store them in the largest form that you can. Of course, this isn't always possible, and some herbs are easier to store in the whole form than others, such as roots, seeds, or whole flower buds.

2. Make Sure Your Herbs Are Dry

When you are preparing to store dried herbs, it's important to make sure that they are totally dry first. This applies if you are wildcrafting or harvesting fresh herbs from your backyard and then drying them for later use. You will want to make sure that there is absolutely no moisture left when they are finished drying. A good way to check is to rub a bit between your fingers—it should crumble easily and be almost crispy to the touch. A great way to dry your herbs is with a homemade drying screen, in a dehydrator, or by simply hanging them upside down.

3. Store In Airtight Containers

Oxygen will degrade herbs over time, so storing your dried herbs in airtight containers is best. Glass jars or metal tins with screw top lids work well, as do jars with clamp-on lips (Fido style). Avoid using plastic if possible, as it may leach chemicals into your herbs.

4. Keep Out Of Direct Sunlight

While those rays of sunlight hitting your jars of herbs might look pretty, they are doing damage to the potency of the herbs. For this reason, it's best to store them out of direct sunlight. Using dark-colored glass jars is even better for blocking all potential light. Keep them in a closed cabinet or make a curtain to cover them if need be.

5. Keep In A Cool And Dry Location

You want your herbs to stay cool and dry for maximum shelf life. Do not store them near a hot stove or in a steamy bathroom. A root cellar is ideal if you have one, or in a bedroom that is on the coolest side of your house.

6. Be Sure To Label Harvest Or Purchase Date

Keeping track of how old your herbs are is an important habit to develop. Whenever you put a new herb on the shelf, label what it is and when it was harvested or purchased.

Here Is A Good List To Follow When Labeling:

- Name
- Botanical name
- Harvest date (if known)
- Purchase date (if applicable)
- Discard date

Having the highest quality herbs is something that all herbalists should strive for, and it isn't hard if a little care is taken. Besides knowing that it's what is best for your herbs, it's also a good feeling to have a clean and organized apothecary. Labels with names and dates take all guesswork out of it, and you can get into a system of replenishing when the need arises. Make your herbal apothecary your space, treat it like a special place, and your dried herbs will last for quite a while. If you follow these 6 tips for storing dried herbs, you will have the freshest herbs possible in your herbal apothecary!

Herbal Preparation Methods

Infusion

This is often referred to as a "tea". An infusion is used to draw out the most fragile of healing properties of plants. Water is used to extract vitamins, some volatile oils, sugars, enzymes and other proteins, tannins, saponins, glycosides, bitter compounds, polysaccharides (when hot water used), pectins, and some alkaloids. Infusions are most often used with the softer parts of a plant – leaves, and flowers. There are a few exceptions, like Goldenseal root and Valerian root.

Infusions Can Be Done Hot Or Cold.

For a cold infusion, place the plant material in the cold water (I prefer steam distilled water) and allow it to "steep" for 4 to 8 hours, depending on the herb. This can be done at room temperature or in the fridge.

For a hot infusion, place 1 tsp. of the dried herb, or 2 tbsp. of the fresh herb in a cup pour 1 cup of boiling water over the herb cover and allow to steep for 10 minutes, or until cool enough to drink. These are very general guidelines and can be adjusted according to need or taste. If you are going to make a pint of infusion, adjust the amount of herb. If you need a stronger infusion, use more herbs.

Somewhere between the two is "sun tea" prepare the herbs as you would for a hot infusion, but pour room temperature water in the container. Tightly cover the container (a mason jar is great for this) and leave on a sunny window sill or outside in the sun for 4 to 8 hours. This works well. Herb "teas" can be soothing, refreshing, invigorating, and very healthful. They are the easiest of preparations and are quickly absorbed into your system.

Decoction

A decoction is used most often with more woody, resinous material, like roots, bark, seeds, and nuts. To make a decoction, use approximately the same amount of herb to water as for an infusion. You can either place the herbs in boiling water (at a very low boil, or simmer) or put the herbs in cold water and bring it up to a boil over low heat. The pot (NEVER use aluminum!) should have a tight-fitting lid. Once the water is simmering, cover and allow to simmer for approximately 20 minutes (some herbs need longer). Take off the heat, allow to cool, strain, and drink. Or, you can allow the decoction to steep all night, strain, and drink in the morning.

Juice

Some plants are best used for juicing the fresh plant. Fresh, spring picked nettles or wheatgrass is very nutritious this way. If you have a wheatgrass juicer, it can be used with other herbs. A Champion

Juicer can be used if you combine the herb with some vegetables, like celery or carrot. Or, you can put the plant material in a blender with some pineapple juice, but some oxidation happens with this method, and you need to strain the liquid before drinking. If you happen to have a hydraulic press, you can also try pressing the plants to get the juice.

Fomentation

A fomentation is taking an infusion or decoction (often double or quadruple strength) and dipping some natural material (cotton, wool, silk) in the liquid, wringing out the excess liquid, and placing the soaked cloth over the affected area. You can also place a dry towel or cloth over the fomentation to keep it warm as long as possible, and some plastic wrap over that helps keep the liquid from dripping out.

Poultice

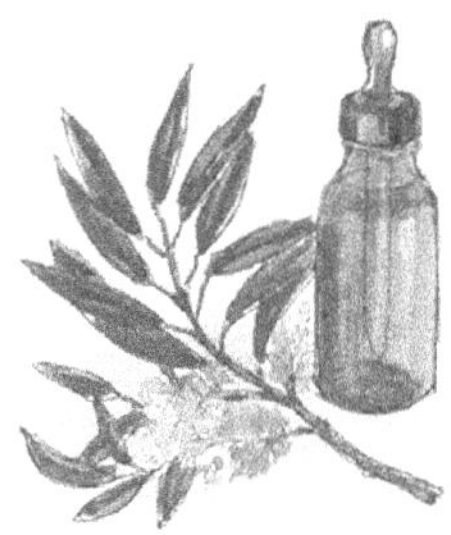

A poultice is the plant material itself placed over an affected area. Usually, the herb is bruised or macerated and placed over the injury or affected area, and covered with a bandage. It can be as simple as tearing up and bruising some yarrow leaves, and placing them over a cut, or putting some plantain leaves in your mouth, chewing them until they are a soft mass, and placing that over a bee sting. You can also use something like flaxseed to hold the herb in place. Grind up some flaxseed, mix in some of the powdered, fresh, or tinctured herb, and apply to the problem area. The ground flaxseed makes a sticky mass and may need nothing to hold it in place. If the flax seeds have been warmed up, this can be a warm poultice.

Oils

Extra virgin, cold-pressed olive oil is my oil of choice for making herbal oils. Olive oil takes a long time to go rancid at room temperature, and it is very nutritive in its own right. You can also use cold-pressed almond oil, grape seed oil, or apricot oil. These are especially good for facial products (considered cosmetic grade oils). Be sure to use the freshest, highest grade of oil.

You can use dried herbs or fresh herbs in your oil. If you use fresh herbs, make sure there is no excess moisture on the plant material. You can "wilt" the plants (let them dry in a warm place out of direct sunlight) for a few hours to be sure that there is no excess moisture.

Place your herbs in the container either a mason jar or a non-aluminum pan with a tight lid. Pour enough oil to cover the herbs and, in a mason jar, add 2 to 3 inches more of oil, or, in a non-aluminum pot, add another inch of oil. This keeps the herbs from poking out of the oil and attracting bacteria, which would spoil the oil.

If you wish to infuse the oil, place a tight lid (for dried herbs) or a clean cloth held on with a rubber band (for fresh herbs) on the jar and put the jar in a sunny window for two weeks.

You can place your mason jar of herbs and oil in the oven as is, or in a pan of water so that the water comes halfway up the side of the jar in the oven. Turn the oven onto the lowest heat setting, and leave the jar in there for 1 to 3 hours. The temperature of the oil should never go above 120 degrees Fahrenheit.

For a faster oil, place the dried, fresh herbs in the top of a double boiler (glass or stainless steel) and cover with oil as instructed above. Cover, and bring the water up to a slow simmer. Keep it there for 30 minutes to 3 hours, depending on how hot the oil gets. As warned above, the oil should never get over

120 degrees Fahrenheit. Around 100 degrees is preferable. Keeping the oil at a lower temperature, longer, gives a better quality of the oil. Cool the oil and strain.

Store this in a dark bottle in a cool place.

Ointment / Salve

Once you've made the oil as above, making the ointment is fairly easy. For every cup of herbal oil, use 1/4 cup of grated beeswax. Bring your oil back up to temperature (not over 120 degrees) over a double boiler. I like to meet the bee's wax separately because it melts at a higher temperature. Melt the beeswax, and slowly pour it into your heated herbal oil, while stirring. Keep stirring until the liquid is consistent color, and is clear. To test the consistency, put a spoonful of the mixture in the freezer for a few minutes. If it is the hardness you want, then finish the preparation. If it is too soft, add a little more melted beeswax. If it is a little too hard, add a little more heated herbal oil.

Before cooling the mixture, you may add 8 drops of tincture of Benzoin for every cup of herbal oil you used, as a natural preservative. Take the mixture off the double boiler to cool. Add a few drops (don't go overboard!) of essential oil for a more pleasant aroma. Keep stirring the mixture until it just starts getting cloudy. This means it is ready to set up. Pour into small glass jars and seal. These can be kept in a cool, dark place, or even in the fridge. They should last for several months. If you start to see signs of spoilage or mold, throw them out.

Tincture / Liniment

Tinctures are an infusion in a menstruum of alcohol, vinegar, or glycerin. There are almost as many ways to make tinctures as there are herbalists. Most alcohol tinctures are made with grain alcohol – 80 to 100 proof vodka (this is 40 to 50% alcohol). You can use other things like wine, brandy, etc. to add a different flavor, but those have other ingredients in them. For some herbs, stronger alcohol needs to be used – in the range of 60 to 90% alcohol. You can adjust the alcohol level by adding some distilled water to the mix if you don't want 90% alcohol.

I fill a mason jar 1/2 to 3/4 full with dried or fresh herb material. Then I fill the jar to the top with the alcohol. I put a tight lid on the jar and shake it well. Leave this in a dark place for a minimum of 2 weeks shaking the bottle at least once a day, and preferably 3 times a day or more. Some herbalists leave the tinctures for up to 6 weeks. Some start the tinctures at the dark phase of the moon and strain it at the full moon. Try it in different ways.

When you are ready, strain the herbs through several layers of clean, cotton cloth or cheesecloth – I like to use flour sackcloth. Strain it several times, if need be, so there is no sediment. You want a clean tincture, so no bacteria will grow in it.

Pour the strained tincture into dark bottles and cap tightly. Keep them in a cool, dark place, and they should last for years.

Dosages of tinctures vary greatly depending on what herbs are used, on the age of the person, and if the health complaint is chronic or acute. It can be anywhere from 15 – 30 drops 3 times a day, to a teaspoon or more every hour. Tinctures can be taken straight. The healing properties will begin being absorbed into the system through the blood vessels in the mouth, especially if you drop the tincture under the tongue. Some people don't wish to take the alcohol or give it to children, so the tincture can be put into a cup of boiled water. Let it sit until the liquid is cool enough to drink, and most of the alcohol will have dissipated.

A vinegar tincture is made the same way using raw, apple cider vinegar. Use the same proportions of herbs to vinegar as in the alcohol tincture, and allow to infuse for 2 to 6 weeks. This makes a good tonic remedy, but it won't be as strong as an alcohol tincture. And you should start checking to see if it is still good after 6 to 8 months. A lot depends on where it is stored.

A glycerin tincture (a glycerite) is made the same way, using equal parts of pure vegetable glycerin to water, or using 2 parts glycerin to one part water. Make it the same as the alcohol tincture. This will draw out some healing properties from the herbs, but not as much as the alcohol. This is often used for children's formulas because glycerin is sweet.

Now, liniments are essentially the same as a tincture but can be made with either rubbing alcohol (PLEASE be sure to mark the bottle for external use only!!!) or vinegar. Liniments are used as antiseptics on minor scrapes and wounds, or as a rub for sour muscles and joints.

Macerations

This method of preparation is certainly the easiest. The fresh or dried plant material is simply covered in cool water and soaked overnight. The herb is strained out and the liquid is taken. Normally this is used for very tender plants and/or fresh plants, or those with delicate chemicals that might be harmed by heating or which might be degraded in strong alcohol. This is also the easiest to adapt to western methods since tablets or capsules can be used instead. Alternatively, just stir the ground plant powder into juice, water, or smoothies and drink.

Syrup

This is a great way to prepare a formula for a child to take – or, for an adult, if the herbs are particularly bad tasting! I have seen several different ways of making syrups. Most of the old recipes use sugar... lots of it.

Start with 2 oz. of dried herb mix to 1 quart of water in a double boiler. Simmer this until you have 1 pint of liquid. Strain and pour the liquid back into the double boiler. For each pint of liquid, add a cup of raw honey. Heat this just enough so that the honey is mixed in with the herb decoction. Don't "cook" the honey.

When this is ready, take it off the heat to cool. Now, you can add a little fruit brandy (3 to 4 tbsp. per cup of syrup), or a few drops of essential oil, or a fruit concentrate for flavoring. The brandy is relaxing to the throat muscles, but if you are concerned about giving alcohol to children, then go with the essential oil or fruit concentrate. Peppermint, spearmint, or wintergreen essential oils are great.

Pour this into dark bottles, and keep it in the refrigerator. They will keep for several weeks to several months.

Powder / Capsules

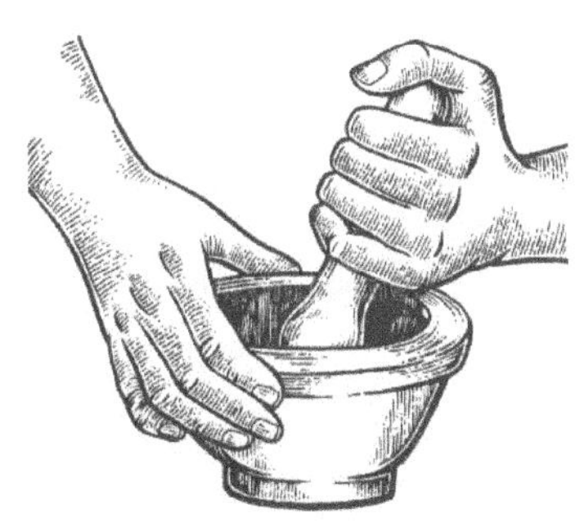

This is an easy one... you can buy most herbs already powdered. Or, you can powder them, yourself, using a small coffee grinder (don't use one that has been used to grind the coffee, however!). If you grind your herbs, be sure to sift them to get any larger pieces out before encapsulating them. You can take the powdered herbs straight, swallowing it down with some herbal tea. However, I don't know of too many herbs that taste good enough for me to want to do this. I like to use the Capsule Machine for making my capsules.

Now, you can use the gelatin capsules, or, if you are vegetarian, you can get plant-based capsules. Why take capsules? Well, it takes longer for the herbs to get into your system with capsules, but you aren't losing any of the herbs, either. If you want to use the whole plant, capsules are the way to go. Take the capsules with warm, herbal tea. (Be careful with cayenne capsules, however – they can start to disintegrate in the throat, and you will feel the heat!)

Pills / Lozenge / Suppository

These are all made in similar ways – powdered herbs are added to a liquid until a stiff dough is formed. Then the mixture is shaped as needed.

For pills or lozenges, powdered herbs (usually for the throat or for a cough) are mixed with water and honey to make a paste. To this, add a few drops of essential oil, like peppermint or wintergreen. Thicken the mixture with enough Slippery elm, comfrey root, or marshmallow root powder to make the mixture's consistency like dough. Pinch off enough to make a small pill or a larger lozenge. Roll it into a ball and press between your fingers to flatten (they dry through faster in this shape, but you can leave them as balls). Then cover it with a little more Slippery elm powder or some carob powder. Place these pills/lozenges in a very low oven, in a dryer set on low, or in the sun for a day. Once they are dry, they will keep for a long time.

A suppository is similar, but the powdered herbs are mixed into melted cocoa butter. Cocoa butter is a hard fat at room temperature, but it melts at body temperature. This is a very good way to get herbs directly into the vagina, the rectum, or even in the nasal passages. Use about 1/2 oz. of powdered herbs to 3/4 to 1 oz. of melted cocoa butter. Stir until the mixture starts to thicken. Form the mixture into small cylinders, about 1/4″ by 1″ for the rectum or vagina. Put these on a plate and cover with a paper towel. When they are hardened, they can be used. Usually, the suppository is placed in the vaginal or rectal area just before going to bed, and it is wise to wear a pad in case any of the melted cocoa butter runs out.

For the nasal passages, form them into 1/8″ by 1/4 to 1/2″ cylinders. Harden them the same way. Place the suppository up into the nose. Prepare for running and sneezing as the cocoa butter melts and the herbs start to work.

Importance of Medicinal Plants And Herbs

Medicinal plants are considered as rich resources of ingredients that can be used in drug development either pharmacopoeial, non- pharmacopoeial, or synthetic drugs. Apart from that, these plants play a critical role in the development of human cultures around the whole world. Moreover, some plants are considered an important source of nutrition, and as a result that they are recommended for their therapeutic values. Some of these plants include ginger, green tea, walnuts, aloe, pepper, and turmeric, etc. Some plants and their derivatives are considered as an important source for active ingredients which are used in aspirin and toothpaste etc.

Apart from the medicinal uses, herbs are also used in natural dye, pest control, food, perfume, tea, and so on. In many countries, different kinds of medicinal plants/ herbs are used to keep ants, flies, mice, and flee away from homes and offices. Nowadays medicinal herbs are important sources for pharmaceutical manufacturing.

Recipes for the treatment of common ailments such as diarrhea, constipation, hypertension, low sperm count, dysentery and weak penile erection, piles, coated tongue, menstrual disorders, bronchial asthma, leucorrhoea, and fevers are given by the traditional medicine practitioners very effectively.

Importance of Some Herbs With Their Medicinal Values

1. Herbs such as black pepper, cinnamon, myrrh, aloe, sandalwood, ginseng, red clover, burdock, bayberry, and safflower are used to heal wounds, sores, and boils.

2. Basil, Fennel, Chives, Cilantro, Apple Mint, Thyme, Golden Oregano, Variegated Lemon Balm, Rosemary, Variegated Sage are some important medicinal herbs and can be planted in the kitchen garden. These herbs are easy to grow, look good, taste and smell amazing and many of them are magnets for bees and butterflies.

3. Many herbs are used as blood purifiers to alter or change a long-standing condition by eliminating the metabolic toxins. These are also known as 'blood cleansers'. Certain herbs improve the immunity of the person, thereby reducing conditions such as fever.

4. Some herbs are also having antibiotic properties. Turmeric is useful in inhibiting the growth of germs, harmful microbes, and bacteria. Turmeric is widely used as a home remedy to heal cuts and wounds.

5. Sandalwood and Cinnamon are great astringents apart from being aromatic. Sandalwood is especially used in arresting the discharge of blood, mucus, etc.

6. Some herbs are used to neutralize the acid produced by the stomach. Herbs such as marshmallow root and leaf. They serve as antacids. The healthy gastric acid needed for proper digestion is retained by such herbs.

7. Herbs like Cardamom and Coriander are renowned for their appetizing qualities. Other aromatic herbs such as peppermint, cloves, and turmeric add a pleasant aroma to the food, thereby increasing the taste of the meal.

8. Some herbs like aloe, sandalwood, and turmeric are commonly used as antiseptic and are very high in their medicinal values.

9. Ginger and cloves are used in certain cough syrups. They are known for their expectorant property, which promotes the thinning and ejection of mucus from the lungs, trachea, and bronchi. Eucalyptus, Cardamom, Wild cherry, and cloves are also expectorants.

10. Herbs such as Chamomile, Calamus, Ajwain, Basil, Cardamom, Chrysanthemum, Coriander, Fennel, Peppermint, and Spearmint, Cinnamon, Ginger, and Turmeric help promote good blood circulation. Therefore, they are used as cardiac stimulants.

11. Certain medicinal herbs have disinfectant property, which destroys disease-causing germs. They also inhibit the growth of pathogenic microbes that cause communicable diseases.

12. Certain aromatic plants such as Aloe, Goldenseal, Barberry, and Chirayata are used as mild tonics. The bitter taste of such plants reduces toxins in the blood. They help destroy infection as well.

13. A wide variety of herbs including Giloe, Goldenseal, Aloe, and Barberry are used as tonics. They can also be nutritive and rejuvenate a healthy as well as the diseased individual.

14. Honey, turmeric, marshmallow, and licorice can effectively treat a fresh cut and wound. They are termed as vulnerable herbs.

Misuse of Medicinal Plants And Herbs

Misuse refers to patient overdosing and concomitant drug consumption. Kava, for example, is used as an anxiolytic and a mild tranquilizer in dosing ranging from 60 to 120mg of kava pyrones daily. Some users may consume as much as triple this amount for extended periods without concern for the potentially dangerous effects, which include malnutrition, liver, and renal dysfunction, and pulmonary hypertension.

Some Other Common Misuses Of Medicinal Herbs/Products

- Carelessness with prescriptions and medical drugs
- Nonprofessionals making prescriptions and selling, unaware of harmful side effects
- Uneducated people using medicinal plants.
- Alternative medicine- a common misconception is that they are safer than man-made drugs because they are natural.
- Only certified doctors and professionals have regulated the strength and dosage of the medicinal ingredients.

Tips For Using Medicinal Herbs Safely

- Buy or use herbal products from a qualified practitioner or reputable supplier.
- Ask for products that are clearly labeled in English with your name, batch number, date, quantity, dosage, directions, safety information (if applicable), and your practitioner's contact details.
- Avoid using over-the-counter products from a health food shop, pharmacy, or the internet.
- Make sure you know how to prepare and take your herbs. Like conventional medicine, taking the correct dose at the right time is important for herbal remedies to work safely.
- Talk to your doctor and complementary health practitioner
- Ask the practitioner for ways to mask the taste of the herbs if you find them bitter.

Essential Tools And Useful Instruments

1. Felco Pruners

Pruners are the tool I use most often when gathering and processing foraged herbs. They snip right through herbaceous stems, twigs, small branches, and roots. I reach for them so often that I keep them in a leather holster on a belt at my hip. If you can only purchase one tool to get started, pruners are the way to go!. Felco pruners come in a wide variety of models. Look for a pair that will reduce hand fatigue and strain. The pruner handles, when fully opened, should not exceed the width of your extended grasp.

2. Hori-Hori, Or Weeding Knife, Or Japanese Garden Knife

This tool looks like it sounds. Heavy duty and compact, it's a sturdy wildcrafting tool and excellent weeding implement. I use my hori-hori to break up soils and dig small- to medium-sized roots from the earth. These garden "knives" cut through most clay soils and can even pry rocks out of the ground. You can also use it for transplanting and dividing roots.

3. Digging Fork

This is the tool of choice for digging most roots. The tines of the fork effectively loosen soils and lift branching roots free from the earth. Digging forks are much less likely to damage roots than a shovel or spade. I also use my digging fork in the garden to weed, loosen soil, and harvest medicinal roots.

4. Shovel

You likely already have this tool hanging out in your garage or garden shed. Having a couple of different types is useful. Make sure you have at least one long-handled shovel with a pointed blade (as opposed to flat). It is used primarily to help begin the excavation process of large, tap-rooted plants like burdock (Arctium lappa, A. minus), or digging in heavily compacted soils.

5. Kitchen Scissors

A sharp pair of kitchen scissors is my go-to tool for gathering tender-stemmed greens like chickweed (Stellaria media), violet (Viola spp.), and cleavers (Galium aparine). Pruners can make a muck of this job as they're meant for tougher stems and the reach of their blades is limited.

6. Pruning Saw

A foldable pruning saw is handy for cutting small- to medium-sized tree limbs and branches. I use mine most often in the spring when I'm gathering medicinal tree barks like wild cherry (Prunus serotina) and black birch (Betula lenta).

7. Assorted Baskets

Baskets will reward you in more ways than one. They're handy for gathering and drying herbs, and they are beautiful to behold. It's helpful to have an assortment of baskets on hand. You can typically find used baskets in thrift stores. Look for a few that have an open weave and are broad and flattish (helpful for increasing ventilation when drying loose herbs).

9. Gloves

Foraging can be hard on the hands, and your fingertips will thank you for stashing a pair of gloves in your pack for prickly situations (think: picking stinging nettles or wading through a berry bramble). I keep two pairs of gloves on hand a thin, supple pair for delicate tasks and thicker leather and/or canvas pair for moments when I need more protection.

10. Hand Lens Or Loupe

I highly recommend purchasing a hand lens, also called a jeweler's loupe preferably 10x to 20x (10 to 20 times magnification). These nifty little tools allow you to gaze at wee botanical parts (helpful for plant ID) and have a much higher magnification ability than plain magnifying lenses (the kind used for enlarging print). Many have an LED attached, which is ideal because the increased lighting makes it much easier to spy on flowers.

CHAPTER 3 : NATIVE AMERICAN HERBS

1. Aloe - Aloe Doctrina

Aloe is a cactus-like plant that grows in hot, dry climates. In the United States, aloe is grown in Florida, Texas, and Arizona. Aloe produces two substances, gel, and latex, which are used for medicines. Aloe gel is the clear, jelly-like substance found in the inner part of the aloe plant leaf. Aloe latex comes from just under the plant's skin and is yellow. Some aloe products are made from the whole crushed leaf, so they contain both gel and latex. The aloe that is mentioned in the Bible is an unrelated fragrant wood used as incense.

Aloe medications can be taken by mouth or applied to the skin. People take aloe products by mouth for conditions such as obesity, diabetes, osteoarthritis, and many others, but there is no good scientific evidence to support these uses. People apply aloe gel to the skin for conditions such as acne, dandruff, wound healing, and many others, but there is no good scientific evidence to support these uses.

How Does It Work?

The useful parts of aloe are the gel and latex. The gel is obtained from the cells in the center of the leaf, and the latex is obtained from the cells just beneath the leaf skin. Aloe gel might cause changes in the skin that might help diseases like psoriasis. Aloe seems to be able to speed wound healing by improving blood circulation through the area and preventing cell death around a wound. It also appears that aloe gel has properties that are harmful to certain types of bacteria and fungi. Aloe latex contains chemicals that work as a laxative.

Uses & Effectiveness

Possibly Effective For

- Acne.
- Burns
- Constipation.
- Diabetes.
- Genital herpes.
- Scaly, itchy skin (psoriasis).
- Possibly Ineffective for
- Burning pain in the mouth.
- HIV/AIDS.

Special Precautions & Warnings:

1. Pregnancy Or Breast-Feeding: Aloe either gel or latex is POSSIBLY UNSAFE when taken by mouth. There is a report that aloe was associated with miscarriage. It might also increase the risk of birth defects. Do not take aloe by mouth if you are pregnant or breast-feeding.

2. Children: Aloe gel is POSSIBLY SAFE when applied to the skin appropriately. Aloe latex and aloe whole leaf extracts are POSSIBLY UNSAFE when taken by mouth in children. Children younger than 12 years-old might have stomach pain, cramps, and diarrhea.

3. Diabetes: Some research suggests that aloe might lower blood sugar. If you take aloe by mouth and you have diabetes, monitor your blood sugar levels closely.

4. Hemorrhoids: Do not take aloe latex if you have hemorrhoids. It could make the condition worse. Remember, products made from whole aloe leaves will contain some aloe latex.

5. Kidney Problems: High doses of aloe latex have been linked to kidney failure and other serious conditions.

6. Surgery: Aloe might affect blood sugar levels and could interfere with blood sugar control during and after surgery. Stop taking aloe at least 2 weeks before a scheduled surgery.

Interactions

Major Interaction

- Do not take this combination
- Digoxin (Lanoxin) interacts with ALOE

When taken by mouth aloe latex is a type of laxative called a stimulant laxative. Stimulant laxatives can decrease potassium levels in the body. Low potassium levels can increase the risk of side effects of digoxin (Lanoxin).

Moderate Interaction

Be cautious with this combination

1. Medications Taken By Mouth (Oral Drugs) Interacts With ALOE

When taken by mouth aloe latex is a laxative. Laxatives can decrease how much medicine your body absorbs. Taking aloe latex along with medications you take by mouth might decrease the effectiveness of your medication.

2. Sevoflurane (Ultane) Interacts With ALOE

Aloe might decrease the clotting of the blood. Sevoflurane is used as anesthesia during surgery. Sevoflurane also decreases the clotting of the blood. Taking aloe before surgery might cause increased bleeding during the surgical procedure. Do not take aloe by mouth if you are having surgery within 2 weeks.

3. Stimulant Laxatives Interact With ALOE

When taken orally aloe latex is a type of laxative called a stimulant laxative. Stimulant laxatives speed up the bowels. Taking aloe latex along with other stimulant laxatives could speed up the bowels too much and cause dehydration and low minerals in the body.

4. Warfarin (Coumadin) Interacts With ALOE

When taken orally, aloe latex is a type of laxative called a stimulant laxative. Stimulant laxatives speed up the bowels and can cause diarrhea in some people. Diarrhea can increase the effects of warfarin and increase the risk of bleeding. If you take warfarin, do not take excessive amounts of aloe latex.

5. Water Pills (Diuretic Drugs) Interacts With ALOE

When taken by mouth aloe latex is a laxative. Some laxatives can decrease potassium in the body. "Water pills" can also decrease potassium in the body. Taking aloe latex along with "water pills" might decrease potassium in the body too much. Some "water pills" that can decrease potassium include chlorothiazide (Diuril), chlorthalidone (Thalitone), furosemide (Lasix), hydrochlorothiazide (HCTZ, HydroDIURIL, Microzide), and others.

Dosing

The following doses have been studied in scientific research:

1. Adults

By Mouth:

1. For Constipation: 100-200 mg of aloe or 50 mg of aloe extract taken in the evening has been used. Also, a 500 mg capsule containing aloe, starting at a dose of one capsule daily and increasing to three capsules daily as required, has been used.

2. For Diabetes: The most effective dose and form of aloe for diabetes is unclear. Multiple doses and forms of aloe have been used for 4-14 weeks, including powder, extract, and juice. Doses of powder range from 100-1000 mg daily. Doses of juice range from 15-150 mL daily.

3. For Obesity: A specific aloe gel product containing 147 mg of aloe twice daily for 8 weeks has been used.

4. For A Painful Mouth Disease That Reduces One's Ability To Open The Mouth (Oral Submucous Fibrosis): Pure aloe vera juice 30 mL twice daily along with applying pure aloe vera gel to lesions three times daily for 3 months has been used.

Applied To The Skin:

1. For Acne: A 50% aloe gel has been applied in the morning and evening after washing the face, along with a prescription called tretinoin gel in the evening.

2. For Burns: Aloe and olive oil cream, applied twice daily for 6 weeks, has been used. Also, aloe gel or cream applied twice or three times daily after changing a wound dressing, or every three days until the burn heals, has been used.

3. For Genital Herpes: A cream containing 0.5% aloe extract, applied three times daily for 5 consecutive days once or twice over 2 weeks, has been used.

4. For An Inflammatory Condition That Causes Rash Or Sores On The Skin Or Mouth (Lichen Planus): Aloe gel, applied two to three times daily for 8 weeks has been used. Two tablespoons of aloe mouthwash swished for 2 minutes and then spit, four times daily for one month has been used.

5. For Scaly, Itchy Skin (Psoriasis): Aloe extract 0.5% cream applied three times daily for 4 weeks has been used. A cream containing aloe applied twice daily for 8 weeks, has been used.

Children

Applied To The Skin:

1. For Acne: A 50% aloe gel has been applied in the morning and evening after washing the face, along with a prescription called tretinoin gel in the evening.

2. For A Painful Mouth Disease That Reduces One's Ability To Open The Mouth (Oral Submucous Fibrosis): 5 mg of an aloe gel, applied on each side of the cheeks three times daily for 3 months, has been used.

2. Arsesmart - Polygonum Hydropiper

What Is Smartweed?

Smartweed is an herb. The entire plant is used to make medicine. People take smartweed tea to stop bleeding from hemorrhoids, as well as menstrual bleeding and another uterine bleeding. They also use it to treat diarrhea. Some people put smartweed directly on the skin to wash bloody wounds.

Insufficient Evidence To Rate Effectiveness For

- Stopping bleeding.
- Diarrhea.
- Cleansing bloody wounds, when applied directly.
- Other conditions.

How Does Smartweed Work?

Smartweed contains chemicals that are thought to stop bleeding.

Are There Safety Concerns?

It is not known if smartweed is safe. It can cause side effects such as stomach irritation when taken by mouth. When the fresh plant is handled it can cause skin irritation and swelling (inflammation).

Special Precautions & Warnings:

1. Pregnancy And Breast-Feeding: Not enough is known about the use of smartweed during pregnancy and breast-feeding. Stay on the safe side and avoid use.

Ulcers Or Other Stomach And Intestinal (Gastrointestinal, GI) Disorders: Smartweed can irritate the tissues that line the stomach and intestines, making ulcers and GI problems worse. Avoid using smartweed if you have ulcers or another GI disorder.

Are There Any Interactions With Medications?

Warfarin (Coumadin)Interaction Rating: Moderate Be cautious with this combination. Talk with your health provider.

Smartweed contains large amounts of vitamin K. Vitamin K is used by the body to help blood clot. Warfarin (Coumadin) is used to slow blood clotting. By helping the blood clot, smartweed might decrease the effectiveness of warfarin (Coumadin). Be sure to have your blood checked regularly. The dose of your warfarin (Coumadin) might need to be changed.

Dosing Considerations For Smartweed

The appropriate dose of smartweed depends on several factors such as the user's age, health, and several other conditions. At this time there is not enough scientific information to determine an appropriate range of doses for smartweed. Keep in mind that natural products are not always necessarily safe and dosages can be important. Be sure to follow relevant directions on product labels and consult your pharmacist or physician or other healthcare professional before using.

3. Black Cohosh - Cimicifuga Racemosa

Generic Name: Black Cohosh

Drug Class: Women's Health, Herbals

What Is Black Cohosh (Vasostrict, Adh) And How Does It Work?

Black Cohosh suggested uses include cough, sore throat, painful menstrual periods (dysmenorrhea), indigestion/heartburn, labor induction, menopausal symptoms, nervous tension, premenstrual syndrome, and rheumatism.

Black Cohosh is likely effective for menopausal vasomotor symptoms. Black Cohosh is possibly effective for premenstrual syndrome (PMS) and painful menstrual periods (dysmenorrhea). Black Cohosh is available under the following different brands and other names: Actaea racemosa, baneberry, black snakeroot, bugbane, bugwort, Cimicifuga racemosa, rattle root, rattlesnake root, rattleweed, rheumatism weed, and squawroot.

Dosages Of Black Cohosh:

Suggested Dosing

Dried Root: 300-2000 mg orally three times daily

Extract: 0.3-2 mL orally daily; 1:1, 90% alcohol

Tincture: 2-4 mL orally daily; 1:10, 60% alcohol

Tablet: 20-80 mg orally twice daily; standardized to 1 mg triterpene glycosides/20 mg tablet

What Are Side Effects Associated With Using Black Cohosh?

Side effects of Black Cohosh include:

- Cramping
- Dizziness
- Gastrointestinal (GI) upset
- Headache
- Sweating
- Weight gain
- Rash

- Fast heart rate (overdose)
- CNS disturbances
- Nausea
- Vomiting
- Visual disturbances

This document does not contain all possible side effects and others may occur. Check with your physician for additional information about side effects.

What Other Drugs Interact With Black Cohosh?

If your doctor has directed you to use this medication, your doctor or pharmacist may already be aware of any possible drug interactions and may be monitoring you for them. Do not start, stop, or change the dosage of any medicine before checking with your doctor, health care provider, or pharmacist first.

Black Cohosh has no known severe interactions with other drugs.

Serious interactions of black cohosh include:

- Daclizumab
- Black cohosh has no known moderate interactions with other drugs.

Mild interactions of black cohosh include:

- Nevirapine
- Tamoxifen
- Tenofovir df
- Zidovudine

This document does not contain all possible interactions. Therefore, before using this product, tell your doctor or pharmacist of all the products you use. Keep a list of all your medications with you, and share the list with your doctor and pharmacist. Check with your physician if you have health questions or concerns.

What Are Warnings And Precautions For Black Cohosh (Vasostrict, Adh)?

Warnings

This medication contains black cohosh. Do not take Actaea racemosa, baneberry, black snakeroot, bugbane, bugwort, Cimicifuga rattle root, rattlesnake root, rattleweed, rheumatism weed, or squawroot if you are allergic to black cohosh or any ingredients contained in this drug. Keep out of reach of children. In case of overdose, get medical help or contact a Poison Control Center immediately.

Contraindications

Breast cancer, endometrial cancer, endometriosis, hormone-sensitive conditions, ovarian cancer, pregnancy, lactation, uterine fibroids

Cautions

It May be associated with liver damage

Pregnancy And Lactation

Black cohosh is considered unsafe to use during pregnancy or while breastfeeding.

4. Black Root - Veronicastrum Virgin Icum

What Is Black Root?

Blackroot is a plant. It grows in the US and Canada and has a bitter and nauseating taste. People use the underground stem (rhizome) and the root as medicine. Blackroot is used for ongoing constipation and disorders of the liver and gallbladder. It is also used to cause vomiting.

Insufficient Evidence To Rate Effectiveness For

- Constipation.
- Liver problems.
- Gallbladder problems.
- Causing vomiting.
- Other conditions.

How Does Black Rootwork?

Blackroot might increase bile flow from the gallbladder into the intestine.

Are There Safety Concerns?

There isn't enough information to know if taking black root is safe. However, there have been reports of stomach pain or cramps, changes in stool color or odor, drowsiness, headache, nausea, and vomiting after taking black root. Large doses have been linked to reports of liver damage.

Special Precautions & Warnings:

1. **Pregnancy And Breast-Feeding:** It might be UNSAFE to take the fresh root by mouth. There is a concern that it might cause miscarriages and birth defects, but this hasn't been proven so far. Stay safe and don't take black root if you are pregnant. It's also best to avoid black roots if you are breast-feeding. Not enough is known about how it might affect the nursing infant.

2. **Gallbladder Problems Such As Gallstones Or A Blocked Bile Duct:** Don't take black root if you have gallbladder problems. It might make your condition worse.

3. **Hemorrhoids:** Don't use black roots if you have hemorrhoids. It can act as a laxative and make hemorrhoids more bothersome.

4. **Menstruation:** Don't take black root if you are having your period. It can act as a laxative and add to the discomfort.

Are There Any Interactions With Medications?

1. **Digoxin (Lanoxin)Interaction Rating:** Moderate Be cautious with this combination. Talk with your health provider.

2. Blackroot Is High In Fiber: Fiber can decrease the absorption and decrease the effectiveness of digoxin (Lanoxin). As a general rule, any medications taken by mouth should be taken one hour before or four hours after the black root to prevent this interaction.

3. Warfarin (Coumadin)Interaction Rating: Moderate Be cautious with this combination. Talk with your health provider.

4. Water Pills (Diuretic drugs)Interaction Rating: Moderate Be cautious with this combination. Talk with your health provider.

5. Blackroot Is A Laxative: Some laxatives can decrease potassium in the body. "Water pills" can also decrease potassium in the body. Taking black root along with "water pills" might decrease potassium in the body too much.

Dosing Considerations For Black Root

The appropriate dose of black root depends on several factors such as the user's age, health, and several other conditions. At this time there is not enough scientific information to determine an appropriate range of doses for black root. Keep in mind that natural products are not always necessarily safe and dosages can be important. Be sure to follow relevant directions on product labels and consult your pharmacist or physician or other healthcare professional before using.

5. Black Walnut - Juglans Nigra

What Are Black Walnuts?

Black walnuts, or Juglans nigra, grow wild across the United States and are the second most cultivated walnut in North America, following English walnuts. They consist of a kernel, a dry outer covering known as a hull, and a hard shell. The kernel is the part of the walnut that's commonly eaten raw or roasted and can be pressed for oil. The hulls contain antioxidants and are used in extracts and supplements for medicinal purposes, such as to treat parasitic infections or decrease inflammation. Black walnuts have a unique flavor and aroma, making them bolder and earthier than English walnuts. They're a popular addition to recipes like baked goods and desserts. Black walnuts are the second most common walnut and prized for their bold and earthy flavor. The nutrients in the hulls are extracted and used in supplements.

Black Walnut Nutrition

Black walnuts are high in protein, healthy fats, and many vitamins and minerals. A 1-ounce (28-gram) serving of black walnuts contains:

- Calories: 170
- Protein: 7 grams
- Fat: 17 grams
- Carbs: 3 grams
- Fiber: 2 grams
- Magnesium: 14% of the Reference Daily Intake (RDI)
- Phosphorus: 14% of the RDI
- Potassium: 4% of the RDI
- Iron: 5% of the RDI

- Zinc: 6% of the RDI
- Copper: 19% of the RDI
- Manganese: 55% of the RDI
- Selenium: 7% of the RDI

Potential Health Benefits Of Black Walnut

The fiber, omega-3 fatty acids, and antioxidants in black walnuts provide various health benefits. Also, black walnut hulls have unique antibacterial properties and are used in herbal medicine extracts and supplements. Black walnuts are nutritionally similar to English walnuts, which have been studied extensively for their health benefits.

May Benefit Heart Health

Black walnuts contain various nutrients and compounds that benefit heart health, including:

- Omega-3 fatty acids. May improve certain heart disease risk factors like high blood pressure and cholesterol levels.
- Tannins. Help lower blood pressure and decrease blood lipid levels, potentially improving heart health.
- Ellagic acid. May help prevent a narrowing of the arteries caused by plaque buildup that can lead to heart disease.

May Have Anticancer Properties

Black walnuts contain an antitumor compound called juglone. Test-tube studies have found this compound to significantly reduce tumor growth Several test-tube studies indicate that juglone can cause cell death in certain cancerous cells, including the liver and stomach Also, black walnuts contain flavonoid antioxidants that have been shown to have beneficial effects against lung, breast, prostate, and colon cancer.

Have Antibacterial Properties

Black walnut hulls are high in tannins compounds with antibacterial properties. Tannins in black walnuts have antibacterial effects against, for example, Listeria, Salmonella, and E. coli bacteria that commonly cause foodborne illnesses. A test-tube study found that black walnut hull extracts have antioxidant and antibacterial activities, preventing the growth of Staphylococcus aureus, a bacteria that can cause infections.

May Aid Weight Loss

Studies show that eating nuts particularly walnuts may help you lose weight Though walnuts are high in calories, most of these calories come from healthy fats. Fats can help increase feelings of fullness and fend off hunger. Walnuts have been found to keep you fuller for longer, which can help you naturally eat less, potentially promoting weight loss. In one 3-month study, people who ate 1/4 cup (30 grams) of walnuts daily experienced greater weight loss than the control group despite the additional calories of the walnuts

Black Walnut Uses

Plant compounds in black walnut hulls are extracted and used as supplements in the form of capsules or liquid drops. Due to its antibacterial properties, the black walnut extract is used in wormwood complex supplements. Wormwood complex is a tincture made from black walnut hulls, a plant called wormwood, and cloves. It's a natural remedy against parasitic infections.

Safety Of Black Walnut

Although black walnuts have many health benefits, there are some safety aspects to consider when eating them or taking them as a supplement. People with any nut or tree nut allergy should not eat black walnuts or use supplements that contain them. Supplements are not regulated by the Food and Drug Administration (FDA). Therefore, you should purchase them from reputable brands that offer products that are independently tested for safety and potency.

Research on the effects of black walnut supplements during pregnancy or while breastfeeding is insufficient, and it's unknown whether it's safe to take these supplements during pregnancy or lactation. Additionally, the tannins in black walnuts may interact with certain medications. It's best to consult with your healthcare provider before taking black walnut extract if you take medications or are pregnant or breastfeeding

6. Bloodroot - Sanguinaria Canadensis

Bloodroot is a plant. People use the underground stem (rhizome) to make medicine. People sometimes use bloodroot by mouth or apply it to the skin for a long list of conditions, but there is no scientific evidence to support these uses, and using it can be unsafe.

How Does It Work?

Bloodroot contains chemicals that might help fight bacteria, inflammation, and plaque.

Uses & Effectiveness?

Possibly Effective For

- Dental plaque.
- Swelling of the gums (gingivitis).
- Insufficient Evidence for
- Coughs.
- Spasms.
- Emptying the bowels.
- Causing vomiting.
- Wound cleaning.
- Other conditions.

Side Effects & Safety

Bloodroot is POSSIBLY SAFE for most people when taken by mouth, short-term. Side effects include nausea, vomiting, drowsiness, and grogginess.

Long-term use by mouth in high amounts is POSSIBLY UNSAFE. At high doses, it can cause low blood pressure, shock, coma, and an eye disease called glaucoma. Also, bloodroot is POSSIBLY UNSAFE when used as a toothpaste, mouthwash, or applied to the skin. Don't let bloodroot get into your eyes because it can irritate. It may also cause white patches on the inside of the mouth. Skin contact with the fresh plant can cause a rash. Bloodroot can also burn and erode the skin, leaving an uneven scar.

Special Precautions & Warnings:

1. Pregnancy And Breast-Feeding: Bloodroot is LIKELY UNSAFE when taken by mouth during pregnancy and POSSIBLY UNSAFE when taken by mouth while breast-feeding; avoid use.

2. An Eye Disease Called Glaucoma: Bloodroot might affect glaucoma treatment. If you have glaucoma, don't use bloodroot unless a healthcare professional recommends it and monitors your eye health.

Dosing

The appropriate dose of bloodroot depends on several factors such as the user's age, health, and several other conditions. At this time there is not enough scientific information to determine an appropriate range of doses for bloodroot. Keep in mind that natural products are not always necessarily safe and dosages can be important. Be sure to follow relevant directions on product labels and consult your pharmacist or physician or other healthcare professional before using.

7. Bearberry - Uva Urst

Uva ursi is a shrub that grows flowers and berries. The leaves are used to make medicine. Bears are particularly fond of uva ursi berries. This explains the Latin name, "uva ursi," which means "bear's grape." Most authorities refer to Arctostaphylos uva-ursi as uva ursi. Do not confuse this plant with Arctostaphylos adentricha and Arctostaphylos coactylis, which have also been referred to as uva ursi. Uva ursi is used for infections of the kidney, bladder, or urethra (urinary tract infections or UTIs) and swelling (inflammation) of the urinary tract, but there is no good scientific evidence to support these uses.

How Does It Work?

Uva ursi can reduce bacteria in the urine. It can also reduce swelling (inflammation), and have a drying (astringent) effect on the tissues.

Uses & Effectiveness?

Insufficient Evidence For

- Swelling of the bladder and urethra.
- Swelling of the urinary tract.
- Constipation.
- Kidney infections.
- Bronchitis.
- Other conditions.

Side Effects & Safety

When taken by mouth: Uva ursi is POSSIBLY SAFE for most adults when taken for up to one month. It can cause nausea, vomiting, stomach discomfort, and a greenish-brown discoloration of the urine. But uva ursi is POSSIBLY UNSAFE when taken in high doses for more than one month. It can cause liver damage, breathing problems, convulsions, and death when used in high doses. When used for a long time, it might increase the risk of cancer.

Special Precautions & Warnings:

1. Pregnancy And Breast-Feeding: Using uva ursi during pregnancy is LIKELY UNSAFE because it might start labor. There isn't enough reliable information to know if uva ursi is safe to use when breastfeeding. Stay on the safe side and avoid use.

2. Children: Uva ursi is POSSIBLY UNSAFE in children when taken by mouth. Uva ursi contains a chemical that might cause severe liver problems. Do not give uva ursi to children.

3. Retinal Thinning: Uva ursi contains a chemical that can thin the retina in the eye. This could worsen the condition of people whose retinas are already too thin. Avoid use if you have this problem.

Dosing

The appropriate dose of uva ursi depends on several factors such as the user's age, health, and several other conditions. At this time there is not enough scientific information to determine an appropriate range of doses for uva ursi. Keep in mind that natural products are not always necessarily safe and dosages can be important. Be sure to follow relevant directions on product labels and consult your pharmacist or physician or other healthcare professional before using.

8. Capsicum - Capsicum Minimum, C. Frutescens

Capsicum

Capsicums, available in a multitude of colors, is an excellent source of vitamins A and C. This versatile vegetable can be stuffed, roasted, used in stir-fries, or simply eaten raw. In Victoria, capsicums are at their peak between March and November.

Also Called: peppers, sweet peppers, red pepper, green pepper, red capsicum, green capsicum, bell pepper, red bell pepper, green bell pepper, banana capsicum, Capsicum annuum L. (botanical name)

What Is Capsicum?

The rainbow of colors in which capsicum appears in Australia hints at the versatility of this vegetable – stuff it with herbs, meat, and rice, roast and use the smoky flesh in dips or simply eat it raw as a crudité, a traditional French appetizer. First prepared by herdsman as a hearty meal, the delicious Hungarian goulash wouldn't be the same without the addition of capsicum. The Capsicum species originated in South and Central America, and Christopher Columbus brought it back to Europe when he returned from the Americas. Records show that capsicum has been used in cooking since 6000 BC. In Australia, capsicum became popular thanks to European and Asian immigrants who use it extensively.

Why Capsicum Is Good To Eat

- Capsicums are an excellent source of vitamin A and C (red contain more than green capsicums).
- They are also a good source of dietary fiber, vitamin E, B6, and folate.

- The sweetness of capsicums is due to their natural sugars (green capsicums have less sugar than red capsicums).
- Energy 100 g of green capsicum supplies 90 kJ (105 kJ from red capsicum).

How Are They Grown And Harvested?

- Capsicums grow on a flowering bush that can reach up to 60 or 80 cm. Capsicum plants prefer stable, warm climates and are usually planted as seedlings.
- The seedlings take from 11 to 13 weeks to grow into mature plants with the capsicums ready to harvest. Red capsicums start green but if left on the bush to ripen they eventually turn red. Other types of capsicum turn yellow, orange, brown, or purple/black.
- Take care when you harvest capsicums. Rough treatment can injure the plant as the stems are very brittle and can snap off easily.

Choosing Capsicum

When choosing capsicums you should select ones with the firm, glossy skins. Avoid those with shriveled skins, soft spots, or other visible damage.

How To Store And Keep Capsicum

Store capsicums in the crisper section of your fridge. Ordinary plastic bags cause capsicums to sweat, so only use fridge storage bags. Capsicum should be used within five days.

How To Use

- To help remove the blackened skin of roasted peppers, place them in a plastic bag and allow them to cool for 10 minutes.
- For a Mediterranean flavor remove the stem and stuff red and green capsicums with a mixture of rice, tomato, pine nuts, and fresh herbs and bake until soft and tender.
- For a fresh, tangy salsa to accompany grilled fish mix chopped roasted red and yellow peppers, a small chili, coriander leaf, red onion, and dress with red wine vinegar oil and lime.
- Make a delicious savory dip by pureeing roasted peppers, garlic, capers, and fresh herbs with oil and lemon juice.

9. Catnip - Nepeta Cataria

Catnip, (Nepeta cataria), also called catmint, herb of the mint family (Lamiaceae), noted for its aromatic leaves, which are particularly exciting to cats. Catnip is commonly grown by cat owners for their pets, and the dried leaves are often used as a stuffing for cat playthings. The herb is native to Eurasia and is used as a seasoning and as a medicinal tea for colds and fever in some places. Catnip (nepeta cataria) is a fun plant for cats. Most cats are attracted to the plant and will roll around near it since its aroma acts as a stimulant. These medicinal plants also act as a sedative for cats if consumed.

For humans, on the other hand, it is normally used as a stress reliever, sleep aid, and a solution for skin issues. The majority of its health benefits come from the presence of nepetalactone, thymol, and other compounds that make this plant great for you and your furry friend.

Catnip Health Benefits:

- Repels bugs and relieves irritation from bug bites
- Calms restlessness, anxiety, and stress
- Relieves stomach discomfort
- Accelerates recovery from colds and fevers

Common uses:

- Brew leaves for a tea
- Dry leaves and burn to release the aroma
- Apply essential oils or leaves topically

10. Chamomile - Chamaemelum Nobile

Chamaemelum Nobile has daisy-like white flowers and procumbent stems; the leaves are alternate, bipinnate, finely dissected, and downy to glabrous. The solitary, terminal flowerheads, rising 20–30 cm (8–12 in) above the ground, consist of prominent yellow disk flowers and silver-white ray flowers. The flowering time in the Northern Hemisphere is June and July, and its fragrance is sweet, crisp, fruity, and herbaceous. Although the plant is often confused with German chamomile (M. chamomilla), its morphology, properties, and chemical composition are markedly different

Uses

- Chamaemelum Nobile has been used traditionally in hair care and skin care products. The plant may be used to flavor foods, in herbal teas, perfumes, and cosmetics. It is used in aromatherapy; its practitioners believe it to be a calming agent to reduce stress and aid in sleep.
- It can be used to create a fragrant chamomile lawn. A chamomile lawn needs light soil, adequate moisture, and sun to thrive. Each square meter contains 83-100 plants. The lawn is only suitable for light foot traffic or in places where mower access is difficult.

Chamomile health benefits:

- Improves overall skin health
- Relieves pain
- Aids sleep
- Reduces inflammation and swelling
- Rich source of antioxidants
- Relieves congestion

11. Centaury - Centaurium Ervtraea

What Is Centaury?

Centaury is a small, annual herb, native to Europe and naturalized in the United States. It thrives in boggy meadows as well as in dry dunes. The root is fibrous and woody. The plant has pale green, oval leaves, a capsule fruit, and light pink to red flowers. The whole herb is used in medicine.

Synonyms are Erythraea Centaurium, C. umbellatum, C. minus. Centaurium consists of approximately 40 species (annuals or biennials).

What Is It Used For?

Traditional/Ethnobotanical uses

Genus Erythraea is derived from the Greek erythrose, relating to the red color of the flowers. The genus formerly was called Chironia, from Centaur, Chiron. Hippocrates describes Centaurium, under the Greek Kentareion and according to legend, Chiron (founder of medicine) used centaury to heal a wound inflicted by a poisoned arrow. Historically, centaury has been used as herbal medicine to kill worms, to treat dropsy, as a sedative, to treat snakebite and other wounds, and topically for freckles and spots. It is reputed to be an aromatic bitter and tonic for treating GI complaints such as bloating, dyspepsia, and flatulence, and anorexia. Centaury is said to act on the liver and kidneys to "purify the blood," and for jaundice. Centaury also was used traditionally to treat fever, hence the name "feverwort." This bitter herb enhances the production of gastric secretions, which stimulates appetite and improves digestion. Long-term use of the herb is required for the tonic effects on the stomach to fully develop. Other effects include anti-inflammatory as well as antimutagenic effects. Little research is available to support these traditional uses.

What Is The Recommended Dosage?

There is no recent published clinical evidence to guide dosage of the century. The German Commission E monograph calls for 1 to 2 g of herb daily, while other uses for dyspepsia specify as much as 6.

Contraindications

Contraindications have not yet been identified.

Pregnancy/Lactation

Information regarding safety and efficacy in pregnancy and lactation is lacking.

Interactions

None well documented.

Side Effects

There are no known adverse reactions.

Toxicology

There are no known reports of toxicity. Because the safety of centaury taken during pregnancy has not been established, its use during this time is best avoided.

12. Chaga - Inonotus Obliquus

Chaga is a fungus. It produces a woody growth, called a conk, which is used to make medicine. People take Chaga by mouth for heart disease, diabetes, stomach and intestine cancer, liver disease, parasites, stomach pain, and tuberculosis.

How Does It Work?

Chaga might stimulate the immune system. It contains some chemicals that have antioxidant effects. Chaga might lower blood sugar and cholesterol levels.

Uses & Effectiveness?

Insufficient Evidence For

- Heart disease.
- Diabetes.
- Gastritis.
- Stomach and intestinal cancer.
- Liver disease.
- Tuberculosis.
- Other conditions.

Side Effects & Safety

It isn't known if Chaga is safe or what the possible side effects might be. It contains a chemical called oxalate which can damage the kidneys.

Special Precautions & Warnings:

1. **Pregnancy And Breast-Feeding:** Not enough is known about the use of Chaga during pregnancy and breast-feeding. Stay on the safe side and avoid use.

2. **Bleeding Disorders:** There is concern that Chaga might increase the risk of bleeding. Don't use chaga if you have a bleeding disorder.

3. **Diabetes:** Chaga might lower blood sugar levels in people with diabetes. Watch for signs of low blood sugar (hypoglycemia) and monitor your blood sugar carefully if you have diabetes and use Chaga products. The dose of your diabetes medications may need to be adjusted by your healthcare provider.

4. **Surgery:** Chaga might affect blood sugar control or increase the risk of bleeding during and after surgery. Stop using Chaga at least 2 weeks before a scheduled surgery.

Dosing

The appropriate dose of Chaga depends on several factors such as the user's age, health, and several other conditions. At this time there is not enough scientific information to determine an appropriate range of doses for Chaga. Keep in mind that natural products are not always necessarily safe and dosages can be important. Be sure to follow relevant directions on product labels and consult your pharmacist or physician or other healthcare professional before using.

13. Chickweed - Stellaria Media

What Is Chickweed?

Chickweed is a common plant, particularly throughout Europe and North America. This low-growing annual has a thin hairy stem with pointed oval leaves. It produces small, white, star-shaped flowers throughout much of the year.

What Is It Used For?

Traditional/Ethnobotanical Uses

Chickweed has been used as a folk remedy for centuries for many conditions, including asthma, blood disorders, conjunctivitis, constipation, inflammation, dyspepsia, skin ailments, and obesity. Chickweed extract has been used internally as a demulcent but is more typically used externally for the treatment of rashes and sores. The young shoots are edible and have been used as salad greens. In homeopathy, the plant is used to relieve rheumatic pains and psoriasis. Chickweed is noted as a folk remedy for many conditions, including asthma, blood disorders, conjunctivitis, constipation, inflammation, dyspepsia, skin ailments, and obesity.

What Is The Recommended Dosage?

There is no recent published clinical evidence to guide the dosage of chickweed.

Contraindications

Contraindications have not yet been identified.

Pregnancy/Lactation

Information regarding safety and efficacy in pregnancy and lactation is lacking.

Interactions

None well documented.

Side Effects

Human cases of paralysis have been reported from large amounts of the infusion.

Toxicology

There is no overwhelming evidence to suggest that chickweed is toxic.

14. Damiana - Turnera Dif Usa Var. Aphrodisiac

What Is Damiana?

Damiana is a wild shrub that grows in Mexico, Central America, and the West Indies. The leaf and stem are used to make medicine. Historically, it was used mostly to increase sexual desire (as an aphrodisiac). Damiana is used to treat headaches, bedwetting, depression, nervous stomach, and constipation; for prevention and treatment of sexual problems; boosting and maintaining mental and physical stamina, and as an aphrodisiac. Some people inhale damiana for a slight "high."

Insufficient Evidence To Rate Effectiveness For

- Sexual problems

- ❖ Weight loss
- ❖ Headaches
- ❖ Bedwetting
- ❖ Depression
- ❖ Nervous upset stomach
- ❖ Constipation
- ❖ Boosting mental and physical stamina
- ❖ Other conditions.

How Does Damiana Work?

Damiana contains chemicals that may affect the brain and nervous system.

Are There Safety Concerns?

Damiana is LIKELY SAFE when taken by mouth in amounts commonly found in foods. Damiana is POSSIBLY SAFE when taken by mouth in medicinal amounts, but there have been serious side effects. Convulsions and other symptoms similar to rabies or strychnine poisoning have been reported after taking 200 grams of damiana extract.

Special Precautions & Warnings:

1. Pregnancy And Breast-Feeding: There is not enough reliable information about the safety of taking damiana if you are pregnant or breastfeeding. Stay on the safe side and avoid use.

2. Diabetes: Damiana might affect blood sugar levels in people with diabetes. Watch for signs of low blood sugar (hypoglycemia) and monitor your blood sugar carefully if you have diabetes and use damiana.

3. Surgery: Since damiana seems to affect blood glucose levels, there is a concern that it might interfere with blood glucose control during and after surgery. Stop using damiana at least 2 weeks before a scheduled surgery.

Are There Any Interactions With Medications?

1. Medications For Diabetes (Antidiabetes Drugs)Interaction Rating: Moderate Be cautious with this combination. Talk with your health provider.

2. Damiana Might Decrease Blood Sugar: Diabetes medications are also used to lower blood sugar. Taking damiana along with diabetes medications might cause your blood sugar to go too low. Monitor your blood sugar closely. The dose of your diabetes medication might need to be changed.

Some medications used for diabetes include glimepiride (Amaryl), glyburide (Diabeta, Glynase PresTabs, Micronase), insulin, metformin (Glucophage), pioglitazone (Actos), rosiglitazone (Avandia), and others.

Dosing Considerations For Damiana

The appropriate dose of damiana depends on several factors such as the user's age, health, and several other conditions. At this time there is not enough scientific information to determine an appropriate range of doses for damiana. Keep in mind that natural products are not always necessarily safe and dosages can be important. Be sure to follow relevant directions on product labels and consult your pharmacist or physician or other healthcare professional before using.

15. Dandelion - Taraxacum Of Icinale

Dandelion is an herb that is native to Europe. It is also found throughout mild climates of the northern hemisphere. People use dandelion for conditions such as swelling (inflammation) of the tonsils (tonsillitis), infections of the kidney, bladder, or urethra (urinary tract infections or UTIs), and many others, but there is no good scientific evidence to support these uses.

How Does It Work?

Dandelion contains chemicals that may increase urine production, prevent crystals from forming in the urine, and decrease swelling (inflammation).

Uses & Effectiveness?

Insufficient Evidence For

- Arthritis-like pain.
- Bruises.
- Constipation.
- Eczema.
- Heart failure.
- Loss of appetite.
- Upset stomach.
- Intestinal gas (flatulence).
- Other conditions.

Side Effects & Safety

When taken by mouth: Dandelion is LIKELY SAFE for most people when taken by mouth in the amounts commonly found in food. It is POSSIBLY SAFE when taken by mouth in medicinal amounts (larger amounts than those found in food). Taking dandelion by mouth might cause allergic reactions, stomach discomfort, diarrhea, or heartburn in some people.

Special Precautions & Warnings:

1. Pregnancy And Breast-Feeding: There isn't enough reliable information to know if dandelion is safe to use when pregnant or breast-feeding. Stay on the safe side and avoid use.

2. Eczema: People with eczema seem to have a higher chance of having an allergic reaction to dandelion. If you have eczema, be sure to check with your healthcare provider before taking dandelion.

3. Bleeding Disorders: Dandelion might slow blood clotting. In theory, taking dandelion might increase the risk of bruising and bleeding in people with bleeding disorders.

4. Ragweed Allergy: People who are allergic to ragweed and related plants (daisies, chrysanthemums, marigolds) might be more likely to be allergic to dandelion. But conflicting data exists. If you have allergies, be sure to check with your healthcare provider before taking dandelion.

5. Kidney Failure: Dandelion might reduce how much oxalate is released through urine. In theory, this might increase the risk of complications in people with kidney problems.

Interactions

Moderate Interaction

Be cautious with this combination

1. Antibiotics (Quinolone Antibiotics) Interacts With DANDELION

Dandelion might decrease how much antibiotic the body absorbs. Taking dandelion along with antibiotics might decrease the effectiveness of some antibiotics. Some antibiotics that might interact with dandelion include ciprofloxacin (Cipro), enoxacin (Penetrex), norfloxacin (Chibroxin, Noroxin), sparfloxacin (Zagam), trovafloxacin (Trovan), and grepafloxacin (Raxar).

2. Lithium Interacts With DANDELION

Dandelion might affect a water pill or "diuretic." Taking dandelion might decrease how well the body gets rid of lithium. This could increase how much lithium is in the body and result in serious side effects. Talk with your healthcare provider before using this product if you are taking lithium. Your lithium dose might need to be changed. Medications changed by the liver (Cytochrome P450 1A2 (CYP1A2) substrates) interacts with DANDELION

3. Some Medications Are Changed And Broken Down By The Liver.

Dandelion might decrease how quickly the liver breaks down some medications. Taking dandelion along with some medications that are broken down by the liver can increase the effects and side effects of some medications. Before taking dandelion, talk to your healthcare provider if you take any medications that are changed by the liver.

4. Water Pills (Potassium-Sparing Diuretics) Interacts With DANDELION

Dandelion contains significant amounts of potassium. Some "water pills" can also increase potassium levels in the body. Taking some "water pills" along with dandelion might cause too much potassium to be in the body. Some "water pills" that increase potassium in the body include amiloride (Midamor), spironolactone (Aldactone), and triamterene (Dyrenium).

Dosing

The appropriate dose of dandelion depends on several factors such as the user's age, health, and several other conditions. At this time there is not enough scientific information to determine an appropriate range of doses for dandelion. Keep in mind that natural products are not always necessarily safe and dosages can be important. Be sure to follow relevant directions on product labels and consult your pharmacist or physician or other healthcare professional before using

16. Echinacea - Echinacea Angustifolia

What Is Echinacea?

Echinacea is an herb that is native to areas east of the Rocky Mountains in the United States. It is also grown in western States, as well as in Canada and Europe. Several species of the echinacea plant are used to make medicine from its leaves, flower, and root. Echinacea was used in traditional herbal remedies by the Great Plains Indian tribes. Later, settlers followed the Indians' example and began using echinacea for medicinal purposes as well. For a time, echinacea enjoyed official status as a result of being listed in the US National Formulary from 1916-1950. However, the use of echinacea fell out of favor in the United States with the discovery of antibiotics. But now, people are becoming interested in echinacea again because some antibiotics don't work as well as they used to against certain bacteria.

Echinacea is widely used to fight infections, especially the common cold, the flu, and other upper respiratory infections. Some people take echinacea at the first sign of a cold, hoping they will be able to keep the cold from developing. Other people take echinacea after cold symptoms have started, hoping they can make symptoms less severe.

Echinacea is also used against many other infections including urinary tract infections, vaginal yeast infections, herpes, HIV/AIDS, human papillomavirus (HPV), bloodstream infections (septicemia), tonsillitis, streptococcus infections, syphilis, typhoid, malaria, ear infection, swine flu, warts, and nose and throat infections called diphtheria. Other uses include anxiety, low white blood cell count, chronic fatigue syndrome (CFS), rheumatoid arthritis, migraines, acid indigestion, pain, dizziness, rattlesnake bites, attention deficit-hyperactivity disorder (ADHD), and improving exercise performance.

Sometimes people apply echinacea to their skin to treat boils, gum disease, abscesses, skin wounds, ulcers, burns, eczema, psoriasis, sun-related skin damage, herpes simplex, yeast infections, bee stings, snake and mosquito bites, and hemorrhoids. Echinacea is also used as an injection to treat vaginal yeast infections and urinary tract infections (UTIs). Commercially available echinacea products come in many forms including tablets, juice, and tea.

There are concerns about the quality of some echinacea products on the market. Echinacea products are frequently mislabeled, and some may not even contain echinacea, despite label claims. Don't be fooled by the term "standardized." It doesn't necessarily indicate accurate labeling. Also, some echinacea products have been contaminated with selenium, arsenic, and lead.

Possibly Effective For

Common cold. Many scientific studies show that taking some echinacea products when cold symptoms are first noticed can modestly reduce symptoms of the common cold in adults. But other scientific studies show no benefit. The problem is that scientific studies have used different types of echinacea plants and different methods of preparation. Since the studies have not been consistent, it is not surprising that different studies show different results. If it helps for TREATING a cold, the benefit will likely be modest at best. Research on the effects of echinacea for PREVENTING the common cold is also mixed. Some research shows that taking echinacea can reduce the risk of catching a cold by 45% to 58%. But other research shows that taking echinacea does not prevent the common cold when you are exposed to cold viruses.

Insufficient Evidence To Rate Effectiveness For

1. **Anxiety:** Early research suggests that taking 40 mg of a specific echinacea extract (ExtractumPharma ZRT, Budapest, Hungary) per day for 7 days reduces anxiety. But taking less than 40 mg per day does not seem to be effective.

2. **Exercise Performance:** Early research shows that taking echinacea (Puritan's Pride, Oakdale, NY) four times daily for 28 days increases oxygen intake during exercise tests in healthy men.

3. Gingivitis: Early research suggests that using a mouth rinse containing echinacea, Gotu kola, and elderberry (HM-302, Izum Pharmaceuticals, New York, NY) three times daily for 14 days might prevent gum disease from worsening. Using a specific mouth patch containing the same ingredients (PerioPatch, Izun Pharmaceuticals, New York, NY) also seems to reduce some symptoms of gum disease, but it is not always effective.

4. Herpes Simplex Virus (HSV): Evidence on the effect of echinacea for the treatment of HSV is unclear. Some research shows that taking a specific echinacea extract (Echinaforce, A Vogel Bioforce AG) 800 mg twice daily for 6 months does not seem to prevent or reduce the frequency or duration of recurrent genital herpes. However, other research shows that taking a combination product containing echinacea (Esberitox, Schaper & Brummer, Salzgitter-Ringelheim, Germany) 3-5 times daily reduces itchiness, tension, and pain in most people with cold sores (herpes labialis).

5. Human Papillomavirus (HPV): Early research shows that taking a combination product containing echinacea, Andrographis, grapefruit, papaya, pau d'arco, and cat's claw (Immune Act, Erba Vita SpA, Reppublica San Marino, Italy) daily for one month reduces the recurrence of anal warts in people who had surgical removal of anal warts. But this study was not of high quality, so the results are questionable.

6. Influenza (Flu): Early research shows that taking a specific echinacea product (Monoselect Echinacea, PharmExtracta, Pontenure, Italy) daily for 15 days might improve the response to the flu vaccine in people with breathing problems such as bronchitis or asthma.

7. Middle Ear Infection: Early research suggests that taking a specific liquid echinacea extract three times daily for 3 days at the first sign of a common cold does not prevent ear infection in children 1-5 years-old with a history of ear infections. Ear infections seemed to increase.

8. Eye Inflammation (Uveitis): Early research suggests that taking 150 mg of an echinacea product (Iridium, SOOFT Italia SpA) twice daily, in addition to eye drops and a steroid used to treat inflammation for 4 weeks, does not improve vision any more than eye drops and steroids alone in people with eye inflammation.

How Does Echinacea Work?

Echinacea seems to activate chemicals in the body that decrease inflammation, which might reduce cold and flu symptoms. Laboratory research suggests that echinacea can stimulate the body's immune system, but there is no evidence that this occurs in people. Echinacea also seems to contain some chemicals that can attack yeast and other kinds of fungi directly.

Are There Safety Concerns?

Echinacea is LIKELY SAFE for most people when taken by mouth in the short-term. Various liquid and solid forms of Echinacea have been used safely for up to 10 days. There are also some products, such as Echinaforce (A. Vogel Bioforce AG, Switzerland) that have been used safely for up to 6 months.

Some side effects have been reported such as fever, nausea, vomiting, unpleasant taste, stomach pain, diarrhea, sore throat, dry mouth, headache, numbness of the tongue, dizziness, insomnia, disorientation, and joint and muscle aches. In rare cases, echinacea has been reported to cause inflammation of the liver.

Special Precautions & Warnings:

1. Children: Echinacea is POSSIBLY SAFE when taken by mouth in the short-term. It seems to be safe in most children ages 2-11 years. However, about 7% of these children may experience a rash that could be due to an allergic reaction. There is some concern that allergic reactions to echinacea could be more severe in some children. For this reason, some regulatory organizations have recommended against giving echinacea to children under 12 years of age.

2. Pregnancy: Echinacea is POSSIBLY SAFE when taken by mouth in the short-term. There is some evidence that echinacea might be safe when taken during the first trimester of pregnancy without harming the fetus. But until this is confirmed by additional research, it is best to stay on the safe side and avoid use.

3. Breastfeeding: There is not enough reliable information about the safety of taking echinacea if you are breastfeeding. Stay on the safe side and avoid use.

4. An Inherited Tendency Toward Allergies (Atopy): People with this condition are more likely to develop an allergic reaction to echinacea. It's best to avoid exposure to echinacea if you have this condition.

5. "Auto-immune disorders" such as multiple sclerosis (MS), lupus (systemic lupus erythematosus, SLE), rheumatoid arthritis (RA), a skin disorder called pemphigus Vulgaris or others: Echinacea might affect the immune system that could make these conditions worse. Don't take echinacea if you have an auto-immune disorder.

17. Feverfew - Chrysanthemum Parthenium

Feverfew is a plant that is native to Asia Minor and the Balkans. It is now commonly grown throughout the world. Feverfew leaves are normally dried for use in medicine. Fresh leaves and extracts are also used. People most commonly take feverfew by mouth for migraine headaches. People also take feverfew by mouth for itching, tension headache, and many other conditions, but there is no good scientific evidence to support these uses.

How Does It Work?

Feverfew leaves contain many different chemicals, including one called parthenolide. Parthenolide or other chemicals decrease factors in the body that might cause migraine headaches.

Uses & Effectiveness?

Possibly Effective For

1. Migraine: Some research using feverfew alone or feverfew combined with other ingredients shows that taking feverfew by mouth can reduce the frequency and duration of migraine headaches and might reduce pain, nausea, vomiting, and sensitivity to light and noise when they do occur. Feverfew may be more effective in people with more frequent migraine attacks.

Insufficient Evidence For

- Itching
- Tension headache
- Allergies

- Asthma
- Bone disorders
- Cancer
- Common cold
- Dizziness
- Earache
- Fever
- Intestinal parasites
- Liver disease
- Menstrual irregularities
- Miscarriage prevention
- Muscle tension
- Nausea
- Psoriasis
- Ringing in the ears
- Swollen feet
- Toothaches
- Upset stomach
- Vomiting
- Other conditions

Side Effects & Safety

1. When Taken By Mouth: Dried feverfew leaf or feverfew extract is LIKELY SAFE when taken by mouth appropriately in the short-term (up to 4 months). Side effects might include upset stomach, heartburn, diarrhea, constipation, bloating, flatulence, nausea, and vomiting. Other reported side effects include nervousness, dizziness, headache, trouble sleeping, joint stiffness, tiredness, menstrual changes, rash, pounding heart, and weight gain. The safety of feverfew beyond 4 months' use has not been studied. Feverfew is POSSIBLY UNSAFE when fresh leave is chewed. Chewing fresh feverfew leaves can cause mouth sores, swelling of the mouth, and loss of taste.

Special Precautions & Warnings

1. Pregnancy: Feverfew is POSSIBLY UNSAFE when taken by mouth during pregnancy. There is concern that it might cause early contractions and miscarriage. Don't use feverfew if you are pregnant.

2. Breast-Feeding: There is not enough reliable information about the safety of feverfew if you are breast-feeding. Stay on the safe side and avoid use.

3. Bleeding Disorders: Feverfew might slow blood clotting. In theory, taking feverfew could increase the risk of bleeding in some people. Until more is known, use feverfew cautiously if you have a bleeding disorder.

4. Allergy to ragweed and related plants: Feverfew may cause an allergic reaction in people who are sensitive to the Asteraceae/Compositae plant family. Members of this family include ragweed, chrysanthemums, marigolds, daisies, and many others. If you have allergies, be sure to check with your healthcare provider before taking feverfew.

5. Surgery: Feverfew might slow blood clotting. It might cause bleeding during and after surgery. Stop taking feverfew at least 2 weeks before a scheduled surgery.

Dosing

The following doses have been studied in scientific research:

1. **By Mouth:**

For migraine: 50-150 mg of feverfew powder taken once daily for up to 4 months. A dose of 2.08-18.75 mg of a carbon dioxide extract of feverfew (MIG-99, Schaper & Brümmer GmbH & Co) taken three times daily for 3 to 4 months.

The following combination products have been used for 3 months for preventing migraines: a combination of feverfew 300 mg and white willow 300 mg, taken twice daily (Mig-RL, Naturveda-Vitro-Bio Research Institute); a combination of feverfew 100 mg, coenzyme Q10, magnesium, and vitamin B6, taken daily (Antemig, PiLeJe); a combination of feverfew (containing Tanacetum parthenium 150 mg), 5-HTP, and magnesium, taken daily (Aurastop, Aesculapius Farmaceutici).

Specific combination products containing feverfew and ginger (GelStat Migraine, GelStat Corporation; LipiGesic M, PuraMed BioScience, Inc.) have been used to treat migraines after a migraine starts for up to 1 month. Two 2-mL doses have been given under the tongue, 5 minutes apart. Each dose has been held under the tongue for 60 seconds before swallowing.

18. Gravel Root - Eutrochium Purpureum

Gravel root is an herb. The bulb, root, and parts that grow above the ground are used to make medicine. Despite safety concerns, people use gravel root for conditions such as bladder infections, kidney stones, arthritis pain, fever, and many others, but there is no good scientific evidence to support these uses.

How Does It Work?

Gravel root might work for certain conditions by reducing swelling (inflammation).

Uses & Effectiveness?

Insufficient Evidence For

- Arthritis-like pain.
- Fever.
- Gout.
- Urinary and kidney stones.
- Urinary tract infections.
- Other conditions.

Side Effects & Safety

1. When Taken By Mouth: There's a lot of concern about using gravel root as medicine, because it contains chemicals called hepatotoxic pyrrolizidine alkaloids (PAs). These chemicals may block blood flow in the veins and cause liver or lung damage. Gravel root preparations that are not certified and labeled "hepatotoxic PA-free" are considered LIKELY UNSAFE. There isn't enough reliable information to know if it's safe to take "hepatotoxic PA-free" gravel root by mouth. It's best to avoid use.

2. When Applied To The Skin: It is LIKELY UNSAFE to apply gravel root to broken skin. The dangerous chemicals in gravel root can be absorbed quickly through broken skin and can lead to dangerous body-wide toxicity. Steer clear of skin products that aren't certified and labeled "hepatotoxic PA-free." There isn't enough reliable information to know if it's safe to apply "hepatotoxic PA-free" gravel root to the skin. It's best to avoid use.

Special Precautions & Warnings:

1. Pregnancy: It's LIKELY UNSAFE to use gravel root preparations that might contain hepatotoxic PAs during pregnancy. These products might cause birth defects and liver damage. It's not known whether products that are certified "hepatotoxic PA-free" are safe to use during pregnancy. Stay on the safe side and avoid using any gravel root preparation.

2. Breast-Feeding: It's LIKELY UNSAFE to use gravel root preparations that might contain hepatotoxic PAs if you are breast-feeding. These chemicals can pass into breast milk and might harm the nursing infant. It's not known whether products that are certified "hepatotoxic PA-free" are safe to use when breastfeeding. Stay on the safe side and avoid using any gravel root preparation.

3. Allergy To Ragweed And Related Plants: Gravel root may cause an allergic reaction in people who are allergic to the Asteraceae/Compositae plant family. Members of this family include ragweed, chrysanthemums, marigolds, daisies, and many others. If you have allergies, be sure to check with your healthcare provider before taking gravel root.

4. Liver Disease: There is concern that the hepatotoxic PAs in gravel root might make liver disease worse.

Dosing

The appropriate dose of gravel root depends on several factors such as the user's age, health, and several other conditions. At this time there is not enough scientific information to determine an appropriate range of doses for gravel root. Keep in mind that natural products are not always necessarily safe and dosages can be important. Be sure to follow relevant directions on product labels and consult your pharmacist or physician or other healthcare professional before using.

19. Hops - Humulus Lupulus

Hops are the dried, flowering part of the hop plant. They are commonly used in brewing beer and as flavoring components in foods. Hops are also used to make medicine. Hops are commonly used orally for anxiety, sleep disorders such as the inability to sleep (insomnia) or disturbed sleep due to rotating or nighttime work hours (shift work disorder), restlessness, tension, excitability, attention deficit-hyperactivity disorder (ADHD), nervousness, irritability, and symptoms of menopause among other uses. But there is limited scientific evidence to support using hopes for any of these conditions.

How Does It Work?

The chemicals in hops seem to have weak effects similar to the hormone estrogen. Some chemicals in hops also seem to reduce swelling, prevent infections, and cause sleepiness.

Uses & Effectiveness?

Insufficient Evidence For

- Anxiety
- Attention deficit-hyperactivity disorder (ADHD)
- Body odor
- Breast-feeding
- Breast cancer
- Excitability
- High levels of cholesterol or other fats (lipids) in the blood (hyperlipidemia)
- Improving appetite
- Indigestion (dyspepsia)
- Insomnia
- Intestinal cramps
- Irritability
- Leg sores are caused by weak blood circulation (venous leg ulcers)
- Nerve pain
- Nervousness
- Ovarian cancer
- Pain and swelling (inflammation) of the bladder
- Prostate cancer
- Restlessness
- Tension
- Tuberculosis

Side Effects & Safety

1. **When Taken By Mouth:** Hops are LIKELY SAFE when consumed in amounts commonly found in foods. Hops are POSSIBLY SAFE when taken for medicinal uses, short-term. Hops might cause dizziness and sleepiness in some people. Women taking hops might notice changes in their menstrual cycle.

Special Precautions & Warnings

1. **Pregnancy And Breast-Feeding:** There isn't enough reliable information to know if hops are safe to use when pregnant or breast-feeding. Stay on the safe side and avoid use.

2. **Depression:** Hops may make depression worse. Avoid use.

3. **Hormone-Sensitive Cancers And Conditions:** Some chemicals in hops act like the hormone estrogen. People who have conditions that are sensitive to hormones should avoid hops. Some of these conditions including breast cancer and endometriosis.

4. **Surgery:** Hops might cause too much sleepiness when combined with anesthesia and other medications during and after surgical procedures. Stop taking hops at least 2 weeks before a scheduled surgery.

Interactions?

Moderate Interaction

Alcohol Interacts With HOPS

Alcohol can cause sleepiness and drowsiness. Hops might also cause sleepiness and drowsiness. Taking large amounts of hops along with alcohol might cause too much sleepiness.

Dosing

The appropriate dose of hops depends on several factors such as the user's age, health, and several other conditions. At this time there is not enough scientific information to determine an appropriate range of doses for hops. Keep in mind that natural products are not always necessarily safe and dosages can be important. Be sure to follow relevant directions on product labels and consult your pharmacist or physician or other healthcare professional before using.

20. Mullein - Verbascum

What Is Mullein?

Mullein is a plant. The flower is used to make medicine. Mullein is used for cough, whooping cough, tuberculosis, bronchitis, hoarseness, pneumonia, earaches, colds, chills, flu, swine flu, fever, allergies, tonsillitis, and sore throat. Other uses include asthma, diarrhea, colic, gastrointestinal bleeding, migraines, joint pain, and gout. It is also used as a sedative and as a diuretic to increase urine output. Mullein is applied to the skin for wounds, burns, hemorrhoids, bruises, frostbite, and skin infections (cellulitis). The leaves are used topically to soften and protect the skin. In manufacturing, mullein is used as a flavoring ingredient in alcoholic beverages.

Insufficient Evidence To Rate Effectiveness For

- Ear infections (otitis media)
- Wounds
- Hemorrhoids
- Colds
- Flu
- Asthma
- Diarrhea
- Migraines
- Gout
- Tuberculosis
- Croup
- Cough
- Sore throat
- Inflammation of the airways (bronchitis)
- Other conditions

How Does Mullein Work?

The chemicals in mullein might be able to fight influenza and herpes viruses, and some bacteria that cause respiratory infections.

Are There Safety Concerns?

Mullein is POSSIBLY SAFE for when applied to the ear, short-term. A specific product (Otikon Otic Solution, Healthy-On Ltd.) that contains mullein, garlic, calendula, and St. John's wort has been used in the ear for up to 3 days.

Special Precautions & Warnings:

1. Children: Mullein is POSSIBLY SAFE when applied to the ear, short-term. A specific product (Otikon Otic Solution, Healthy-On Ltd.) that contains mullein, garlic, calendula, and St. John's wort has been used in the ear for up to 3 days.

2. Pregnancy And Breast-Feeding: There is not enough reliable information about the safety of taking mullein if you are pregnant or breast-feeding. Stay on the safe side and avoid use.

Dosing Considerations For Mullein

The appropriate dose of mullein depends on several factors such as the user's age, health, and several other conditions. At this time there is not enough scientific information to determine an appropriate range of doses for mullein. Keep in mind that natural products are not always necessarily safe and dosages can be important. Be sure to follow relevant directions on product labels and consult your pharmacist or physician or other healthcare professional before using.

21. Nettle - Urtica Dioica

Stinging Nettle

Stinging nettle is a plant. The root and above-ground parts are used as medicine. Stinging nettle is used for diabetes and osteoarthritis. It is sometimes used for urinary tract infections (UTIs), kidney stones, enlarged prostate (benign prostatic hyperplasia or BPH), muscle pain, and other conditions, but there is no good scientific research to support these uses. In foods, young stinging nettle leaves are eaten as a cooked vegetable.

In manufacturing, stinging nettle extract is used as an ingredient in hair and skin products. Stinging nettle leaf has a long history of use. It was used primarily as a diuretic and laxative in ancient Greek times. Don't confuse stinging nettle (Urtica dioica) with white dead nettle (Lamium album).

How Does It Work?

Stinging nettle contains ingredients that might decrease inflammation and increase urine output.

Uses & Effectiveness?

Possibly Effective For

1. Diabetes: Taking stinging nettle leaf preparations for 8-12 weeks seems to reduce blood sugar in people with type 2 diabetes. The effect of stinging nettle on A1c in people with diabetes is unclear.

2. Osteoarthritis: Taking stinging nettle leaf preparations by mouth or applying it to the skin might reduce pain in people with osteoarthritis. Taking stinging nettle leaf preparations by mouth might also reduce the need for pain medications.

Insufficient Evidence For

- Hay fever
- A mild form of gum disease (gingivitis)
- Anemia
- Asthma
- Bleeding
- Cancer
- Diarrhea
- Eczema (atopic dermatitis)
- Heart failure
- Infections of the kidney, bladder, or urethra (urinary tract infections or UTIs)
- Joint pain
- Kidney stones
- Male-pattern baldness (androgenic alopecia)
- Muscle pai
- Poor circulation
- Rough, scaly skin on the scalp and face (seborrheic dermatitis)
- Water retention
- Wound healing
- Other conditions

Side Effects & Safety

1. When Taken By Mouth: Stinging nettle is POSSIBLY SAFE when taken by mouth for up to 2 years. It might cause diarrhea, constipation, and upset stomach in some people.

2. When Applied To The Skin: Stinging nettle is POSSIBLY SAFE when applied to the skin in appropriate amounts. Touching the stinging nettle plant can cause skin irritation.

Special Precautions & Warnings:

1. Pregnancy And Breast-Feeding: Stinging nettle is LIKELY UNSAFE to take during pregnancy. It might stimulate uterine contractions and cause a miscarriage. It's also best to avoid stinging nettle if you are breast-feeding.

2. Diabetes: There is some evidence that stinging nettle above-ground parts can decrease blood sugar levels. This might increase the chance of blood sugar levels becoming too low in people being treated for diabetes. Monitor your blood sugar carefully.

3. Low Blood Pressure: Stinging nettle above ground parts might lower blood pressure. In theory, stinging nettle might increase the risk of blood pressure dropping too low in people prone to low blood pressure. If you have low blood pressure, discuss stinging nettle with your healthcare provider before starting it.

4. Kidney Problems: The above-ground parts of stinging nettle seem to increase urine flow. If you have kidney problems, discuss stinging nettle with your healthcare provider before starting it.

Dosing

The following doses have been studied in scientific research:

Adults

By Mouth:

1. For Diabetes: 500 mg of stinging nettle leaf extract has been taken three times per day for 12 weeks. Also, 3.3 grams of stinging nettle leaf has been taken three times daily for 8 weeks. A combination product containing 200 mg of stinging nettle, 200 mg of milk thistle, and 200 mg of frankincense taken three times per day for 3 months has also been used.

2. For Osteoarthritis: 9 grams of crude stinging nettle leaf has been used daily. Also, an infusion containing 50 mg of stinging nettle leaf has been taken along with 50 mg of diclofenac daily for 14 days.

Applied To The Skin:

For osteoarthritis: Fresh stinging nettle leaf has been applied to painful joints for 30 seconds once per day for one week. Also, a specific cream containing stinging nettle leaf extract (Liquid Phyto-Caps Nettle Leaf by Gaia Herbs) has been applied twice daily for 2 weeks.

22. Oregon Grape - Mahonia Aquifolium

The Oregon grape (Mahonia aquifolium) is a broadleaf evergreen shrub that grows well in shadier spots. It originated in western North America and is the state flower of Oregon. It will provide color throughout all four seasons with its green and burgundy foliage, yellow flowers, and purplish-blue fruit.

Hardiness And Growing Tips

The soil needs to be moist with good drainage for optimal growth. It needs to be acidic or at least neutral as alkaline soils can be problematic. Change your soil to be more acidic if the pH is not too much above neutral.

This shrub is best suited for USDA Zones 5-9. It is native to western North America. Partial shade is ideal for this species. It can also be grown in full shade or full sun, though too much light can cause foliage scorching. Try to find a planting location that offers some shelter from the wind. Since these are evergreen and do not drop in the fall, the leaves may dry out in the winter if the shrub is hit by wind often.

Propagation can be performed through the use of seed germination, taking cuttings, and dividing existing plants. The plant will also naturally propagate itself through cloning.

Size And Design Tips

Oregon grape will be 3 to 10 feet tall and 2 to 5 feet wide. Look for the 'Compactum' cultivar if you want a shrub that is shorter, at 3 feet tall. Or, if you want a similar looking shrub that is more of a groundcover, choose the creeping mahonia (Mahonia repens). This species only is about a foot tall at maturity.

The fruit is a berry that does resemble a grape in shape and color. They are edible but are quite tart and can be used to make jams, jellies, and preserves. Oregon grape can be used as part of a wildlife garden to attract butterflies, bees, hummingbirds, and other birds to your yard.

This shrub can clone itself and spread. On one hand, this can be a useful feature as you can use it to populate a native garden or divide to create new plants. However, this tendency can also lead to the species being invasive in some locations. Your local extension service will know if it is a problem in your area.

Foliage

The evergreen leaves are sharply toothed like members of the holly genus as noted in the species name. It can be used as a privacy screen to keep unwanted visitors out since the leaves are sharp. These are pinnately compound leaves that are up to 12" long and made up of several leaflets. When they first appear, they are red. As time passes they turn into a shiny green hue. During autumn, they become burgundy but do not fall off.

Health Benefits

The root of Oregon grape has been used as herbal medicine to treat many maladies including colds, flu, herpes, hepatitis, syphilis, stomach upset, cancer, skin disorders, yeast infections, and more. Herbalists have touted the use of Oregon grape, claiming that it is effective in stimulating liver function, treating infections, and supporting digestive health.

It's important to note that there are limited clinical research study results available on the safety and health benefits of the Oregon grape. Most of the published clinical research study results on Oregon grape involved the use of the root of the herb in a topical (administered on the skin) cream, for the treatment of a skin condition called psoriasis. Oregon grape has also been used for its digestive stimulant properties (relieving spasms in the intestinal tract), antimicrobial properties (including its anti-fungal, antibacterial, and anti-parasitic action), immune-boosting, and anti-inflammatory properties.

Medical Uses

Oregon grape has been demonstrated to help lower blood sugar in patients with insulin resistance. It also has some cholesterol-lowering effects. The herb has traditionally been used for maladies including, eye infections, acne, athlete's foot, gastrointestinal issues, skin conditions, and more, though there is limited scientific research on these claims.

Some studies have shown that Oregon grape may be effective for the treatment of giardia (a type of infectious diarrhea), eczema (an inflammatory skin condition), and as an herbal treatment for urinary tract infections. The primary medicinal component of Oregon grape, berberine, has been shown to have anti-bacterial properties that are helpful in the treatment of several infections including, throat, intestinal, and urinary tract infections. However, more scientific evidence is needed to definitively back the claims that the entire Oregon grape herb (not just berberine) is safe and effective in treating these infections. Extensive medical research data has shown that Oregon grape may be safe and effective for the treatment of psoriasis (a common skin condition that causes skin cells to form scales and itchy, sometimes painful red patches).

23. Primrose (Evening) Oil - Oenothera Biennis

Evening primrose is a plant native to North and South America. It also grows throughout Europe and parts of Asia. It has yellow flowers which open at sunset and close during the day. The oil from the seeds of evening primrose is used to make medicine. Evening primrose is used for premenstrual syndrome (PMS), symptoms of menopause, arthritis, swelling, and other conditions, but there is no good scientific evidence to support its use. In foods, the oil from evening primrose is used as a source of essential fatty acids. In manufacturing, the oil from evening primrose is used in soaps and cosmetics.

How Does It Work?

Evening primrose oil contains "fatty acids." Some women with breast pain might not have high enough levels of certain "fatty acids." Fatty acids also seem to help decrease inflammation related to conditions such as arthritis and eczema.

Uses & Effectiveness?

Possibly Effective For

1. Nerve Damage Caused By Diabetes: Research shows that taking evening primrose oil daily for 6-12 months improves symptoms of nerve damage caused by diabetes.

2. Osteoporosis: Taking evening primrose oil with fish oil and calcium seems to decrease bone loss and increase bone density in elderly people with osteoporosis.

Possibly Ineffective For

1. Asthma: Several small studies show that taking 15-20 mL or 4-6 grams of evening primrose daily for up to 16 weeks doesn't improve asthma symptoms.

2. Breast Pain (Mastalgia): High-quality research shows that evening primrose is no more effective than a placebo (sugar pill) for reducing breast pain.

Insufficient Evidence For

1. Eczema (Atopic Dermatitis): Research evaluating evening primrose for eczema shows conflicting results. Some research shows that taking evening primrose, up to 6 grams per day by mouth for 3-5 months, reduces the severity and symptoms of eczema in adults and children. However, other studies show that taking evening primrose, 6-8 grams per day in adults or 2-4 grams per day in children for 12-16 weeks, has no benefit. Other early research shows that applying a cream containing evening primrose for 2 weeks may improve symptoms of eczema.

2. Chronic Fatigue Syndrome (CFS): One early study shows that taking a specific combination of evening primrose and fish oil might reduce CFS-like symptoms that occurred after a viral infection. However, in another study in people with a confirmed diagnosis of CFS, the same product was no better than a placebo (sugar pill).

3. Nerve Pain In People With Diabetes (Diabetic Neuropathy): Evidence on the effectiveness of evening primrose for treating nerve damage in people with diabetes is conflicting. One study shows that taking up to 6 grams of evening primrose daily for up to 12 months improves how well the nerves work in people with nerve damage caused by diabetes. Other research shows that taking a similar amount of evening primrose does not improve nerve function in people with this condition.

4. Dry Eye: Early research shows that taking a specific evening primrose product 3 grams daily for 6 months improves dry eye symptoms in women wearing soft contact lenses.

5. Swelling (inflammation) of the liver caused by the hepatitis B virus (hepatitis B). Early research shows that taking 4 grams per day of evening primrose for 12 months does not improve liver damage in people with hepatitis B.

6. High levels of cholesterol or other fats (lipids) in the blood (hyperlipidemia). Some research shows that taking evening primrose oil can decreases total cholesterol and blood fats called triglycerides while increasing good (HDL) cholesterol. But not all research agrees.

7. An inherited skin disorder that causes dry, scaly skin (ichthyosis). Early research shows that taking evening primrose, 3 grams per day in adults or 2 grams per day in children, does not improve symptoms of ichthyosis.

8. Liver Cancer: Early research shows that taking 18 grams of evening primrose per day does not affect liver size or survival in people with liver cancer.

9. Symptoms Of The Menopause: In most studies, taking evening primrose does not reduce hot flashes or night sweats any more than a placebo (sugar pill). But taking evening primrose oil might help to improve mood.

10. Multiple Sclerosis (MS): Some early research shows that taking evening primrose for 6 months improves disability scores in some people with MS. But other research shows that using a specific evening primrose product for 2 years may increase the likelihood of symptom worsening compared with a placebo (sugar pill).

11. Childbirth: However, another study did not show this effect. Other early research shows that taking evening primrose from week 37 of pregnancy until delivery doesn't improve childbirth. It might prolong labor and increase the need for contraction-inducing medicine (oxytocin).

12. Rheumatoid Arthritis (RA): One early study shows that taking 6 grams per day of evening primrose for 12 months improves self-reported symptoms of RA. However, other research has found evening primrose to be no better than a placebo (sugar pill).

- A motor skill disorder marked by clumsiness (developmental coordination disorder or DCD).
- Water warts.
- Diabetes.
- A learning disorder marked by difficulty reading (dyslexia).
- Low bone mass (osteopenia).
- A hormonal disorder that causes enlarged ovaries with cysts (polycystic ovary syndrome or PCOS).
- Scaly, itchy skin (psoriasis).
- Joint swelling (inflammation) in people with psoriasis.
- A type of inflammatory bowel disease (ulcerative colitis).
- Alzheimer disease.
- Heart disease.
- Infant development.
- Schizophrenia.
- Other conditions.

Side Effects & Safety

1. When Taken By Mouth: Evening primrose is LIKELY SAFE for most people when taken by mouth in doses up to 6 grams daily. It may cause mild side effects including upset stomach, nausea, diarrhea, and headache in some people.

2. When Applied To The Skin: Evening primrose is LIKELY SAFE for most people when applied to the skin.

Special Precautions & Warnings

1. Pregnancy And Breast-Feeding: Taking evening primrose by mouth is POSSIBLY SAFE during pregnancy. Taking up to 4 grams daily for up to 10 weeks during pregnancy seems to be safe. But until this is confirmed by additional research, it is best to stay on the safe side and avoid use. Taking evening primrose during the last weeks of pregnancy might delay labor. Don't use this product close to the end of pregnancy.

2. Children: Evening primrose is LIKELY SAFE for most people when taken by mouth in doses up to 6 grams daily. It is also LIKELY SAFE when applied to the skin.

3. Bleeding Disorders: There is a concern that evening primrose might increase the chance of bruising and bleeding. Don't use it if you have a bleeding disorder.

4. Epilepsy Or Another Seizure Disorder: There is a concern that taking evening primrose might make seizures more likely in some people.

5. Schizophrenia: Seizures have been reported in people with schizophrenia treated with phenothiazine drugs, GLA (a chemical found in evening primrose oil), and vitamin E. Get your healthcare provider's opinion before starting evening primrose.

6. Surgery: Evening primrose might increase the chance of bleeding during or after surgery. Stop using it at least 2 weeks before a scheduled surgery.

Dosing

The following doses have been studied in scientific research:

By Mouth:

For breast pain: 3-4 grams daily.

24. Purslane - Portulaca Oleracea

Purslane

Use

Purslane has been used as a vegetable source of omega-3 fatty acids and is high in vitamins and minerals. It possesses marked antioxidant activity. Roles in abnormal uterine bleeding, asthma, type 2 diabetes, and oral lichen planus are suggested; however, clinical studies are limited and diverse.

Dosing

Limited clinical studies are available to provide dosage guidelines; however, 180 mg/day of purslane extract has been studied in diabetic patients, and powdered seeds have been taken at 1 to 30 g daily in divided doses, as well as both ethanol and aqueous purslane extracts. Traditional Chinese Medicine recommendations of 9 to 15 g of dried aerial parts, and 10 to 30 g fresh herb, have been reported for a variety of indications. One hundred grams of fresh purslane leaves yields approximately 300 to 400 mg of alpha-linolenic acid.

Contraindications

Contraindications have not been identified.

Pregnancy/Lactation

Information regarding safety and efficacy in pregnancy and lactation is lacking.

Interactions

None well documented.

Adverse Reactions

Limited clinical studies have not reported clinically important adverse effects. Effects on uterine contractions are contradictory.

Health Benefits Of Purslane

Health Benefits Nutrition How To Eat Purslane

Purslane, also known as little hogweed, is a common weed worldwide. But just because it's considered a weed doesn't mean it's worthless. This salty, slightly sour plant, is completely edible and provides some impressive health benefits. Purslane is a succulent that offers a juicy bite. This allows it to be grown in conditions that would kill even the hardiest lettuce. Its sturdy nature makes purslane a great garden-vegetable option for dry, hot regions or gardeners who don't trust themselves to water regularly. Purslane's health benefits are an added benefit for this hearty, gardener's treasure.

Health Benefits

Purslane has vitamins, minerals, and antioxidants that can provide important health benefits. For example, vitamin A helps your eyes remain healthy as well as improve your immune system. Vitamin A is also critical to the health of your organs because it supports healthy cell division. Purslane is also rich in vitamin C, which is important to keep your collagen and blood vessels in good shape, as well as helping injuries heal.

Also, Purslane Can Provide Other Health Benefits, Like:

1. Lower Risk Of Cancer

Purslane is full of beta-carotene, the pigment responsible for the reddish color of its stems and leaves. Beta-carotene is one of many antioxidants s found in purslane. These antioxidants have been found to reduce the number of free radicals in your body. Free radicals are oxygen by-products given off by all cells in the body. Lowering the number of free radicals can help reduce the risk of cellular damage. This, in turn, lowers your risk of cancer.

2. Heart Health

Purslane is also helpful for supporting your cardiovascular system. It is one of the few vegetables that are rich in omega-3 fatty acids, which are important to support healthy arteries and can help prevent strokes, heart attacks, and other forms of heart disease. Purslane has the highest recorded levels of omega-3 fatty acids of any land-based plant.

3. Bone Health

Purslane is also a great source of two minerals that are important to bone health: calcium and magnesium. Calcium is the most common mineral in your body, and failing to eat enough of it can slowly weaken your bones, leading to osteoporosis. On the other hand, magnesium indirectly affects skeletal health by affecting the growth of bone cells. Getting enough of both of these minerals can improve skeletal health and prevent complications from osteoporosis and aging.

Nutrition

Purslane is rich in folate, which aids in safe cell division and promotes DNA duplication. Doctors recommend that people who can become pregnant consume at least 400 mcg of folate daily because it helps avoid birth defects.

Purslane is also an excellent source of:

- Vitamin A
- Vitamin C
- Potassium
- Calcium
- Iron
- Folate
- Choline
- Magnesium

How To Eat Purslane

Purslane can easily be found outdoors during the spring and summer in most parts of the world. The plant reproduces easily and can survive harsh growing environments, so it's often spotted between cracks in the sidewalk or untended gardens. Any purslane plant can be harvested and eaten, as the leaves, stems, and flowers are completely edible. When preparing wild purslane, it's important to wash the plant carefully to ensure that no pesticides are on the leaves. Purslane is tart and a little salty, making it a great addition to salads and other dishes. It can be eaten raw or cooked. When added to soups and stew, it thickens the broth nicely.

Here Are Some Ways You Can Include Purslane In Your Diet:

- Add purslane to soups
- Sauté purslane as a side dish
- Chop purslane and add it to salads for color
- Mix purslane into grilled vegetables

- Use purslane as a garnish
- Sprinkle purslane flowers on fish as a point of interest

25. Passionflower - Passiflora Incarnata

Passionflower is a climbing vine that is native to the southeastern United States, and Central and South America. The above-ground parts are used to make medicine. Passionflower is used for anxiety, including anxiety before surgery. Some people take passionflower for insomnia, stress, attention deficit-hyperactivity disorder (ADHD), pain, and many other conditions. But there is no good scientific research to support these uses. In foods and beverages, passionflower extract is used as a flavoring.

How does it work?

The chemicals in passionflower have to calm, sleep-inducing, and muscle spasm relieving effects. Passionflower is a climbing vine that is native to the southeastern United States, and Central and South America. The above-ground parts are used to make medicine.

Uses & Effectiveness?

Possibly Effective For

1. **Anxiety:** Some research shows that taking passion flower by mouth can reduce symptoms of anxiety. It might work as effectively as some prescription medications.

2. **Anxiety Before Surgery:** Some research shows that taking passion flower by mouth can reduce anxiety before surgery when taken 30-90 minutes before surgery. It might work as effectively as some other treatments for pre-operative anxiety such as melatonin or midazolam.

Insufficient Evidence For

- Attention deficit-hyperactivity disorder (ADHD)
- Insomnia
- Alcohol use disorder
- Asthma
- Burns
- Diarrhea
- Fibromyalgia
- Heart failure and fluid build up in the body (congestive heart failure or CHF)
- Hemorrhoids
- Inability to cope or adjust to a stressful event (adjustment disorders)
- Indigestion (dyspepsia)
- Irregular heartbeat (arrhythmia).
- Menstrual cramps (dysmenorrhea)
- Muscle cramps
- Pain
- Premenstrual syndrome (PMS)
- Seizures are not caused by epilepsy
- Stress

- Symptoms of the menopause
- Other conditions

Side Effects & Safety

1. When Taken By Mouth: Passionflower is LIKELY SAFE for most people when used in food-flavoring amounts. It is POSSIBLY SAFE for most people when taken as a tea nightly for 7 nights, or as a medicine for up to 8 weeks. It may cause side effects such as drowsiness, dizziness, and confusion.

It is POSSIBLY UNSAFE for most people when taken by mouth in large amounts, such as 3.5 grams of a specific extract (Sedacalm by Bio plus Healthcare) over 2 days.

2. When Applied To The Skin: There isn't enough reliable information to know if passionflower is safe or what the side effects might be when applied to the skin.

Special Precautions & Warnings:

1. Children: Passionflower is POSSIBLY SAFE for most children when taken by mouth for short periods. A specific passionflower product (Pasipay by Iran Darouk Pharmaceutical Company) has been used safely in children aged 6-13 years at a dose of 0.04 mg per kg body weight daily for up to 8 weeks.

2. Pregnancy: Passionflower is POSSIBLY UNSAFE when taken by mouth during pregnancy. There are some reports of early labor and other problems when passionflower has been used in pregnancy. There are some chemicals in the passionflower plant that might cause the uterus to contract. Don't use passionflower if you are pregnant.

3. Breast-feeding: There isn't enough reliable information to know if passionflower is safe to use when breastfeeding. Stay on the safe side and avoid use.

4. Surgery: Passionflower might cause drowsiness. It might increase the effects of anesthesia and other medications on the brain during and after surgery. Talk to your healthcare provider if you are taking passion flower within 2 weeks of scheduled surgery.

Dosing

The following doses have been studied in scientific research:

Adults

By Mouth:

1. For Anxiety: Capsules containing 400 mg of passionflower extract twice daily for 2-8 weeks has been used. Also, 45 drops of a liquid extract of passionflower have been used daily for up to one month.

2. For Reducing Anxiety Before Surgery: 20 drops of a specific passionflower extract taken the evening before surgery and 90 minutes before the start of surgery has been used. Passionflower 260-1000 mg has been taken 30-90 minutes before dental surgery. Also, a syrup containing 700 mg of passionflower extract (Passiflora syrup by Sandoz) has been taken 30 minutes before surgery.

26. Red Clover - Trifolium Pratense

Red clover is a plant. The flowers are used to make medicine. Red clover is used for symptoms of menopause, weak and brittle bones, high levels of cholesterol, and many other conditions, but there is no good scientific evidence to support these uses. In foods and beverages, red clover is used as a flavoring ingredient. Red clover (Trifolium pratense) is an herb that belongs to the legume family, which also includes peas and beans. In herbal medicine, red clover is typically used to treat respiratory issues (such as asthma, whooping cough, and bronchitis), skin disorders (such as eczema and psoriasis), inflammatory conditions like arthritis, and women's health problems1 (such as menopausal and menstrual symptoms).

Red clover's brightly colored flowers contain many nutrients including calcium, chromium, magnesium, niacin, phosphorus, potassium, thiamine, and vitamin C. They're also a rich source of isoflavones. These are compounds that act as phytoestrogens plant chemicals similar to the female hormone estrogen. Isoflavone extracts are touted as dietary supplements for high cholesterol and osteoporosis in addition to menopausal symptoms.

Health Benefits

In alternative medicine, red clover is said to help with the following conditions. Note, however, that research hasn't shown that the herb is conclusively effective for these or any other health concerns.

1. Menopausal Symptoms

Several small studies have been done to see if red clover may help relieve the discomforts of menopause, especially hot flashes. Though you may hear some anecdotal support for this, there has been no conclusive evidence to back it up. A research review conducted in 2013 notes that phytoestrogen treatments (including red clover) are not proven to effectively alleviate menopausal symptoms.

2. Bone Loss

Research is ongoing as to whether isoflavones lower the loss of bone mineral density in postmenopausal women. Red clover is one source of supplements used in some studies. A review done in 2016 concluded there may be some beneficial effects on bone health, while a 2017 review found that different formulations of red clover may be effective or ineffective.

3. Cancer

Preliminary research suggests that red clover may help reduce the risk of prostate cancer. In a 2009 study of prostate cancer cells, scientists found that treatment with red clover led to a decrease in the prostate-specific antigen (PSA), a protein found at elevated levels in men with prostate cancer.

4. Heart Disease

A few clinical trials have looked at the effects of red clover on the development of risk factors for heart disease in postmenopausal women, with no strong evidence that it helps, reports Memorial Sloan Kettering Cancer Center. Keep in mind that, due to the lack of long-term studies, it's too soon to recommend red clover for any condition. It's also important to note that self-treating a condition and avoiding or delaying standard care may have serious consequences.

5. Selection And Preparation

Red clover is available in a variety of preparations, including teas, tinctures, tablets, capsules, liquid extract, and extracts standardized to specific isoflavone contents. It's not always clear, however, that a product contains the promised isoflavone content.

Making Red Clover Tea

You can also make tea from dried flower heads. Some proponents claim that to get the full benefit of red clover you need to use the whole flower, and not commercial red clover isoflavones, which many studies use. To make a tea, use one to three teaspoons of dried red clover flowers for every cup of simmering (not boiling) water. Let steep for 15 minutes. Drink up to three cups of tea a day.

How Does It Work?

Red clover contains chemicals called phytoestrogens that are similar to the hormone estrogen.

Uses & Effectiveness?

Possibly Ineffective For

Weak and brittle bones (osteoporosis). Most research shows that taking red clover daily does not improve the density of bones in women.

Insufficient Evidence For

1. **Male-Pattern Baldness (Androgenic Alopecia):** Early research shows that applying a combination product containing red clover flower extract might increase hair growth in people with hair loss.

2. **Enlarged Prostate (Benign Prostatic Hyperplasia Or BPH):** Some early research suggests that red clover supplements might improve some symptoms of an enlarged prostate. It seems to reduce nighttime urination.

3. **Breast Pain (Mastalgia):** There is some early evidence that red clover might help relieve cyclic breast pain and tenderness.

4. **High Cholesterol:** Most research shows that taking red clover extracts by mouth for 3 months to a year does not seem to reduce low-density lipoprotein (LDL or "bad") cholesterol or increase high-density lipoprotein (HDL or "good") cholesterol in women who have moderately elevated cholesterol levels.

- Symptoms of the menopause.
- Asthma.
- Eczema (atopic dermatitis).
- Breast cancer.
- Swelling (inflammation) of the main airways in the lung (bronchitis).
- Burns.
- Cough.
- Indigestion (dyspepsia).Cancer of the lining of the uterus (endometrial cancer).
- Premenstrual syndrome (PMS).
- Sexually transmitted diseases (STDs).
- Scaly, itchy skin (psoriasis).
- Whooping cough (pertussis).
- Wound healing.

Side Effects & Safety

1. When Taken By Mouth: Red clover is LIKELY SAFE for most people when used in the amounts found in food. It is POSSIBLY SAFE when used in medicinal amounts. Red clover can cause rashes, muscle aches, headache, nausea, and vaginal bleeding (spotting) in some women.

2. When Applied To The Skin: Red clover is POSSIBLY SAFE when applied in medicinal amounts.

Special Precautions & Warnings:

1. Pregnancy And Breast-Feeding: Red clover is LIKELY SAFE when taken by mouth in amounts commonly found in food. However, it is LIKELY UNSAFE when used in medicinal amounts. Red clover acts like estrogen and might disturb important hormone balances during pregnancy or breast-feeding. Don't use it.

2. Bleeding Disorders: Red clover might increase the chance of bleeding. Avoid large amounts and use with caution.

3. Protein S Deficiency: People with protein S deficiency have an increased risk of forming blood clots. There is some concern that red clover might increase the risk of clot formation in these people because it has some of the effects of estrogen. Don't use red clover if you have protein S deficiency.

4. Surgery: Red clover might slow blood clotting. It might increase the chance of bleeding during and after surgery. Stop taking red clover at least 2 weeks before a scheduled surgery.

Dosing

The appropriate dose of red clover depends on several factors such as the user's age, health, and several other conditions. At this time there is not enough scientific information to determine an appropriate range of doses for red clover. Keep in mind that natural products are not always necessarily safe and dosages can be important. Be sure to follow relevant directions on product labels and consult your pharmacist or physician or other healthcare professional before using

27. Sassafras Sassafras Albidum

What Is Sassafras?

Sassafras is a plant. The root bark is used to make medicine. Despite serious safety concerns, sassafras is used for urinary tract disorders, swelling in the nose and throat, syphilis, bronchitis, high blood pressure in older people, gout, arthritis, skin problems, and cancer. It is also used as a tonic and "blood purifier." Some people apply sassafras directly to the skin to treat skin problems, achy joints (rheumatism), swollen eyes, sprains, and insect bites or stings. Sassafras oil is also applied to the skin to kill germs and head lice.

In beverages and candy, sassafras was used in the past to flavor root beer. It was also used as a tea. But sassafras tea contains a lot of safrole, the chemical in sassafras that makes it poisonous. One cup of tea made with 2.5 grams of sassafras contains about 200 mg of safrole.

Insufficient Evidence To Rate Effectiveness For

- Urinary tract problems
- Gout
- Arthritis
- Skin problems
- Eye swelling
- Sprains
- Insect bites and stings
- Purifying the blood

How Does Sassafras Work?

There isn't enough information available to know how sassafras works.

Are There Safety Concerns?

Sassafras seems safe in foods and beverages if it is "safrole-free."

However, it is UNSAFE for use as a medicine. Don't take it by mouth or put it on your skin. The safrole in sassafras root bark and oil can cause cancer and liver damage. Consuming just 5 mL of sassafras oil can kill an adult. Even "safrole-free" sassafras used in medicinal amounts has been linked with tumors. Sassafras can cause sweating and hot flashes. High amounts can cause vomiting, high blood pressure, hallucinations, and more severe side effects. It can cause skin rashes when used on the skin.

Special Precautions & Warnings:

It is UNSAFE for anyone to use sassafras in medicinal amounts, but some people have extra reasons not to use it:

1. Pregnancy And Breast-Feeding: Don't use sassafras if you are pregnant. There is evidence that sassafras oil might cause a miscarriage.

2. Children: Sassafras is UNSAFE for children. A few drops of sassafras oil may be deadly.

3. Surgery: In medicinal amounts, sassafras can slow down the central nervous system. This means it can cause sleepiness and drowsiness. When combined with anesthesia and other medications used during and after surgery, it might slow down the central nervous system too much. Stop using sassafras at least 2 weeks before a scheduled surgery.

4. Urinary Tract Conditions: Sassafras might make these conditions worse.

Are There Any Interactions With Medications?

Sedative medications (CNS depressants)Interaction Rating: Moderate Be cautious with this combination. Talk with your health provider.

Sassafras might cause sleepiness and drowsiness. Medications that cause sleepiness are called sedatives. Taking sassafras along with sedative medications might cause too much sleepiness.

Some sedative medications include clonazepam (Klonopin), lorazepam (Ativan), phenobarbital (Donnatal), zolpidem (Ambien), and others.

Dosing Considerations For Sassafras.

The appropriate dose of sassafras depends on several factors such as the user's age, health, and several other conditions. At this time there is not enough scientific information to determine an appropriate range of doses for sassafras. Keep in mind that natural products are not always necessarily safe and dosages can be important. Be sure to follow relevant directions on product labels and consult your pharmacist or physician or other healthcare professional before using.

28. Skullcap Scutellaria Lateriflora

Skullcap is a plant. The above-ground parts are used to make medicine. Skullcap is used for many conditions, but so far, there isn't enough scientific evidence to determine whether or not it is effective for any of them. Skullcap is used for trouble sleeping (insomnia), anxiety, stroke, and paralysis caused by stroke. It is also used for fever, high cholesterol, "hardening of the arteries" (atherosclerosis), rabies, epilepsy, nervous tension, allergies, skin infections, inflammation, and spasms.

Skullcap products are not always what the labels claim. The plant's germander and teucrium are often unwanted and unlabeled ingredients in skullcap products. Secondly, you may think you are buying Scutellaria lateriflora, the species of skullcap that has been studied for medicinal use, but the product may contain a different species of skullcap instead. The most often substituted species are Western Skullcap (Scutellaria canescens), Southern Skullcap (Scutellaria cordifolia), or Marsh Skullcap (Scutellaria galericulatum). These species contain different chemicals, so they are not considered interchangeable.

How Does It Work?

The chemicals in the skullcap might work by preventing swelling (inflammation). Other chemicals in the skullcap are thought to cause sedation (drowsiness).

Uses & Effectiveness?

Insufficient Evidence For

- Anxiety.
- Seizures.
- Trouble sleeping (insomnia).
- Stroke.

Side Effects & Safety

There is not enough information available to know if a skullcap is safe to take for medical conditions.

Special Precautions & Warnings

1. Pregnancy And Breast-Feeding: There is not enough reliable information about the safety of taking a skullcap is you are pregnant or breastfeeding. Stay on the safe side and avoid use.

2. Surgery: Skullcap may slow down the central nervous system. Healthcare providers worry that anesthesia and other medications during and after surgery might increase this effect. Stop taking skullcap at least 2 weeks before a scheduled surgery.

Dosing

The appropriate dose of skullcap depends on several factors such as the user's age, health, and several other conditions. At this time there is not enough scientific information to determine an appropriate range of doses for skullcap. Keep in mind that natural products are not always necessarily safe and dosages can be important. Be sure to follow relevant directions on product labels and consult your pharmacist or physician or other healthcare professional before using.

29. Turkey Corn Dicentra Canadensis

What Is Turkey Corn?

Turkey corn is a plant. The fleshy root (tuber) is used to make medicine. Despite serious safety concerns, people take turkey corn for digestion problems, urinary tract diseases, and skin rashes. Women take it for menstrual disorders.

Insufficient Evidence To Rate Effectiveness For

- Digestive problems.
- Menstrual disorders.
- Urinary tract diseases.
- Skin rashes.

How Does Turkey Corn Work?

Turkey corn might help the body get rid of extra fluids by increasing urine production.

Are There Safety Concerns?

Turkey corn seems to be UNSAFE. It may cause poisoning.

Special Precautions & Warnings

Pregnancy and breast-feeding: Since turkey corn seems to be UNSAFE, it's best to avoid use, especially if you are pregnant or breast-feeding.

Are There Any Interactions With Medications?

1. Lithium Interaction Rating: Moderate Be cautious with this combination. Talk with your health provider.

2. Turkey corn might affect a water pill or "diuretic." Taking turkey corn might decrease how well the body gets rid of lithium. This could increase how much lithium is in the body and result in serious side effects. Talk with your healthcare provider before using this product if you are taking lithium. Your lithium dose might need to be changed.

Dosing Considerations For Turkey Corn

The appropriate dose of turkey corn depends on several factors such as the user's age, health, and several other conditions. At this time there is not enough scientific information to determine an appropriate range of doses for turkey corn. Keep in mind that natural products are not always necessarily safe and dosages can be important. Be sure to follow relevant directions on product labels and consult your pharmacist or physician or other healthcare professional before using.

30. Valerian - Valeriana Officinalis

What Is Valerian?

Valerian is an herb. Medicine is made from the root. Valerian is most commonly used for sleep disorders, especially the inability to sleep (insomnia). It is frequently combined with hops, lemon balm, or other herbs that also cause drowsiness. Some people who are trying to withdraw from the use of "sleeping pills" use valerian to help them sleep after they have tapered the dose of the sleeping pill. There is some scientific evidence that valerian works for sleep disorders, although not all studies are positive. Valerian is also used for conditions connected to anxiety and psychological stress including nervous asthma, hysterical states, excitability, fear of illness (hypochondria), headaches, migraine, and stomach upset.

Some people use valerian for depression, mild tremors, epilepsy, attention deficit-hyperactivity disorder (ADHD), and chronic fatigue syndrome (CFS). Valerian is used for muscle and joint pain. Some women use valerian for menstrual cramps and symptoms associated with menopause, including hot flashes and anxiety. Sometimes, valerian is added to bathwater to help with restlessness and sleep disorders. In manufacturing, the extracts and oil made from valerian are used as a flavoring in foods and beverages.

Is Valerian Effective?

There is some scientific evidence that valerian can help people who have trouble sleeping. It seems to help people fall asleep faster and get a better night's rest. Valerian might work about as well as some low-dose sleeping pills, but it may take up to a month of nightly use before sleeping improves. There is also some evidence that valerian can improve mood and the ability to concentrate.

There isn't enough information to know whether or not valerian is effective for the other conditions people use it for, including depression, convulsions, mild tremors, epilepsy, attention-deficit hyperactivity disorder (ADHD), muscle and joint pain, headache, stomach upset, menstrual pains, menopausal symptoms including hot flashes and anxiety, and many others. Do not use valerian for these conditions until more is known.

Possibly Effective For

Inability to sleep (insomnia). Some research suggests that valerian does not relieve insomnia as fast as "sleeping pills." Continuous use for several days, even up to four weeks, maybe needed before an effect is noticeable. Valerian seems to improve the sleep quality of people who are withdrawing from the use of sleeping pills. Not all evidence is positive, however. Some studies have found that valerian doesn't improve insomnia any better than a "sugar pill" (placebo).

Insufficient Evidence To Rate Effectiveness For

- Anxiety

- Depression
- Restlessness
- Menstrual disorders (dysmenorrhea)
- Stress
- Convulsions
- Mild tremors
- Epilepsy
- Attention-deficit hyperactivity disorder (ADHD)
- Chronic fatigue syndrome (CFS)
- Muscle and joint pain
- Headache
- Stomach upset
- Menopausal symptoms including hot flashes and anxiety.

How Does Valerian Work?

Valerian seems to act as a sedative on the brain and nervous system.

Are There Safety Concerns?

Valerian can cause some side effects such as headache, excitability, uneasiness, and even insomnia in some people. A few people feel sluggish in the morning after taking valerian, especially at higher doses. It's best not to drive or operate dangerous machinery after taking valerian. The long-term safety of valerian is unknown. To avoid possible side effects when discontinuing valerian after long-term use, it's best to reduce the dose slowly over a week or two before stopping completely.

Special Precautions & Warnings

1. Pregnancy Or Breast-Feeding: There isn't enough information about the safety of valerian during pregnancy or breast-feeding. Stay on the safe side and avoid use.

2. Surgery: Valerian slows down the central nervous system. Anesthesia and other medications used during surgery also affect the central nervous system. The combined effects might be harmful. Stop taking valerian at least two weeks before a scheduled surgery.

Are There Any Interactions With Medications?

Alcoholinteraction Rating: Major Do Not Take This Combination.

Alcohol can cause sleepiness and drowsiness. Valerian might also cause sleepiness and drowsiness. Taking large amounts of valerian along with alcohol might cause too much sleepiness. However, some research has found that combining valerian with alcohol does not increase sleepiness.

Alprazolam (Xanax)Interaction Rating: Moderate Be cautious with this combination. Talk with your health provider. Valerian can decrease how quickly the liver breaks down alprazolam (Xanax). Taking valerian with alprazolam (Xanax) might increase the effects and side effects of alprazolam (Xanax) such as drowsiness.

Some medications are changed and broken down by the liver. Valerian might decrease how quickly the liver breaks down some medications. Taking valerian along with some medications that are broken down by the liver can increase the effects and side effects of some medications. Before taking valerian, talk to your healthcare provider if you are taking any medications that are changed by the liver.

Sedative medications (Benzodiazepines)Interaction Rating: Moderate Be cautious with this combination. Talk with your health provider.

Valerian might cause sleepiness and drowsiness. Drugs that cause sleepiness and drowsiness are called sedatives. Taking valerian along with sedative medications might cause too much sleepiness.

Some of these sedative medications include alprazolam (Xanax), clonazepam (Klonopin), diazepam (Valium), lorazepam (Ativan), midazolam (Versed), temazepam (Restoril), triazolam (Halcion), and others.

Sedative medications (CNS depressants)Interaction Rating: Moderate Be cautious with this combination. Talk with your health provider.

Some sedative medications include pentobarbital (Nembutal), phenobarbital (Luminal), secobarbital (Seconal), thiopental (Pentothal), fentanyl (Duragesic, Sublimaze), morphine, propofol (Diprivan), and others.

Some medications are changed and broken down by the liver. Valerian might decrease how quickly the liver breaks down some medications. Taking valerian along with some medications that are broken down by the liver can increase the effects and side effects of some medications. Before taking valerian, talk to your healthcare provider if you are taking any medications that are changed by the liver.

Dosing Considerations For Valerian.

The following doses have been studied in scientific research:

By Mouth:

For The Inability To Sleep (Insomnia):

- 400-900 mg valerian extract up to 2 hours before bedtime for as long as 28 days, or
- Valerian extract 120 mg, with lemon balm extract 80 mg 3 times daily for up to 30 days, or
- A combination product containing valerian extract 187 mg plus hops extract 41.9 mg per tablet, 2 tablets at bedtime for 28 days.
- Take valerian 30 minutes to 2 hours before bedtime.

31. Wormwood - Artemisia Absinthium

What Is Wormwood?

Wormwood is an herb. The above-ground plant parts and oil are used for medicine. Wormwood is used for various digestion problems such as loss of appetite, upset stomach, gall bladder disease, and intestinal spasms. Wormwood is also used to treat fever, liver disease, and worm infections; to increase sexual desire; as a tonic; and to stimulate sweating. Wormwood oil is also used for digestive disorders, to increase sexual desire, and to stimulate the imagination. Some people apply wormwood directly to the skin for healing wounds and insect bites. Wormwood oil is used as a counterirritant to reduce pain. In manufacturing, wormwood oil is used as a fragrance component in soaps, cosmetics, and perfumes. It is also used as an insecticide.

Wormwood is used in some alcoholic beverages. Vermouth, for example, is a wine beverage flavored with extracts of wormwood. Absinthe is another well-known alcoholic beverage made with wormwood. It is an emerald-green alcoholic drink that is prepared from wormwood oil, often along with other dried herbs such as anise and fennel. Absinthe was popularized by famous artists and writers such as Toulouse-Lautrec, Degas, Manet, van Gogh, Picasso, Hemingway, and Oscar Wilde. It is now banned in many countries, including the U.S. But it is still allowed in European Union countries as long as the thujone content is less than 35 mg/kg. Thujone is a potentially poisonous chemical found in wormwood. Distilling wormwood in alcohol increases the thujone concentration.

Insufficient Evidence To Rate Effectiveness For

- Loss of appetite
- Indigestion
- Gallbladder disorders
- Wounds
- Insect bites
- Worm infestations
- Low sexual desire
- Spasms
- Increasing sweating

How Does Wormwood Work?

Wormwood oil contains the chemical thujone, which excites the central nervous system. However, it can also cause seizures and other adverse effects.

Are There Safety Concerns?

Wormwood is LIKELY SAFE when taken by mouth in the amounts commonly found in food and beverages including bitters and vermouth, as long as these products are thujone-free. Wormwood that contains thujone is POSSIBLY UNSAFE when it is taken by mouth. Thujone can cause seizures, muscle breakdown (rhabdomyolysis), kidney failure, restlessness, difficulty sleeping, nightmares, vomiting, stomach cramps, dizziness, tremors, urine retention, thirst, numbness of arms and legs, paralysis, and death.

Special Precautions & Warnings

1. Pregnancy And Breast-Feeding: Wormwood is LIKELY UNSAFE when taken by mouth during pregnancy in amounts greater than what is commonly found in food. The concern is the possible thujone content. Thujone might affect the uterus and endanger the pregnancy. It's also best to avoid topical wormwood since not enough is known about the safety of applying wormwood directly to the skin. If you are breast-feeding, don't use wormwood until more is known about safety.

2. Allergy To Ragweed And Related Plants: Wormwood may cause an allergic reaction in people who are sensitive to the Asteraceae/Compositae family. Members of this family include ragweed, chrysanthemums, marigolds, daisies, and many others. If you have allergies, be sure to check with your healthcare provider before taking wormwood.

3. A Rare Inherited Blood Condition Called Porphyria: Thujone present in wormwood oil might increase the body's production of chemicals called porphyrins. This could make porphyria worse.

4. Kidney Disorders: Taking wormwood oil might cause kidney failure. If you have kidney problems, talk with your healthcare provider before taking wormwood.

5. Seizure Disorders, Including Epilepsy: Wormwood contains thujone, which can cause seizures. There is concern that wormwood might make seizures more likely in people who are prone to them.

Are There Any Interactions With Medications?

Medications used to prevent seizures (Anticonvulsants)Interaction Rating: Moderate Be cautious with this combination. Talk with your health provider.

Medications used to prevent seizures affect chemicals in the brain. Wormwood may also affect chemicals in the brain. By affecting chemicals in the brain, wormwood may decrease the effectiveness of medications used to prevent seizures.

Some medications used to prevent seizures include phenobarbital, primidone (Mysoline), valproic acid (Depakene), gabapentin (Neurontin), carbamazepine (Tegretol), phenytoin (Dilantin), and others.

Dosing Considerations For Wormwood

The appropriate dose of wormwood depends on several factors such as the user's age, health, and several other conditions. At this time there is not enough scientific information to determine an appropriate range of doses for wormwood. Keep in mind that natural products are not always necessarily safe and dosages can be important. Be sure to follow relevant directions on product labels and consult your pharmacist or physician or other healthcare professional before using.

32. Witch Hazel Hamamelis Virginiana

Witch hazel is a plant. The leaf, bark, and twigs are used to make medicine. You may see a product called witch hazel water (Hamamelis water, distilled witch hazel extract). This is a liquid that is distilled from dried leaves, bark, and partially dormant twigs of witch hazel. Witch hazel is taken by mouth for diarrhea, mucus colitis, vomiting blood, coughing up blood, tuberculosis, colds, fevers, tumors, and cancer.

Some people apply witch hazel directly to the skin for itching, pain, and swelling (inflammation), eye inflammation, skin injury, mucous membrane inflammation, vaginal dryness after menopause, varicose veins, hemorrhoids, bruises, insect bites, minor burns, acne, sensitive scalp, and other skin irritations. In manufacturing, witch hazel leaf extract, bark extract, and witch hazel water are used as astringents to tighten the skin. They are also included in some medications to give those products the ability to slow down or stop bleeding. Those medications are used for treating insect bites, stings, teething, hemorrhoids, itching, irritations, and minor pain.

How Does It Work?

Witch hazel contains chemicals called tannins. When applied directly to the skin, witch hazel might help reduce swelling, help repair broken skin, and fight bacteria.

Uses & Effectiveness?

Possibly Effective For

1. Hemorrhoids: Applying witch hazel water to the skin may help to temporarily relieve itching, discomfort, irritation, and burning from hemorrhoids and other anal disorders.

2. Minor Bleeding: Applying witch hazel bark, leaf, or water to the skin reduces minor bleeding.

3. Skin Irritation: Applying witch hazel cream seems to relieve mild skin irritation, but not as well as hydrocortisone. Other research shows that applying a specific witch hazel ointment (Hametum) to the skin appears to improve symptoms of skin injury or irritated skin as effectively as a dexpanthenol ointment in children.

Possibly Ineffective For

1. Itchy And Inflamed Skin (Eczema): Applying a cream containing witch hazel to the skin for 14 days does not seem to improve itchy and inflamed skin in people with moderate eczema. Applying hydrocortisone cream seems to be a more effective treatment option.

Insufficient Evidence For

- Health problems after menopause.
- Bruises.
- Colds.
- Coughing up blood.
- Diarrhea.
- Eye inflammation.
- Fevers.
- Tuberculosis.
- Varicose veins.
- Vomiting blood.

Side Effects & Safety

Witch hazel is LIKELY SAFE for most adults when applied directly to the skin. In some people, it might cause minor skin irritation. Witch hazel is POSSIBLY SAFE for most adults when small doses are taken by mouth. In some people, witch hazel might cause stomach upset when taken by mouth. Large doses might cause liver problems. Witch hazel contains a cancer-causing chemical (safrole), but in amounts that are too small to be of concern.

Special Precautions & Warnings

1. Children: Witch hazel is POSSIBLY SAFE for children when applied directly to the skin.

2. Pregnancy And Breast-Feeding: There is not enough reliable information about the safety of taking witch hazel if you are pregnant or breast-feeding. Stay on the safe side and avoid use.

Dosing

The following doses have been studied in scientific research:

Adults

Applied To The Skin:

For Skin Irritation: An after sun lotion containing 10% witch hazel water has been used.

Applied To The Anus:

For itching and discomfort associated with hemorrhoids and other anal disorders: Witch hazel water has been applied up to 6 times per day or after every bowel movement. Suppositories have been placed in the anus 1-3 times per day.

Children

Applied To The Skin:

For Skin Irritation: An ointment containing witch hazel has been applied several times per day in children aged 2-11 years.

CONCLUSION

As our lifestyle is now getting techno-savvy, we are moving away from nature. While we cannot escape from nature because we are part of nature. As herbs are natural products they are free from side effects, they are comparatively safe, eco-friendly, and locally available. Traditionally there are a lot of herbs used for ailments related to different seasons. There is a need to promote them to save human lives.

Medicinal plants are useful to keep on hand to treat common ailments. You can reach for certain medical plants to relieve headaches, tummy trouble, and even irritation from bug bites. Plants can be consumed in teas, used as a garnish, applied topically as an essential oil, or consumed as a pill.

These herbal products are today are the symbol of safety in contrast to the synthetic drugs, that are regarded as unsafe to human being and environment. Although herbs had been priced for their medicinal, flavoring, and aromatic qualities for centuries, the synthetic products of the modern age surpassed their importance, for a while. However, the blind dependence on synthetics is over and people are returning to the naturals with the hope of safety and security. It's time to promote them globally.

Medicinal plants, also called medicinal herbs, have been discovered and used in traditional medicine practices since prehistoric times. Plants synthesize hundreds of chemical compounds for functions including defense against insects, fungi, diseases, and herbivorous mammals. Numerous phytochemicals with potential or established biological activity have been identified. However, since a single plant contains widely diverse phytochemicals, the effects of using a whole plant as medicine are uncertain. Further, the phytochemical content and pharmacological actions, if any, of many plants having medicinal potential remain unassessed by rigorous scientific research to define efficacy and safety. It's important to remember that you should always double-check with your doctor before consuming or using anything new for your body. If you choose to grow some of these plants, remember to take proper care according to the plant's care guidelines and refrain from using any pesticides or other harmful chemicals on your plants. You don't want any of those chemicals in or on your body!

NATIVE AMERICAN HERBAL REMEDIES

Natural Herbal Remedies, Sacred Medicinal Plants, and Recipes to Heal Common Ailments

Taahira Maskwa

INTRODUCTION

Plants, herbs, and ethnobotanicals have been used since the early days of humankind and are still used throughout the world for health promotion and treatment of disease. Plants and natural sources form the basis of today's modern medicine and contribute largely to the commercial drug preparations manufactured today. About 25% of drugs prescribed worldwide are derived from plants. Still, herbs, rather than drugs, are often used in health care. For some, herbal medicine is their preferred method of treatment.

For others, herbs are used as an adjunct therapy to conventional pharmaceuticals. However, in many developing societies, the traditional medicine of which herbal medicine is a core part is the only system of health care available or affordable. Regardless of the reason, those using herbal medicines should be assured that the products they are buying are safe and contain what they are supposed to, whether this is a particular herb or a particular amount of a specific herbal component.

Consumers should also be given science-based information on dosage, contraindications, and efficacy. To achieve this, global harmonization of legislation is needed to guide the responsible production and marketing of herbal medicines. If sufficient scientific evidence of benefit is available for an herb, then such legislation should allow for this to be used appropriately to promote the use of that herb so that these benefits can be realized for the promotion of public health and the treatment of disease.

Health care is moving into the home increasingly often and involving a mixture of people, a variety of tasks, and a broad diversity of devices and technologies; it is also occurring in a range of residential environments. The factors driving this migration include the rising costs of providing health care; the growing numbers of older adults; the increasing prevalence of chronic disease; improved survival rates of various diseases, injuries, and other conditions (including those of fragile newborns); large numbers of veterans returning from war with serious injuries; and a wide range of technological innovations. The health care that results varies considerably in its safety, effectiveness, and efficiency, as well as it's quality and cost.

Results show that traditional medicine, and especially self-treatment with medicinal plants, prevail as treatment options in both rural and peri-urban populations. Contrary to what is commonly assumed, high income is an important determinant of the use of traditional medicine. Likewise, knowledge of medicinal plants, age, education, gender, and illness chronicity were also significant determinants. The importance of self-treatment with medicinal plants should inform the development of health policy tailored to people's treatment-seeking behavior.

High income and knowledge of medicinal plants are important determinants of the use of traditional medicine. This challenges the common assumption that poor and marginalized people are most reliant on traditional medicine due to its availability. Future health policies shall consider the high reliance on self-treatment and the importance of knowledge held within the household about this

Although many issues related to home health care could not be addressed, applications of human factors principles, knowledge, and research methods in these areas could make home health care safer and more effective and also contribute to reducing costs. The committee chose not to prioritize the recommendations, as they focus on various aspects of health care in the home and are of comparable importance to the different constituencies affected.

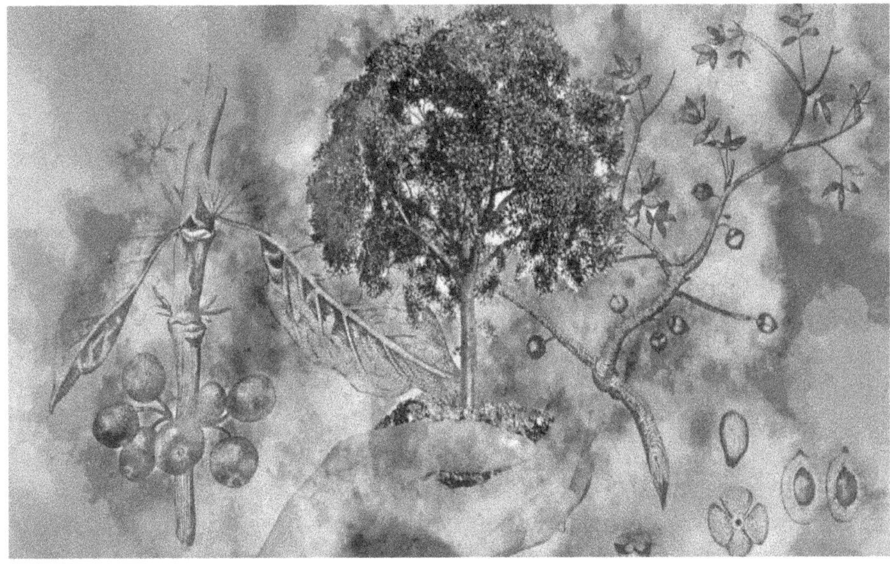

Background: The use of herbal products in children is a concern because little information is available concerning the benefits and risks of these products in the pediatric population.

Objective: This article defines herbal products and reviews the reasons for using such products, the most commonly used herbal products in the United States, their use during pregnancy and breast-feeding, and the adverse effects, drug interactions, and regulatory issues associated with herbal products.

Methods: A literature search was conducted using MEDLINE and references from journal articles.

CHAPTER 1 : NATIVE AMERICAN TRADITIONS

Native American traditions, religious beliefs, and sacramental practices of the indigenous peoples of North and South America. Until the 1950s it was commonly assumed that the religions of the surviving Native Americans were little more than curious anachronisms, dying remnants of humankind's childhood. These traditions lacked sacred texts and fixed doctrines or moral codes and were embedded in societies without wealth, mostly without writing, and without recognizable systems of politics or justice or any of the usual indicators of civilization. Today the situation has changed dramatically. Scholars of religion, students of the ecological sciences, and individuals committed to expanding and deepening their own religious lives have found in these traditions many distinct and varied religious worlds that have struggled to survive but that retain the ability to inspire.

Native American people themselves often claim that their traditional ways of life do not include "religion." They find the term difficult, often impossible, to translate into their languages. This apparent incongruity arises from differences in cosmology and epistemology. Western tradition distinguishes religious thought and action as that whose ultimate authority is supernatural—which is to say, beyond, above, or outside both phenomenal nature and human reason. In most indigenous worldviews there is no such antithesis. Plants and animals, clouds, and mountains carry and embody revelation. Even where native tradition conceives of a realm or world apart from the terrestrial one and not normally visible from it, as in the case of the Iroquois Sky World or the several underworlds of Pueblo cosmologies, the boundaries between these worlds are permeable. The ontological distance between land and sky or between land and underworld is short and is traversed in both directions.

Instead of encompassing a duality of sacred and profane, indigenous religious traditions seem to conceive only of sacred and more sacred. Spirit, power, or something akin moves in all things, though not equally. For native communities religion is understood as the relationship between living humans and other persons or things, however, they are conceived. These may include departed as well as yet-to-be-born human beings, beings in the so-called "natural world" of flora and fauna, and visible entities that are not animate by Western standards, such as mountains, springs, lakes, and clouds. This group of entities also includes what scholars of religion might denote as "mythic beings," beings that are not normally visible but are understood to inhabit and affect either this world or some other world contiguous to it.

Spirituality And Connection

Before delving into more specific information about what native peoples believed, it makes sense to explain that the concept of religion as an organized thing is not a part of most traditions. Religion describes a division between the supernatural, which is ruled by one or multiple deities. Instead of calling their beliefs and practices a set religion, most refer to it as a system of spirituality that permeates every aspect of their lives. Religion is a set doctrine of supernatural beliefs, the ceremonies, and activities associated with it, and includes things like concepts of deities, spirits, or ghosts, what happens to a person after death, and certain special occasions throughout a person's life.

Native American spirituality includes similar ideas, but integrates them more into everyday living rather than reserving them for special occasions. Of course, there are ceremonies for births, deaths, marriages, harvests, and other special times, but daily life was just as filled with beliefs as "holidays" would be. Native American spirituality does not separate the two concepts in any real way. The spiritual or supernatural world is the same thing as the real world. Every supposed division is completely permeable and people can access everything spiritual just as easily as they can wade in a river or feel the sun on their skin.

There also exists a general sense of connection and oneness among a particular tribe of Native American people. The Lakota term "mitakuye oyasin" means that all are related or all beings are relations of each other.[ii] This explains the belief that spirit exists in everything or that everything is connected ins some ways. This does not necessarily encompass an objectified spiritual connection because the concept behind the phrase also pushes for respect for the individual.

Misunderstandings about the purpose behind the word, especially in non-native and non-Lakota communities, carry quite a bit of conflict. Still, the idea that all people and things are part of a whole and should respect and honor each other is not damaging in any way.

No concepts of unattainability or inaccessibility seem to exist for many Native American belief systems. Everything exists about everything else. This concept leads to the belief that tribal people are "one with nature" or similar ideas. Although phrases like that are often used in New Age philosophies, it does, at its core, also pertain to this idea of the spiritual existing firmly in the realm of tangible reality.

Healers

Native American (NA) traditional healing is identified by the National Institutes of Health/National Center for Complementary and Alternative Medicine (NCCAM) as a whole medical system that encompasses a range of holistic treatments used by indigenous healers for a multitude of acute and chronic conditions or to promote health and wellbeing.2 While there are individual tribal differences (i.e., the use of specific healing practices), there are also shared health beliefs and interventional strategies, including a health promotion foundation that embraces bio-psycho-socio-spiritual approaches and traditions. For thousands of years, traditional indigenous medicine has been used to promote health and wellbeing for millions of Native people who once inhabited this continent. Native diets, ceremonies that greet the seasons and the harvests, and the use of native plants for healing purposes have been used to live to promote health by living in harmony with the earth.

Today Native Americans frequently combine traditional healing practices with allopathic medicine to promote health and wellbeing. The ceremony, native herbal remedies, and allopathic medications are used side by side. Spiritual treatments are thus an integral part of health promotion and healing in Native American culture.

Yet, the role of spirituality in health promotion and wellness is uncomfortable for many allopathic providers. Advanced practice nurses with their tradition of holism that embraces the bio-psycho-social-spiritual nature of health have an opportunity to suggest new ways to care modeled on traditional NA practices. The inclusion of family and community in treatment plans decreases the isolation often found in allopathic care. And, thinking about the lack of person-environment harmony and balance may important clues for the diagnostic process.

Symbolic Healing

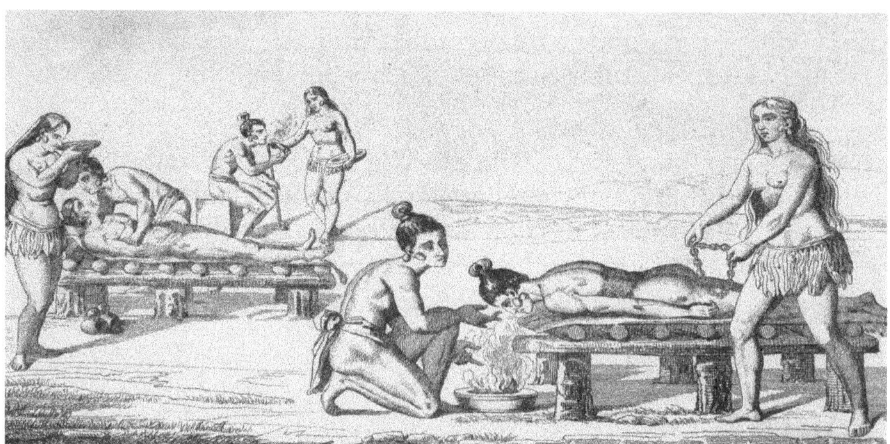

Ceremonies play an important role in the overall wellbeing of traditional Native American people but the healing potential of this practice is typically unappreciated by allopathic health providers. NA ceremonies involve the patient, the family, and the community in the healing process. Ceremonial gatherings may last for days or weeks; the more people that are present, the greater the healing energy. Through their participation in songs, prayer, music, and dance, the family and community contribute healing energy to the patient.

People of all cultures utilize symbolism found in their various religions and spiritual practices to cope with health problems. NA healing ceremonies rely heavily on a combination of traditional and Christian religious symbols, icons, and ritualistic objects. These symbols cue bio-psycho-social-spiritual healing responses by restoring the harmony necessary for health. Symbolism, whether associated with ceremonies or church services, can be incorporated into their treatment plan to create a powerful healing synergy.3

Healing And Ceremony

Many healing practices and spiritual ceremonies that are being practiced today by healing practitioners and metaphysical groups have been adopted from traditions that originated from various Native American tribes. History indicates that each tribe would have one or more elders who were groomed in the healing arts. These individuals would serve as herbalists, healers, and spirit communicators. The duties and types of healing arts and spiritual ceremonies performed would naturally vary from tribe to tribe. Native American healing arts and practices are earth-based, honoring and respectful of the Father Sky, Mother Earth, Grandfather Sun, and Grandmother Moon.

The ceremony is an essential part of traditional Native healing. Because physical and spiritual health is intimately connected, body and spirit must heal together. Traditional healing ceremonies promote wellness by reflecting Native conceptions of Spirit, Creator, and the Universe. They can include prayer, chants, drumming, songs, stories, and the use of a variety of sacred objects. Healers may conduct ceremonies anywhere a sick person needs healing, but ceremonies are often held in sacred places.

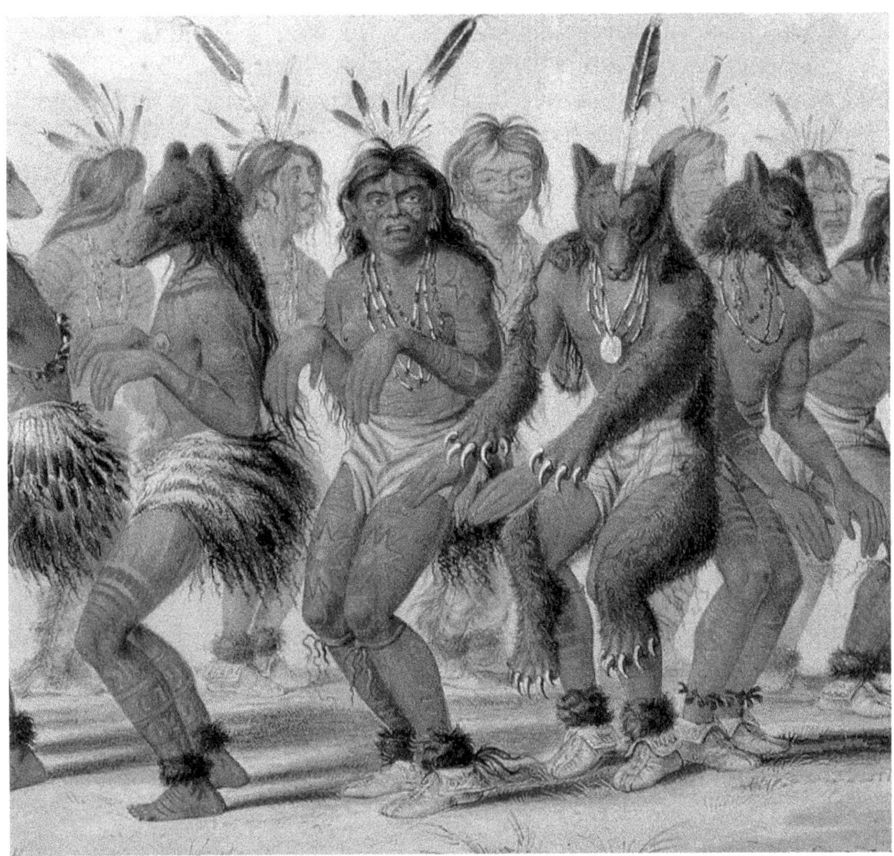

Special structures for healing are often referred to as Medicine Lodges. Wherever they take place, traditional healing ceremonies are considered sacred and are only conducted by Native healers and Native spiritual facilitators. Non-Natives may participate by invitation only.

Indigenous healing practices among Native Americans have been documented in the United States since colonization. Cultural encapsulation has deterred the acknowledgment of Native American medicinal practices as a precursor to folk medicine and many herbal remedies, which have greatly influenced modern medicine.

Understanding Native American healing practices requires helping professionals to know about Native American cultural belief systems about health and wellness, with the many influences that create change in the mind, body, spirit, and natural environment. Native Americans believe their healing practices and traditions operate in the context of relationship to four constructs—namely, spirituality (Creator, Mother Earth, Great Father); community (family, clan, tribe/nation); environment (daily life, nature, balance); and self (inner passions and peace, thoughts, and values).

It is with this in mind, that it's important for today's integrative, complementary medicine practices to become the norm as opposed to the exception. Chief among the ceremonies of Native Americans is the smudging ceremony. Smudging uses the smoking of a variety of herbs and foliage, namely sage and wheatgrass, to be wafted onto the person, belongings, sacred and non-sacred spaces alike. Native Americans differ in their frequency of smudging, but some perform it daily to stay healthy while others only at major life events and when feeling unwell.

While Native American healers' reasonings can vary for why they smudge, from reading many accounts, one of the common reasons is to help others find respect for one another, their environment, and to spend moments in quiet, positive contemplation while practicing this ancient ceremony. In psychology, some of the same tenets of reappraisal and introspection recommended by mental healthcare professionals for greater emotional regulation are given. Here, Native Americans have connected this to their cultural heritage in a way that speaks very meaningfully to the participants

Healing Plants

Native American, Alaska Native, and Native Hawaiian healers all have a long history of using indigenous, or native, plants for a wide variety of medicinal purposes. Medicinal plants and their applications are as diverse as the tribes who use them.

Beyond their medicinal benefits, indigenous plants were a staple of Native people's diet before Western contact. Today, indigenous plants are central to efforts to improve dietary health for current generations. In Hawai'i, the "Waianae Diet" and "Pre-Captain Cook Diet" aim to reduce empty calories, fat, and additives and promote a healthier, more balanced diet by restoring the role of indigenous foods. Alaska Natives and various Indian tribes have similar projects emphasizing traditional foods. Food is medicine.

Native Hawaiian Medicinal Plants

Hawaiian medicinal plants grow in many areas, including in the vicinity of heiaus or temples, sites that are considered sacred. In ancient times, Hawaiian traditional healers would practice La'au Lapa'au, medicinal healing, at some of the heiaus, using plants from around the heiau and in neighboring forests. Most Hawaiian medicinal plants are foods that have additional curative properties. Healers view food as medicine, along with fresh, clean air and water. In all cases, healers offer a prayer to ask permission and give thanks for the medicines before harvesting and preparing them, and ask permission to facilitate medicinal healing on behalf of the Creator

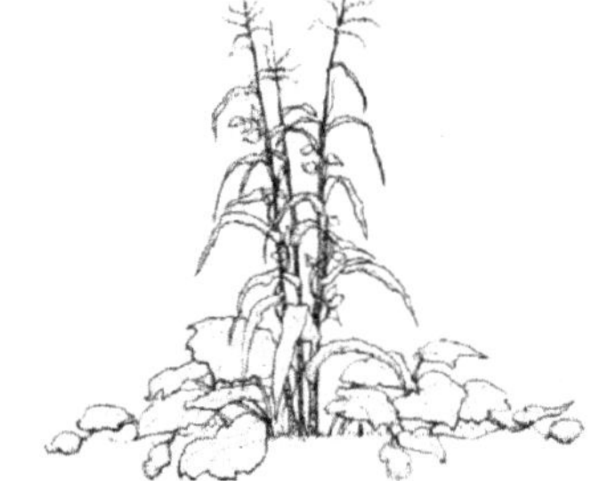

Tools Used In Native American Healing Ceremonies

Well, you are likely to see a modern doctor with a stethoscope hanging on her neck today, the healing implements of the Native American persuasion are equally distinct. Native American healers can be seen with ceremonial headdresses and necklaces of their own making. For healing ceremonies such as those described above, you will find in use a variety of tools from animal totems to peace pipes, prayer ties, and more.

Animal Totems

Since Native American cultures are strongly animistic, animals hold special places in the Native American healing ceremonies and traditions. You can see small animal totems given and used throughout these healing practices, especially during group healing ceremonies, for guidance from their animal spirits.

Dreamcatchers

One of the most iconic Native American healing tools is the dreamcatcher. Representing the Medicine Wheel, or Sacred Hoop, these woven healing instruments are used to help children sleep better, protecting warriors and others traveling away from the tribe, and warding off illness by restoring the balance of mind, emotion, body, and spirit to the person afflicted.

Feather Fetishes

Not what it sounds like, feather fetishes are fans made out of bird feathers, bones, leathered skins of various animals, even seashells, that are used in rituals for prayer and healing. In smudging ceremonies, feather fetishes are used to fan the smoke onto the person being blessed or healed.

Peace Pipes

Peace pipes are a ceremonial tool used usually by elders of a village for major events, but they are also used to smoke a variety of different plants (e.g., peyote, ayahuasca, and other entheogenic herbs). These peace pipes are long-stemmed and typically made of wood or bone, and can be smoked throughout the evening until dawn in healing rituals.

Prayer Ties

Next, prayer ties–small, bound cloth flags–are used as offerings to the Spirit World entities. These colorful little items are laid out to pay homage and thanks to the spirits needed to heal a person.

Smudge Sticks

Finally, but most often used in Native American healing ceremonies, smudge sticks are ribbon-bound herbs used to handily carry and purpose in the smudging ceremonies wherever one might be. Smudge sticks are disassembled to take what herbs are needed for a specific healing ceremony, then the remaining is rebound for later use. Herbs used vary based on the available plant life indigenous to the various Native American nations' regions.

Native American Healing Ceremonies

In addition to the tools mentioned above healers of every Native American tribe extend their toolkit to the knowledge of plant-based medicine. Herbalists didn't simply use smudge sticks to heal afflicted individuals. They had an arsenal of remedies cultivated over generations to handle a variety of ailments that became the source of many modern medicines.

If you would like to gain greater insights into Native American herbalism, in Sacred Plant Medicine: The Wisdom in Native American Herbalism by Stephen Harrod Buhner, he reveals that the Native American cultures not only had spiritual and religious beliefs connected to their herbalism, but an in-depth method for planting, gathering, and harvesting, storing, converting plants to medicine, and uses.

You can find many herbs, such as milkweed, echinacea, wild ginger, and elder in various forms in your local natural foods stores in the supplements section. And, you can thank Native Americans mostly for that!

These herbs are used in many rituals and ceremonies as teas and other concoctions that not only the afflicted person would drink, but many times the family and other members of the tribe, as a means to bond the healing process to the community. Healing is culturally a communal practice and the use of herbs together reinforces that premise.

Death Ceremonies: Native Americans celebrated death, knowing that it was an end to life on Earth, but, believing it to be the start of life in the Spirit World. Most tribes also believed that the journey might be long, so afterlife rituals were performed to ensure that the spirits would not continue to roam the earth. Various tribes honored the dead in several ways, by giving them food, herbs, and gifts to ensure a safe journey to the afterlife.

Green Corn Festivals: Also called the Green Corn Ceremonies, this both a celebration and religious ceremony, primarily practiced by the peoples of the Eastern Woodlands and the Southeastern tribes including the Creek, Cherokee, Seminole, Yuchi, Iroquois, and others. The ceremony typically coincides in the late summer and is tied to the ripening of the corn crops. Marked with dancing, feasting, fasting, and religious observations, the ceremony usually lasts for three days. Activities varied from tribe to tribe, but the common thread is that the corn was not to be eaten until the Great Spirit has been given his proper thanks. During the event, tribal members give thanks for the corn, rain, sun, and a good harvest. Some tribes even believe that they were made from corn by the Great Spirits. The Green Corn Festival is also a religious renewal, with various religious ceremonies. During this time, some tribes hold council meetings where many of the previous year's minor problems or crimes are forgiven. Others also signify the event as the time of year when youth come of age and babies are given their names. Several tribes incorporate ball games and tournaments in the event. Cleansing and purifying activities often occur, including cleaning out homes, burning waste, and drinking emetics to purify the body. At the end of each day of the festival, feasts are held to celebrate the good harvest. Green Corn festivals are still practiced today by many different native peoples of the Southeastern Woodland Culture.

CHAPTER 2: TRADITIONAL REMEDIES FOR COMMON AILMENTS

Native American Medicine Today

Definition

According to Ken "Bear Hawk" Cohen, "Native American medicine is based on widely held beliefs about healthy living, the repercussions of disease-producing behavior, and the spiritual principles that restore balance." These beliefs are shared by all tribes; however, the methods of diagnosis and treatment vary greatly from tribe to tribe and healer to healer.

Origins

The healing traditions of Native Americans have been practiced in North America since at least 12,000 years ago and possibly as early as 40,000 years ago. Although the term Native American medicine implies that there is a standard system of healing, there are approximately 500 nations of indigenous people in North America, each representing a diverse wealth of healing knowledge, rituals, and ceremonies. Many aspects of Native American healing have been kept secret and are not written down. The traditions are passed down by word of mouth from elders, from the spirits in vision quests, and through initiation. It is believed that sharing healing knowledge too readily or casually will weaken the spiritual power of the medicine.

There are, however, many Native American healers who recognize that writing down their healing practices is a way to preserve these traditions for future generations. Many also believe that sharing their healing ways and values may help all people to come into a healthier balance with nature and all forms of life.

Benefits

Native American medicine can benefit anyone who sincerely wishes to live a life of wholeness and balance. These benefits may be physical, emotional, or spiritual. There is, however, the understanding that "the diseases of civilization," or white man's diseases, often need white man's medicine. In those cases, Native American medicine can be an important part of an integrative approach to healing. For example, the most successful programs for treating alcohol addiction in Native communities have combined Western approaches to psychological counseling, social work, and traditional Native American healing practices.

Such inherited conditions as birth defects or retardation are not easily treatable with Native American medicine. Native healers also believe that some illnesses are the result of a patient's behavior. Sometimes they will not treat a person because they do not want to interfere with the life lessons the patient needs to learn. Other illnesses are not treated because they are "callings" or initiation diseases.

Description

Native American medicine is based upon a spiritual view of life. A healthy person is someone who has a sense of purpose and follows the guidance of the Great Spirit. This guidance is written upon the heart of every person. To be healthy, a person must be committed to a path of beauty, harmony, and balance. Gratitude, respect, and generosity are also considered to be essential for a healthy life. Ken Cohen writes, "Health means restoring the body, mind, and spirit to balance and wholeness: the balance of life energy in the body; the balance of ethical, reasonable, and just behavior; balanced relations within family and community; and harmonious relationships with nature."

Theories of disease causation and even the names of diseases vary from tribe to tribe. Diseases may be thought to have internal or external causes or sometimes both. According to Cherokee medicine man Rolling Thunder, negative thinking is the most important internal cause of disease. Negative thinking includes not only negative thoughts about oneself but also feelings of shame, blame, low self-esteem, greed, despair, worry, depression, anger, jealousy, and self-centeredness.

Diseases have external causes too. "Germs are also spirits," according to Shabari Bird of the Lakota Nation. A person is particularly susceptible to harmful germs if they live an imbalanced life, have a weak constitution, engage in negative thinking, or are under a lot of stress. Other people or spirits may also be responsible for an illness. Another external source of the disease is environmental poisons. These poisons include alcohol, impure air, water, and some types of food.

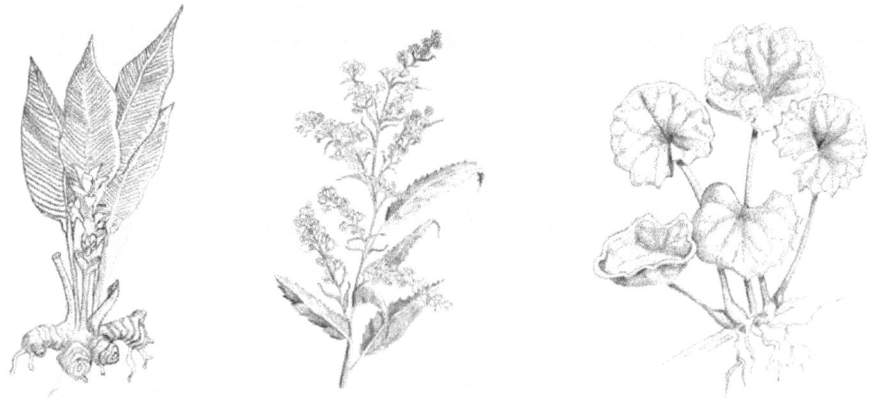

Native American healers believe that disease can also be caused by physical, emotional, or spiritual trauma. These traumas can lead to mental and emotional distress, loss of soul, or loss of spiritual power. In these cases, the healer must use ritual and other ways to physically return the soul and power to the patient. Some diseases are caused when people break the "rules for living." These rules may include ways of showing respect for animals, people, places, ritual objects, events, or spirits.

Native American medicine is not covered by insurance unless perhaps the practitioner is a licensed health care provider. Most Native healers do not charge a set fee for their services. Healing is considered to be "a gift from the Great Spirit." Gifts to the healer are welcomed, however. The offering of a gift "ensures the success of treatment because healing spirits appreciate the generosity."

Gifts may include groceries, cloth, money, or another personal expression of respect and appreciation. Frequently the only gift that is required is a pouch of tobacco.

Native Americans used herbs to purify the spirit and bring balance to people who are unhealthy in spirit, mind, or body. They learned about the healing powers of herbs by watching sick animals. Tobacco, one of the most sacred plants to Native Americans, is used in some way in nearly every cure. It is smoked pure and is not mixed with chemicals. Sage, an abundant and pretty plant with blue flowers and light white or grayish leaves, is believed to protect against bad spirits and to draw them out of the body or the soul. Native Americans use sage for many purposes: to heal problems of the stomach, colon, nasal passages, kidneys, liver, lungs, pores of the skin, bones, and sex organs; on the hair and scalp; to heal burns and grazes; as an antiseptic for allergies, colds, and fever; as a gargle for sore throat; and as a tea to calm the nerves. Cedar, a tall evergreen tree, is a milder medicine than sage. It is combined with sage and sweetgrass, a plant that grows in damp environments like marshes or near water, to make a powerful concoction used in the scared smudging ceremony. Cedar fruit and leaves are boiled and then drunk for coughs. Forehead colds, cedar is burned and inhaled.

Traditional Medicine For

Abscess

1. **Burdock:** Roots and leaves utilized internally and externally. Avoid if pregnant or nursing.

2. **Devil's Claw:** Used in teas and tonics internally and in poultices externally. Should not be used by women who are or may be pregnant.

3. **Chamomile:** Commonly used in teas it is best known to help with sleep.

4. **Pau d'arco:** Long used for a wide range of conditions.

5. **Poke:** Though parts of this plant are highly toxic to livestock and humans, it has long been used as food and medicine by Native Americans.

6. **White Pine:** The inner bark, young shoots, twigs, pitch, and leaves have long been used by Native Americans in medical remedies.

7. **Slippery Elm:** The tree had many traditional uses by Native Americans.

8. **Wild Yam:** Traditionally used as both food and medicine.

Acne

1. **Mint:** Dried leaves used in teas and food, found helpful in several remedies.

2. **Red Clover:** Traditionally used for several conditions.

3. **Sarsaparilla:** Used for centuries in a wide variety of medicinal remedies.

4. Witch Hazel: Widely used for medicinal purposes by American Indians.

5. Yellow Dock: Native Americans as traditional medicine and food.

6. Buffaloberry: Used as food and in herbal remedies. Overindulgence can cause severe problems including death.

7. Burdock: Roots and leaves utilized internally and externally. Avoid if pregnant or nursing.

Allergies

1. Dong Quai: Used for more than a thousand years to treat several conditions.

2. Mint: Dried leaves used in teas and food, found helpful in several remedies.

3. Rooibos: Used in teas to help with a variety of conditions.

4. Goldenrod: Long used for a variety of ailments.

5. Spirulina: A type of blue-green algae that is rich in protein, vitamins.

Anxiety

1. Kola Nut – Long used in medicinal remedies, spiritual practices, and ceremonies. Should not be used by pregnant or nursing women, or those with intestinal or stomach ulcers, blood pressure, insomnia, or heart disorders.

2. Lavender – Dating back to Roman times, Lavender has been used in teas, balms, food, and medicinal remedies.

3. Lemon Balm – A calming herb that has been used since the Middle Ages.

4. Passion Flower – Has a long history of use among Native Americans that and were adapted by early European colonists. Do not take passionflower if you are pregnant or breastfeeding.

5. Peppermint – in addition to flavoring, long used in traditional medicine for its calming and numbing effects. Should not be used or given to infants or small children.

6. Rhodiola – Best known for improving physical and mental performance.

7. Skullcap – A powerful medicinal herb, it was cultivated by Native Americans for use in several remedies. Pregnant women should not take Skullcap.

8. St John's Wort – Most commonly known as an anti-depressant, it also has other medical uses.

9. Valerian Root – Has been used as a medicinal herb since at least the time of ancient Greece and Rome.

10. Wild Lettuce – Indigenous to North American, it was used for sedative purposes, especially in nervous complaints.

Asthma

1. Damiana – Used internally for a variety of medical issues.

2. Eastern Skunk Cabbage – Dried leaves used as a seasoning in remedies, and as a magical talisman by various tribes.

3. Evening Primrose – Used for both food and medicinal remedies, decoctions were used for internal and external ailments.

4. Feverfew – Used for a variety of internal medical problems. Should not be used by women who are pregnant.

5. Goldenrod – Long used for a variety of ailments.

6. Honeysuckle – Used in traditional herbal remedies for thousands of years.

7. Horehound – Whole plant used internally and externally. People with gastritis or peptic ulcer disorders should use it cautiously.

8. Indian Hemp – A type of marijuana it was used to make clothes, rope, and paper as well as boiling the roots into teas for medicinal problems.

9. Kola Nut – Long used in medicinal remedies, spiritual practices, and ceremonies. Should not be used by pregnant or nursing women, or those with intestinal or stomach ulcers, blood pressure, insomnia, or heart disorders.

10. Lemongrass – Having anti-fungal properties, it has not only been used as herbal medicine but, also as a pesticide and preservative.

11. Mullein – A tobacco-like plant and one of the oldest herbs, it has a long history of use as a medicine

12. Poke – Though parts of this plant are highly toxic to livestock and humans, it has long been used as food and medicine by Native Americans.

13. Rabbit Tobacco – Was thought to have had spiritual or mystic powers by many Indians.

14. Rooibos – Used in teas to help with a variety of conditions.

15. Sumac – Viewed by some tribes as a sacred plant, Sumac was used for both food and medicine.

Backache

1. Arnica – Used externally only for aches, pains, and wounds. Poison if taken internally.

2. Devil's Claw – Used in teas and tonics internally and in poultices externally. Should not be used by a woman who is or may be pregnant. Feverwort – Used internally and externally in herbal medicine.

3. Gentiana – Extremely bitter herb used for both internal and external problems. may irritate persons who have ulcers, and may also cause headaches, nausea, or vomiting.

4. Horsemint – leaves and flowering stems are used in teas, tonics, and salves for a variety of medical issues. Should not be used by pregnant women.

5. Milkweed – Though it can be toxic if not prepared properly, Milkweed was used as a food and medicine, as well as in making cords, ropes, and coarse cloth. Warning: Milkweed may be toxic when taken internally, without sufficient preparation.

Boils

1. Buffaloberry – Used as food and in herbal remedies. Overindulgence can cause severe problems including death.

2. Burdock – Roots and leaves utilized internally and externally. Avoid if pregnant or nursing.

3. Cattail – Utilized as a food, as well as in external and internal medical remedies.

4. Dandelion – Used in both foods and internal and external medical remedies.

5. Devil's Claw – Used in teas and tonics internally and in poultices externally. Should not be used by women who are or may be pregnant.

6. Fenugreek – Used internally and externally for a variety of medicinal purposes.

7. Chamomile – Commonly used in teas it is best known to help with sleep.

8. Greenbriar – Teas and salves used internally and externally.

9. Marshmallow Root – Dating back thousands of years, this root has been used as a food and medicine.

10. Passion Flower – Has a long history of use among Native Americans that and were adapted by early European colonists. Do not take passionflower if you are pregnant or breastfeeding.

11. Prickly Pear Cactus – Native Americans used the younger pads for food and in teas; while mature pads were used in poultices.

12. Pau d'arco – Long used for a wide range of conditions.

13. Slippery Elm – The tree had many traditional uses by Native Americans.

14. Tobacco – Long been important in Native American culture for social, religious, ceremonial purposes as well as in medicinal remedies.

15. White Pine – The inner bark, young shoots, twigs, pitch, and leaves have long been used by Native Americans in medicinal remedies.

16. Wild Yam – Traditionally used as both food and medicine.

Bronchial Infections/Problems

1. Bloodroot – Primarily used as a medicine for respiratory and digestive problems, it also used externally. Today, we know it is toxic and the FDA has classified it as unsafe.

2. Cardinal Flower – Roots, leaf tea, and poultices were used internally and externally.

3. Echinacea – Roots were chewed, dried in tea, or pulverized for external use.

4. Eucalyptus – Teas and ointments used for a variety of purposes.

5. Ginger Root – Utilized as both a spice and medicine throughout the world.

6. Horehound – Whole plant used internally and externally. People with gastritis or peptic ulcer disorders should use it cautiously.

7. Horsemint – leaves and flowering stems are used in teas, tonics, and salves for a variety of medical issues. Should not be used by pregnant women.

8. Kola Nut – Long used in medicinal remedies, spiritual practices, and ceremonies. Should not be used by pregnant or nursing women, or those with intestinal or stomach ulcers, blood pressure, insomnia, or heart disorders.

9. Marshmallow Root – Dating back thousands of years, this root has been used as a food and medicine.

10. Licorice Root – Used as a flavoring in food and for herbal remedies.

11. Plantain – Considered to be one of the nine sacred herbs by the ancient Saxon people and has a long history of use as an alternative medicine dating back to ancient times.

12. Pleurisy Root – Long been found to be effective for many respiratory disorders.

13. Rabbit Tobacco – Was thought to have had spiritual or mystic powers by many Indians.

14. Senna – A large genus of flowering plants found to be helpful in many remedies.

15. Slippery Elm – The tree had many traditional uses by Native Americans.

16. Spearmint – Teas, poultices, and oils used internally and externally for several remedies.

17. Wheat Grass – The result of centuries of cultivation, it is used for numerous medical conditions.

18. White Pine – The inner bark, young shoots, twigs, pitch, and leaves have long been used by Native Americans in medical remedies.

19. Wild Black Cherry – The dried inner bark was traditionally used in tea or syrups for several health problems.

20. Wild Garlic – Used throughout its history for both culinary and medicinal purposes.

Burns

1. Bloodroot – Primarily used as a medicine for respiratory and digestive problems, it also used externally. Today, we know it is toxic and the FDA has classified it as unsafe.

2. Buck Brush – Applies to several North American shrubs used in herbal medicine.

3. Chokecherry – Used as both a source of food and medicine, it was considered one of the most important herbs in Native American medicine.

4. Cattail – Utilized as a food, as well as in external and internal medical remedies.

5. Cotton – Roots, leaves, and seeds have been used in the treatment of many conditions.

6. Greenbriar – Teas and salves used internally and externally.

7. Lavender – Dating back to Roman times, Lavender has been used in teas, balms, food, and medicinal remedies.

8. Mint – Dried leaves used in teas and food, found helpful in several remedies.

9. Oak – Acorns and bark are used for a variety of medical ailments.

10. Pinon – Used so extensively by Native Americans it was referred to by some tribes as the "tree of life."

11. Prickly Pear Cactus – Native Americans used the younger pads for food and in teas; while mature pads were used in poultices.

12. Rabbit Tobacco – Was thought to have had spiritual or mystic powers by many Indians.

13. Sumac – Viewed by some tribes as a sacred plant, Sumac was used for both food and medicine.

14. Western Skunk Cabbage – This plant with a "skunky" has long been used by Native Americans as a topical medicine.

15. Yellow Spined Thistle – Long been used by Native Americans in medicinal remedies.

Cancer

1. Cat's Claw – Used in teas and tonics for more than 2,000 years.

2. Grapefruit – Seeds, pulp, and inner rind used for internal conditions.

3. Green Tea – Made solely with the leaves of Camellia Sinensis, it is known for its many helpful properties.

4. Jiaogulan – Known for its many health-giving qualities and anti-aging effects.

5. Maca – Used for centuries, Maca is consumed as a food and used for medicinal purposes.

6. Oat Straw – A food source and medical remedy since prehistoric times.

7. Olive Oil – A traditional tree crop long used in foods and medicines.

8. Pau d'arco – Long used for a wide range of conditions.

9. Poke – Though parts of this plant are highly toxic to livestock and humans, it has long been used as food and medicine by Native Americans.

10. Rosemary – Used for culinary purposes and in medicinal remedies.

11. **Red Clover** – Traditionally used for several conditions.

12. **Sarsaparilla** – Used for centuries in a wide variety of medicinal remedies.

13. **Spirulina** – A type of blue-green algae that is rich in protein, vitamins.

14. **Sumac** – Viewed by some tribes as a sacred plant, Sumac was used for both food and medicine.

15. **Thistle** – This flowering plant of the daisy family, has been used for some 2,000 years for medicinal remedies.

Cough

1. **Aspen** – Tea was made from the inner bark of the Quaking Aspen tree.

2. **American Licorice** – Chewed or used in teas for internal issues, in a poultice externally.

3. **Black Cohosh** – Roots of the plant were used in teas for a variety of ailments.

4. **Black Raspberry** – Roots and leaves are boiled into tea or chewed, and washes are used externally.

5. **Bloodroot** – Primarily used as a medicine for respiratory and digestive problems, it also used externally. Today, we know it is toxic and the FDA has classified it as unsafe.

6. **Boneset** – Dried leaves are used in tea. Caution is advised as it is toxic and has side effects.

7. **Broom Snakeweed** – Roots and leaves used in steam therapies, teas, and poultices.

8. **Chokecherry** – Used as both a source of food and medicine, it was considered one of the most important herbs in Native American medicine.

9. **Echinacea** – Roots were chewed, dried in tea, or pulverized for external use.

10. **Eucalyptus** – Teas and ointments used for a variety of purposes.

11. **Evening Primrose** – Used for both food and medicinal remedies, decoctions were used for internal and external ailments.

12. **Fennel** – Seeds, leaves, and roots used in cooking and medicinal remedies.

13. **Gymnema Sylvestre** – Has been used as a natural treatment for diabetes for nearly 2,000 years.

14. **Hibiscus** – Various species used in traditional herbal medicines dating back to Roman times.

15. **Horehound** – Whole plant used internally and externally. People with gastritis or peptic ulcer disorders should use it cautiously.

16. **Horsemint** – leaves and flowering stems are used in teas, tonics, and salves for a variety of medical issues. Should not be used by pregnant women.

17. **Lemongrass** – Having anti-fungal properties, it has not only been used as herbal medicine but, also as a pesticide and preservative.

18. Marshmallow Root – Dating back thousands of years, this root has been used as a food and medicine.

19. Mullein: A tobacco-like plant and one of the oldest herbs, it has a long history of use as a medicine.

20. Osha – Having a wide variety of medicinal properties, Osha was highly valued by Native Americans.

21. Plantain – Considered to be one of the nine sacred herbs by the ancient Saxon people and has a long history of use as an alternative medicine dating back to ancient times.

22. Pleurisy Root – Long been found to be effective for many respiratory disorders.

23. Rabbit Tobacco – Was thought to have had spiritual or mystic powers by many Indians.

24. Rose Hip – The fruit of the rose plant has long been used in teas to soothe a variety of problems.

25. Sage – Used for thousands of years in cooking and like other culinary herbs, it has long been thought to be a digestive aid and appetite stimulant.

26. Saltbush – Many species are used for a variety of conditions.

27. Sarsaparilla – Used for centuries in a wide variety of medicinal remedies.

28. Saw Palmetto – Long prized as a food product, it was also used by Native Americans to make baskets and fans, as well as in medicinal remedies.

29. Schisandra – A genus of a shrub that has many medicinal uses.

30. Senna – A large genus of flowering plants found to be helpful in many remedies.

31. Slippery Elm – The tree had many traditional uses by Native Americans.

32. Star Anise – The fruit of a small tree with a licorice-like flavor long used in medicinal remedies.

33. Sweetflag – Has a very long history of medicinal use in many herbal traditions.

34. Wheat Grass – The result of centuries of cultivation, it is used for numerous medical conditions.

35. White Pine – The inner bark, young shoots, twigs, pitch, and leaves have long been used by Native Americans in medicinal remedies.

Constipation

1. American Ginseng – Used in teas and tonics, it can be an effective laxative.

2. Boneset – Dried leaves are used in tea. Caution is advised as it is toxic and has side effects.

3. Buffaloberry – Used as food and in herbal remedies. Overindulgence can cause severe problems including death.

4. Cascara Sagrada – Dried bark used in teas. Bark must be aged and dried thoroughly before use.

5. Damiana – Used internally for a variety of medical issues.

6. Dong Quai – Used for more than a thousand years to treat several conditions.

7. Devil's Claw – Used in teas and tonics internally and in poultices externally. Should not be used by women who are or may be pregnant.

8. Elder – Ripe elderberries are used as both food and medicinal remedies.

9. Fennel – Seeds, leaves, and roots used in cooking and medicinal remedies.

10. Fenugreek – Used internally and externally for a variety of medicinal purposes.

12. Garcinia Cambogia – Fruit rind used in a variety of remedies. Not recommended for those with diabetes, people suffering any dementia syndrome, or pregnant and lactating women.

13. Glucomannan – A dietary fiber that has long been used in Asia. It is not recommended for use by pregnant or breast-feeding women.

14. Gymnema Sylvestre – Has been used as a natural treatment for diabetes for nearly 2,000 years.

15. Hibiscus – Various species used in traditional herbal medicines dating back to Roman times.

16. Horehound – Whole plant used internally and externally. People with gastritis or peptic ulcer disorders should use it cautiously.

17. Mayapple – Having been long surrounded by folklore, this plant was used for a variety of medical purposes. Because of its toxicity, this herb should only be used by professional Herbalists.

18. Milkweed – Though it can be toxic if not prepared properly, Milkweed was used as a food and medicine, as well as in making cords, ropes, and coarse cloth. **Warning:** Milkweed may be toxic when taken internally, without sufficient preparation.

19. Olive Oil – A traditional tree crop long used in foods and medicines.

20. Persimmon – Long used as food and in traditional medicine.

21. Psyllium Seed Husk – A rich fiber supplement, long used primarily to improve digestion.

22. Senna – A large genus of flowering plants found to be helpful in many remedies.

23. Sumac – Viewed by some tribes as a sacred plant, Sumac was used for both food and medicine.

24. Wheat Grass – The result of centuries of cultivation, it is used for numerous medical conditions.

25. Yellow Dock – Native Americans as traditional medicine and food.

Cramps

1. Blue Cohosh – Root is used in teas and tonics.

2. Cardinal Flower – Roots, leaf tea, and poultices were used internally and externally.

3. Chamomile – Commonly used in teas it is best known to help with sleep.

4. Ginkgo Biloba – One of the most ancient trees in existence, it has been used for both food and medicine.

5. Poke – Though parts of this plant are highly toxic to livestock and humans, it has long been used as food and medicine by Native Americans.

6. St John's Wort – Most commonly known as an anti-depressant, it also has other medical uses.

7. Valerian Root – Has been used as a medicinal herb since at least the time of ancient Greece and Rome.

8. Wild Ginger – Native Americans used the roots as a seasoning as well as a medicinal herb.

Diabetes

1. Allspice – Dried unripe berries have long been used in teas.

2. American Ginseng – Used in teas and tonics, and sometimes smoked by Native Americans.

3. Cat's Claw – Used in teas and tonics for more than 2,000 years.

4. Dandelion – Used in both foods and internal and external medical remedies.

5. Devil's Claw – Used in teas and tonics internally and in poultices externally. Should not be used by a woman who is or may be pregnant.

6. Fenugreek – Used internally and externally for a variety of medicinal purposes.

7. Ginsing – Numerous specifies throughout the world have been used for thousands of years in medical remedies.

8. Goldenrod – Long used for a variety of ailments.

9. Glucomannan – A dietary fiber that has long been used in Asia. It is not recommended for use by pregnant or breast-feeding women.

10. Green Tea – Made solely with the leaves of Camellia Sinensis, it is known for its many helpful properties.

11. Gymnema Sylvestre – Has been used as a natural treatment for diabetes for nearly 2,000 years.

12. Oat Straw – A food source and medical remedy since prehistoric times.

13. Prickly Pear Cactus – Native Americans used the younger pads for food and in teas; while mature pads were used in poultices.

14. Stevia – An herb long used as a sweetener which also has medical remedy properties.

15. Sumac – Viewed by some tribes as a sacred plant, Sumac was used for both food and medicine.

16. Wild Carrot – Used as both food and for health conditions.

17. Yellow Spined Thistle – Long been used by Native Americans in medicinal remedies

Diarrhea

1. American Licorice – Chewed or used in teas for internal issues, in a poultice externally.

2. Blackberry – Tea made from the root-bark is utilized to soothe these types of ailments.

3. Black Raspberry – Roots and leaves are boiled into tea or chewed, and washes are used externally.

4. Boneset – Dried leaves are used in tea. Caution is advised as it is toxic and has side effects.

5. Broom Snakeweed – Roots and leaves used in steam therapies, teas, and poultices.

6. Buckwheat – The fruit seed was used as both a food and in herbal remedies.

7. Cattail – Utilized as a food, as well as in external and internal medical remedies.

8. Cat's Claw – Used in teas and tonics for more than 2,000 years.

9. Chokecherry – Used as both a source of food and medicine, it was considered one of the most important herbs in Native American medicine.

10. Cotton – Roots, leaves, and seeds have been used in the treatment of many conditions.

11. Dandelion – Used in both foods and internal and external medical remedies.

12. Devil's Claw – Used in teas and tonics internally and in poultices externally. Should not be used by women who are or may be pregnant.

13. Dogwood – Bark, berries, and twigs used in decoctions internally and externally.

14. Feverwort – Used internally and externally in herbal medicine.

15. Galangal – Similar to other ginger related herbs, it is primarily used for digestive disorders.

16. Garcinia Cambogia – Fruit rind used in a variety of remedies. Not recommended for those with diabetes, people suffering any dementia syndrome or pregnant and lactating women.

17. Geranium – Scented geranium used in teas for various conditions.

18. Goldenseal – used internally and externally for medicinal issues. Should not be taken by pregnant women.

19. Guarana – Containing caffeine, it has many of the same effects as coffee.

20. Juniper – Used internally and externally for medicinal purposes. Pregnant women should not use this herb as it has been known to cause miscarriage.

21. Marshmallow Root – Dating back thousands of years, this root has been used as a food and medicine.

22. Native Hemlock – Used by Native Americans as a dye, for tanning hides, making baskets and wooden items, as well as medical remedies.

23. Oak – Acorns and bark are used for a variety of medical ailments.

24. Peppermint – In addition to flavoring, long used in traditional medicine for its calming and numbing effects. Should not be used or given to infants or small children.

25. Psyllium Seed Husk – A rich fiber supplement, long used primarily to improve digestion.

26. Rabbit Tobacco – Was thought to have had spiritual or mystic powers by many Indians.

27. Raspberry – Leaves, and fruits used in a wide range of medical issues.

28. Rose Hip – The fruit of the rose plant has long been used in teas to soothe a variety of problems.

29. Sage – Used for thousands of years in cooking and like other culinary herbs, it has long been thought to be a digestive aid and appetite stimulant.

30. Savory – An aromatic herb used as a spice and in folk medicine.

31. Saw Palmetto – Long prized as a food product, it was also used by Native Americans to make baskets and fans, as well as in medical remedies.

32. Sumac – Viewed by some tribes as a sacred plant, Sumac was used for both food and medicine.

33. Uva Ursi – Used medicinally since the second century. Should not be used by pregnant women.

34. Wild Black Cherry – The dried inner bark was traditionally used in tea or syrups for several health problems.

35. Wild Rose – There are hundreds of species that have been used medicinally for thousands of years.

36. Wild Garlic – Used throughout its history for both culinary and medicinal purposes.

37. Willow – The leaves and bark of the willow tree have been used since the times of ancient Egypt and Greece.

Dropsy

1. Blue Cohosh – Root is used in teas and tonics.

2. Eastern Skunk Cabbage – Dried leaves used as a seasoning, in remedies, and as a magical talisman by various tribes.

3. Greenbriar – Teas and salves used internally and externally.

4. Indian Hemp – A type of marijuana it was used to make clothes, rope, and paper as well as boiling the roots into teas for medicinal problems.

5. Milkweed – Though it can be toxic if not prepared properly, Milkweed was used as a food and medicine, as well as in making cords, ropes, and coarse cloth. **Warning:** Milkweed may be toxic when taken internally, without sufficient preparation.

6. Sweetflag – Has a very long history of medicinal use in many herbal traditions.

7. Tobacco – Long been important in Native American culture for social, religious, ceremonial purposes as well as in medicinal remedies.

8. Wild Carrot – Used as both food and for health conditions.

9. Wild Lettuce – Indigenous to North American, it was used for sedative purposes, especially in nervous complaints.

Eye Problems, Irritation, Soreness

1. Black Gum – Used by Native Americans in baths, washes, and tonics.

2. Dandelion – Used in both foods and internal and external medicinal remedies.

3. Fendler's Bladderpod – Used crushed leaves for internal and external use.

4. Fennel – Seeds, leaves, and roots used in cooking and medicinal remedies.

5. Goldenseal – used internally and externally for medicinal issues. Should not be taken by pregnant women.

6. Pennyroyal – Long used to treat medical problems and to eradicate pests. Pennyroyal should not be used in any way by pregnant women. Over ingestion of this herb has caused death.

7. Plantain – Considered to be one of the nine sacred herbs by the ancient Saxon people and has a long history of use as an alternative medicine dating back to ancient times.

8. Sumac – Viewed by some tribes as a sacred plant, Sumac was used for both food and medicine.

9. Wild Black Cherry – The dried inner bark was traditionally used in tea or syrups for several health problems.

10. White Willow – The use of willow bark dates back thousands of years.

Fever

1. American Ginseng – Used in teas and tonics, and sometimes smoked by Native Americans.

2. American Licorice – Chewed or used in teas for internal issues, in a poultice externally.

3. Boswellia – Fragrant resin utilized in a variety of ailments. Should not be used by pregnant, breastfeeding women and children.

4. Broom Snakeweed – Roots and leaves used in steam therapies, teas, and poultices.

5. Buffaloberry – Used as food and in herbal remedies. Overindulgence can cause severe problems including death.

6. Devil's Claw – Used in teas and tonics internally and in poultices externally. Should not be used by women who are or may be pregnant.

7. Dogwood – bark, berries, and twigs used in decoctions internally and externally.

8. Catnip – Stems and leaves make an aromatic tea which is useful for many conditions.

9. Cardinal Flower – Roots, leaf tea, and poultices were used internally and externally.

10. Dandelion – Used in both foods and internal and external medical remedies.

11. Eucalyptus – Teas and ointments used for a variety of purposes.

12. Feverfew – Used for a variety of internal medical problems. Should not be used by women who are pregnant.

13. Feverwort – Used internally and externally in herbal medicine.

14. Ginger Root – Utilized as both a spice and medicine throughout the world.

15. Gymnema Sylvestre – Has been used as a natural treatment for diabetes for nearly 2,000 years.

16. Hibiscus – Various species used in traditional herbal medicines dating back to Roman times.

17. Honeysuckle – Used in traditional herbal remedies for thousands of years.

18. Horsemint – leaves and flowering stems are used in teas, tonics, and salves for a variety of medical issues. Should not be used by pregnant women.

19. Indian Hemp – A type of marijuana it was used to make clothes, rope, and paper as well as boiling the roots into teas for medicinal problems.

20. Native Hemlock – Used by Native Americans as a dye, for tanning hides, making baskets and wooden items, as well as medicinal remedies.

21. Osha – Having a wide variety of medicinal properties, Osha was highly valued by Native Americans.

22. Pau d'arco – Long used for a wide range of conditions.

23. Pennyroyal – Long used to treat medical problems and to eradicate pests. Pennyroyal should not be used in any way by pregnant women. Over ingestion of this herb has caused death.

24. Persimmon – Long used as food and in traditional medicine.

25. Rabbit Tobacco – Was thought to have had spiritual or mystic powers by many Indians.

26. Sarsaparilla – Used for centuries in a wide variety of medicinal remedies.

27. Sassafras – Used extensively for food and medicine by Native Americans long before European settlers arrived.

28. Spearmint – Teas, poultices, and oils used internally and externally for several remedies.

29. Sumac – Viewed by some tribes as a sacred plant, Sumac was used for both food and medicine.

30. Tobacco – Long been important in Native American culture for social, religious, ceremonial purposes as well as in medical remedies.

31. Wild Rose – There are hundreds of species that have been used medicinally for thousands of years.

32. Wheat Grass – The result of centuries of cultivation, it is used for numerous medical conditions.

33. White Pine – The inner bark, young shoots, twigs, pitch, and leaves have long been used by Native Americans in medical remedies.

34. Wild Black Cherry – The dried inner bark was traditionally used in tea or syrups for several health problems.

35. White Willow – The use of willow bark dates back thousands of years.

Flu

1. American Ginseng – Used in teas and tonics, and sometimes smoked by Native Americans.

2. Boneset – Dried leaves are used in tea. Caution is advised as it is toxic and has side effects.

3. Catnip – Stems and leaves make an aromatic tea which is useful for many conditions.

4. Chamomile – Commonly used in teas it is best known to help with sleep.

5. Echinacea – Roots were chewed, dried in tea, or pulverized for external use.

6. Elder – Ripe elderberries are used as both a food and in medicinal remedies.

7. Eleuthero – Dried roots have been used for centuries. People with medicated high blood pressure should consult their doctor, can cause insomnia.

8. Feverwort – Used internally and externally in herbal medicine.

9. Ginger Root – Utilized as both a spice and medicine throughout the world.

10. Goldenrod – Long used for a variety of ailments.

11. Goldenseal – used internally and externally for medicinal issues. Should not be taken by pregnant women.

12. Green Tea – Made solely with the leaves of Camellia Sinensis, it is known for its many helpful properties.

13. Mint – Dried leaves used in teas and food, found helpful in several remedies.

14. Native Hemlock – Used by Native Americans as a dye, for tanning hides, making baskets and wooden items, as well as medicinal remedies.

15. Osha – Having a wide variety of medicinal properties, Osha was highly valued by Native Americans.

16. Pau d'arco – Long used for a wide range of conditions.

17. Pleurisy Root – Long been found to be effective for many respiratory disorders.

18. Rabbit Tobacco – Was thought to have had spiritual or mystic powers by many Indians.

19. Sage – Used for thousands of years in cooking and like other culinary herbs, it has long been thought to be a digestive aid and appetite stimulant.

20. Sassafras – Used extensively for food and medicine by Native Americans long before European settlers arrived.

21. Star Anise – The fruit of a small tree with a licorice-like flavor long used in medicinal remedies.

22. White Pine – The inner bark, young shoots, twigs, pitch, and leaves have long been used by Native Americans in medicinal remedies.

23. Wild Black Cherry – The dried inner bark was traditionally used in tea or syrups for several health problems.

Heartburn

1. Dandelion – Used in both foods and internal and external medical remedies.

2. Ginger Root – Utilized as both a spice and medicine throughout the world.

3. Licorice Root – Used as a flavoring in food and for herbal remedies.

4. Mint – Dried leaves used in teas and food, found helpful in several remedies.

5. Osha – Having a wide variety of medicinal properties, Osha was highly valued by Native Americans.

6. Peppermint – In addition to flavoring, long used in traditional medicine for its calming and numbing effects. Should not be used or given to infants or small children.

7. Rooibos – Used in teas to help with a variety of conditions.

8. Stevia – An herb long used as a sweetener which also has medical remedy properties.

9. White Pine – The inner bark, young shoots, twigs, pitch, and leaves have long been used by Native Americans in medical remedies.

10. Wormwood – The leaves and flowering tops were gathered and dried to use in medicinal tonics.

Infection

1. Cattail – Utilized as a food, as well as in external and internal medical remedies.

2. Echinacea – Roots were chewed, dried in tea, or pulverized for external use.

3. Eucalyptus – Teas and ointments used for a variety of purposes.

4. Grapefruit – Seeds, pulp, and inner rind used for internal conditions.

5. Goldenseal – used internally and externally for medicinal issues. Should not be taken by pregnant women.

6. Spirulina – A type of blue-green algae that is rich in protein, vitamins.

7. Wild Rose – There are hundreds of species that have been used medicinally for thousands of years.

8. Wheat Grass – The result of centuries of cultivation, it is used for numerous medical conditions.

Inflammation/Swelling

1. American Ginseng – Used in teas and tonics, and sometimes smoked by Native Americans.

2. American Licorice – Chewed or used in teas for internal issues, in a poultice externally.

3. Arnica – Used externally only for aches, pains, and wounds. Poison if taken internally.

4. Ashwagandha – The whole plant is used in numerous remedies. Caution is advised in the use of this plant since it is toxic.

5. Blackberry – Tea made from the root-bark is utilized to soothe these types of ailments.

6. Boswellia – Fragrant resin utilized in a variety of ailments. Should not be used by pregnant, breastfeeding women and children.

7. Buck Brush – Applies to several North American shrubs used in herbal medicine.

8. Buffaloberry – Used as food and in herbal remedies. Overindulgence can cause severe problems including death.

9. Cat's Claw – Used in teas and tonics for more than 2,000 years.

10. Cattail – Utilized as a food, as well as in external and internal medical remedies.

11. Chasteberry – Berries and flowers used in teas. Pregnant or breast-feeding women should not take a chaste berry.

12. Dandelion – Used in both foods and internal and external medical remedies.

13. Devil's Claw – Used in teas and tonics internally and in poultices externally. Should not be used by women who are or may be pregnant.

14. Echinacea – Roots were chewed, dried in tea, or pulverized for external use.

15. Elder – Ripe elderberries are used as both a food and in medicinal remedies.

16. Eleuthero – Dried roots have been used for centuries. People with medicated high blood pressure should consult their doctor, can cause insomnia.

17. Eucalyptus – Teas and ointments used for a variety of purposes.

18. Evening Primrose – Used for both food and medicinal remedies, decoctions were used for internal and external ailments.

19. Fenugreek – Used internally and externally for a variety of medicinal purposes.

20. Garcinia Cambogia – Fruit rind used in a variety of remedies. Not recommended for those with diabetes, people suffering any dementia syndrome or pregnant and lactating women.

21. Gentiana – Extremely bitter herb used for both internal and external problems. May irritate persons who have ulcers, and may also cause headache, nausea, or vomiting.

22. Green Tea – Made solely with the leaves of Camellia Sinensis, it is known for its many helpful properties.

23. Horsemint – leaves and flowering stems are used in teas, tonics, and salves for a variety of medical issues. Should not be used by pregnant women.

24. Lavender – Dating back to Roman times, Lavender has been used in teas, balms, food, and medicinal remedies.

25. Marshmallow Root – Dating back thousands of years, this root has been used as a food and medicine.

26. Mullein – A tobacco-like plant and one of the oldest herbs, it has a long history of use as a medicine.

27. Oak – Acorns and bark are used for a variety of medical ailments.

28. Pleurisy Root – Long been found to be effective for many respiratory disorders.

29. Poke – Though parts of this plant are highly toxic to livestock and humans, it has long been used as food and medicine by Native Americans.

30. Raspberry – Leaves, and fruits used in a wide range of medical issues.

31. Rose Hip – The fruit of the rose plant has long been used in teas to soothe a variety of problems.

32. Skullcap – A powerful medicinal herb, it was cultivated by Native Americans for use in several remedies. Pregnant women should not take Skullcap.

33. St John's Wort – Most commonly known as an anti-depressant, it also has other medical uses.

34. Sweetflag – Has a very long history of medicinal use in many herbal traditions.

35. Western Skunk Cabbage – This plant with a "skunky" has long been used by Native Americans as a topical medicine.

36. Wild Rose – There are hundreds of species that have been used medicinally for thousands of years.

37. White Pine – The inner bark, young shoots, twigs, pitch, and leaves have long been used by Native Americans in medical remedies

38. Wild Black Cherry – The dried inner bark was traditionally used in tea or syrups for several health problems.

39. White Willow – The use of willow bark dates back thousands of years.

40. Witch Hazel – Widely used for medicinal purposes by American Indians.

Insect Bites And Stings

1. Bloodroot – Primarily used as a medicine for respiratory and digestive problems, it also used externally. Today, we know it is toxic and the FDA has classified it as unsafe.

2. Broom Snakeweed – Roots and leaves used in steam therapies, teas, and poultices.

3. Buffaloberry – Used as food and in herbal remedies. Overindulgence can cause severe problems including death.

4. Goldenseal – used internally and externally for medicinal issues. Should not be taken by pregnant women.

5. Honeysuckle – Used in traditional herbal remedies for thousands of years.

6. Lavender – Dating back to Roman times, Lavender has been used in teas, balms, food, and medicinal remedies.

7. Lemon Balm – A calming herb that has been used since the Middle Ages.

8. Osha – Having a wide variety of medicinal properties, Osha was highly valued by Native Americans.

9. Plantain – Considered to be one of the nine sacred herbs by the ancient Saxon people and has a long history of use as an alternative medicine dating back to ancient times.

10. Saltbush – Many species are used for a variety of conditions.

11. Stiff Goldenrod – Long been used to stop bleeding and other ailments.

Menstrual Cramps And Pain

1. Allspice – Dried unripe berries have long been used in teas.

2. Black Cohosh – Roots of the plant were used in teas for a variety of ailments.

3. Dong Quai – Used for more than a thousand years to treat several conditions.

4. Ginger Root – Utilized as both a spice and medicine throughout the world.

5. Hibiscus – Various species used in traditional herbal medicines dating back to Roman times.

6. Horehound – Whole plant used internally and externally. People with gastritis or peptic ulcer disorders should use it cautiously.

7. Osha – Having a wide variety of medicinal properties, Osha was highly valued by Native Americans.

8. Partridgeberry – Used as food and medical problems, primarily for women.

9. Peppermint – in addition to flavoring, long used in traditional medicine for its calming and numbing effects. Should not be used or given to infants or small children.

10. Sage – Used for thousands of years in cooking and like other culinary herbs, it has long been thought to be a digestive aid and appetite stimulant.

11. Spearmint – Teas, poultices, and oils used internally and externally for several remedies.

12. Wild Yam – Traditionally used as both food and medicine.

Pneumonia

1. Dogwood – Bark, berries, and twigs used in decoctions internally and externally.

2. Honeysuckle – Used in traditional herbal remedies for thousands of years.

3. Pleurisy Root – Long been found to be effective for many respiratory disorders.

4. Rabbit Tobacco – Was thought to have had spiritual or mystic powers by many Indians.

5. White Pine – The inner bark, young shoots, twigs, pitch, and leaves have long been used by Native Americans in medical remedies.

6. Wild Black Cherry – The dried inner bark was traditionally used in tea or syrups for several health problems.

Stomach Problems

1. Allspice – Dried unripe berries have long been used in teas.

2. American Licorice – Chewed or used in teas for internal issues, in a poultice externally.

3. Blackberry – Root is used in teas, and leaves are used as a gargle.

4. Black Raspberry – Roots and leaves are boiled into tea or chewed, and washes are used externally.

5. Boswellia – Fragrant resin utilized in a variety of ailments. Should not be used by pregnant, breast-feeding women and children.

6. Dandelion – Used in both foods and internal and external medicinal remedies.

7. Devil's Claw – Used in teas and tonics internally and in poultices externally. Should not be used by a woman who is or may be pregnant.

8. Fennel – Seeds, leaves, and roots used in cooking and medicinal remedies.

9. Fenugreek – Used internally and externally for a variety of medicinal purposes.

10. Feverfew – Used for a variety of internal medical problems. Should not be used by women who are pregnant.

11. Ginger Root – Utilized as both a spice and medicine throughout the world.

12. Grapefruit – Seeds, pulp, and inner rind used for internal conditions.

13. Greenbriar – Teas and salves used internally and externally.

14. Pennyroyal – Long used to treat medical problems and to eradicate pests. Pennyroyal should not be used in any way by pregnant women. Over ingestion of this herb has caused death.

15. Peppermint – In addition to flavoring, long used in traditional medicine for its calming and numbing effects. Should not be used or given to infants or small children.

Syphilis

1. Boswellia – Fragrant resin utilized in a variety of ailments. Should not be used by pregnant, breast-feeding women and children.

2. Cardinal Flower – Roots, leaf tea, and poultices were used internally and externally.

3. Geranium – Scented geranium used in teas for various conditions.

4. Pinon – Used so extensively by Native Americans it was referred to by some tribes as the "tree of life."

5. Poke – Though parts of this plant are highly toxic to livestock and humans, it has long been used as food and medicine by Native Americans.

6. Sarsaparilla – Used for centuries in a wide variety of medicinal remedies.

7. Yellow Spined Thistle – Long been used by Native Americans in medicinal remedies.

Wounds

1. Arnica – Used externally only for aches, pains, and wounds. Poison if taken internally.

2. Broom Snakeweed – Roots and leaves used in steam therapies, teas, and poultices.

3. Buck Brush – Applies to several North American shrubs used in herbal medicine.

4. Buffaloberry – Used as food and in herbal remedies

5. Cattail – Utilized as a food, as well as in external and internal medical remedies.

6. Chokecherry – Used as both a source of food and medicine, it was considered one of the most important herbs in Native American medicine.

7. Cotton – Roots, leaves, and seeds have been used in the treatment of many conditions.

8. Dogwood – Bark, berries, and twigs used in decoctions internally and externally.

9. Echinacea – Roots were chewed, dried in tea, or pulverized for external use.

10. Eucalyptus – Teas and ointments used for a variety of purposes.

11. Evening Primrose – Used for both food and medicinal remedies, decoctions were used for internal and external ailments.

12. Fenugreek – Used internally and externally for a variety of medicinal purposes.

13. Gentiana – Extremely bitter herb used for both internal and external problems. May irritate persons who have ulcers, and may also cause headache, nausea.

14. Goldenrod – Long used for a variety of ailments.

15. Goldenseal – Used internally and externally for medicinal issues. Should not be taken by pregnant women.

CONCLUSION

Herbal medicine has its origins in ancient cultures. It involves the medicinal use of plants to treat disease and enhance general health and wellbeing. Some herbs have potent (powerful) ingredients and should be taken with the same level of caution as pharmaceutical medications. Many pharmaceutical medications are based on man-made versions of naturally occurring compounds found in plants. For instance, the heart medicine digitalis was derived from the foxglove plant. Herbal medicines contain active ingredients. The active ingredients of many herbal preparations are as yet unknown. Some pharmaceutical medications are based on a single active ingredient derived from a plant source. Practitioners of herbal medicine believe that an active ingredient can lose its impact or become less safe if used in isolation from the rest of the plant.

There is no question that physicians who spend more time with patients and listen more carefully will see benefits. Novella agreed that a caring, bonding practitioner is more likely to get patients to adopt healthier lifestyles and that these changes lead to better health. And he agrees that many patients do feel better when practitioners actively try to help them deal with vague, hard-to-diagnose complaints such as pain and fatigue, instead of telling them that there's no diagnosis or effective treatment.

But these aspects of a better patient-practitioner relationship should not be uniquely associated with alternative medicine, and such principles should not attempt to discredit the breakthroughs and innovations from the drug and device industry. Instead, we should look to our doctors to be the nurturing caregivers who take the time to listen to us, bond with us, and guide us toward healthier lifestyles and lower levels of stress.

Results: Many of the herbal products that are being given to children in the United States currently do not meet the standards of good manufacturing practices. No high-quality studies have been conducted to determine the efficacy of these products. Their concentrations of active ingredients are unpredictable, their labeling is inadequate, and they can cause toxicity.

Conclusions: The benefit-risk ratio of most herbal products remains unknown. Greater efforts and resources should be devoted to high-quality research to determine the effectiveness and tolerability of these widely used herbal products.

This review article presents important medicinal plants for the treatment and prevention of herbal remedies for the child. These plants can be used for the preparation of new drugs; their active ingredients may also be used in the treatment of herbal remedies for the ld. In future studies, it is better to focus on the classification of herbal laxatives, based on their mechanisms for treating herbal remedies for the old.

Even in the light of the increased sophistication of modern healthcare as enriched by science and technology, the use of herbal medicine will continue to thrive in both poor and rich societies for many and probably different reasons. It is important for stakeholders: governments, farmers, scientists, healthcare providers (physicians, pharmacists, and nurses), and biotechnical engineers to give enough attention to herbal medicines and their challenges in a deliberate effort to create for it an appropriate niche that will ensure that it develops alongside with conventional medicine. The application of science and technology especially in the area of information resources, conservation and cultivation, production, analytical techniques, and quality control, clinical trials, and regulation should be promoted. These efforts will boost benefits, confidence, and safety in the use of HMs and its possible induction into mainstream healthcare. Though there are several pieces of literature on HM, this book nevertheless has stooped to collate in a simple, unambiguous, and readable manner a wide and indebt information that will be useful to all who have a stake in HM: scientist, healthcare professionals, engineers, and the general public.

Herbal remedies are commonly used by patients who access conventional health care. Few have been shown to have beneficial effects beyond those of conventionally regulated products, and they may be costly, adulterated with dangerous additives, inherently toxic, or cause the patient to forgo potentially curative care.

If a patient presents with a problem that might be due to an herb, the physician should discontinue the product and watch for resolution. If patients ask if "herbal medicines" in general are safe or effective, they should be counseled about the lack of regulations for quality, safety, or efficacy, the differences in preparations from different manufacturers, and the lack of a mechanism for reporting adverse effects. Curious patients can be directed to read the books mentioned, and cautioned against biased information that they may receive from health food store employees, pamphlets shelved near herbs, and the Internet.

NATIVE AMERICAN RECIPES

Natural Herbal Remedies, Sacred Medicinal Plants, and Recipes to Heal Common Ailments

Taahira Maskwa

CHAPTER 1: MOST COMMON DIY HERBAL RECIPES

1. Tea

1. Lemon And Elderflower Tea For Fighting Common Flu

Elderflowers and lemon might easily become your most favorite herbal tea in the world. While lemon tea is no stranger to tea drinkers, elderflowers are still not as widely used as they deserve. Some studies showed that elderberry flowers may have help to relieve flu symptoms. However, the best part of elderflower tea is – the flavor. Because of their unique and sweet flavor, these flowers are popular for making syrups and flavoring soft drinks and water. They blend amazingly well with lemon too. You can use both fresh and dry flowers. Wash them before use. Elderflower usually grows freely in nature and start blooming around May.

Blend: (For 1 Cup)

- 1 spoon of elderflowers
- 1-2 teaspoons of lemon juice
- 1 teaspoon of honey

2. Ginger Tea

Fresh, dried, pickled, or powdered, ginger tastes well in any form and in any dish or drink – especially in tea. Ginger tea is the only tea we recommend making with fresh instead of dry ingredients. Peel, wash, and slice ginger into thin slices. Then add it to a small saucepan together with 1 ½ cup of water and a few peppercorns. Bring it to a boil and let it simmer for another 10-15 minutes. Strain, add honey, and drink. Why adding peppercorns to a blend? Both ginger and peppercorns may warm you up, may offer benefits for the digestive system, and positively influence the mood.

Blend: (For One Cup)

- ½ – 1 inch of fresh ginger
- A teaspoon of honey
- A few peppercorns

3. Mint And Lavender

Upgrade the simple mint tea by adding a touch of lavender flowers. Lavender may help with relaxation, and help freshen the breath. Together with mint, it gives a delicious and potent tea with relaxing, antimicrobial, antiviral, and antioxidant properties. To brew mint and lavender tea, use about 1 teaspoon of dry leaves. Bring water to a boil and let it cool for a few minutes. Oversteeped lavender tea may become bitter. You can easily fix this by adding a spoon of honey. Once brewed, you can cool it down and serve it with honey and ice as iced tea.

Blend: (For 2 Cups)

- 1 spoon of mint
- ¼ spoon of lavender flowers
- 1 teaspoon of honey

4. Herbal Chai Tea

Nothing beats a cup of warm chai – in any season. While the real chai is made with strong black tea, herbal chai has no caffeine at all. This warm and soothing drink can be made with powdered or crushed spices. The best base for herbal chai is pure rooibos tea. It's strong enough to hold all the spices and blends well with milk. Rooibos is naturally lightly sweet, and won't have a bitter taste even if over-brewed.

Blend: (For 4-5 Cups)

- 4 spoons of rooibos tea
- 1 teaspoon of ginger powder
- 2 inches of crushed cinnamon bark
- ½ -1 teaspoon of crushed cardamom
- ½ -1 teaspoon of cloves

2. Decoctions

What Is An Herbal Decoction?

So, what precisely is an herbal decoction? A decoction is an herbal preparation created by boiling herbs in liquid, usually water. Herbalist James Green explains, "the object of preparing decoctions is to secure, in aqueous solution, the soluble active principles of herbs that are hard and woody and have a close, dense texture"

1. Roasted Dandelion Root Tea Recipe

Ingredients

- 4½ tsp dried dandelion root (where to buy dandelion root if you can't find it locally)
- 2 cups of water
- 1 to 2 tbsp butter or cream to taste (optional)
- Optional additions - 1 cinnamon stick OR 1/2 teaspoon of dried ginger OR 1 teaspoon fresh minced ginger. OR vanilla extract to taste (or a combination of these)

Instructions

- Place a medium pot over medium heat and place the dried dandelion root in the bottom.
- Toast the root until it becomes fragrant and golden brown, then add water and additional flavorings (if using) and bring to a boil.
- When the water boils, reduce heat and allow to simmer for 30-45 minutes, then strain and serve.
- Blend in a little maple syrup and a tablespoon of butter, or try a dollop of cream and 2-3 drops of vanilla extract.

Marshmallow Decoction Recipe

- 1.5 cups water
- 1 tablespoon cut and sifted marshmallow root

Instructions: Bring water and marshmallow to a boil, then cover and simmer on low for 20 minutes. Remove from heat, strain with a mesh strainer or cheesecloth, and sweeten if desired before serving.

3. Popsicles

Popsicles Made With Chamomile And Hibiscus

Ingredients

- 2 tablespoons dry chamomile
- 1 tablespoon dry hibiscus
- 1 ¼ cups boiling water
- 1 cup greek yogurt
- Honey to taste
- Pinch of salt
- 1 tablespoon lemon juice
- Popsicle molds (you can use paper cups and Popsicle sticks)

Instructions

- Begin your Popsicles by making a tea out of the chamomile and hibiscus. Put the herbs in a cup, pour water over the herbs, and let steep for five minutes. (sometimes waiting is the hardest part)
- Strain into a small bowl
- While the mixture is still hot, add honey to taste. Stir well so the honey combines well with the tea. You will be mixing this with the yogurt so you may want to make it more on the sweet side.
- Add a pinch of salt
- Add the lemon juice. You can use the juice of fresh lemon. We keep this type of fresh lemon juice on hand for convenience.
- Let the mixture cool a little
- Add the yogurt and mix well
- Pour into the Popsicle molds
- Places these in the freezer until frozen solid

Lavender Plus Lemon Balm Popsicles

Ingredients

- 4 cups of water
- 5-6 whole fresh lavender blossoms
- 1 small handful of fresh lemon balm
- 2-4 tbsp honey

Instructions

- ❖ Bring the water to a boil, then pour over the lavender and lemon balm in a quart-sized jar.
- ❖ Steep the tea for 10-15 minutes, then strain out the herbs with a fine-mesh sieve and stir in the honey to your desired sweetness.
- ❖ Let the tea cool down a bit (you can add a few ice cubes if you're impatient like me), then pour it into a popsicle mold. Freeze for several hours or overnight.

Sunshine Pops

Ingredients:

- ❖ 2 tablespoons chamomile
- ❖ 2 tablespoons lemon balm
- ❖ 2 tablespoons milky oats (or oatstraw)
- ❖ 1 teaspoon lavender
- ❖ Peel from ¼ of a lemon
- ❖ Honey to taste
- ❖ Bee pollen to taste (optional)

Directions:

- ❖ Prepare your tea or infusion by pouring 4 cups of boiling water over the herbs and lemon peel.
- ❖ Steep for 30 min and taste. If you would like a stronger brew, steep for an additional 30 minutes and then strain. Mix in honey to taste.
- ❖ Pour liquid into your popsicle mold of choice and freeze for one hour.
- ❖ After one hour, add in the bee pollen to the molds and gently combine and then insert popsicle sticks into each pop and freeze for an additional four hours, or until completely frozen

4. Ice Cubes

Ingredients

- ❖ Herbs, of choice (basil, chives, cilantro, fennel, lovage, mint, oregano, parsley, rosemary, sage, tarragon, thyme)
- ❖ Boiling water

Directions

- ❖ Mince herb (s) of choice.
- ❖ Pack minced herb (s) into an ice cube tray, each 3/4 full.
- ❖ Fill with boiling water, (this will blanch the herbs before freezing and will help them retain their flavor and color).
- ❖ Once the herbal ice cubes are frozen, you can pop them out of their tray and into freezer bags for storage.
- ❖ Use as needed.

Herb Infused Ice Cubes

Ingredients

- Ice Cube Tray
- Fresh herbs
- Water

Directions

- Fill each section of an ice cube tray with fresh herbs.
- Fill the ice cube tray with boiling water. This will blanch the herbs and help them retain their color and flavor.
- Freeze

5. Bath

Spring Tea Bath

Materials:

- Five 5" x 7" sized muslin bags or cheesecloth
- Big mixing bowl
- Spoon for mixing
- Cooking twine or cotton string (if using cheesecloth)

Ingredients

- 1 cup dried lavender flowers
- 1 cup dried rose petals
- 1 cup dried chamomile flowers
- 1 cup dried calendula petals
- 1 cup dried red clover blossoms

Instructions

- Pour flowers into a mixing bowl and blend them.
- Fill each muslin bag with the flour mixture or use cheesecloth and twine to create a small pouch.
- Tie shut and use one bag per bath. The bag can be tied to the water spout for the hot water to run through, or simply placed in the tub to float like a teabag in an infusion.

6. Breast milk

1. Fennel Seeds

Fennel seeds are great for increasing the milk supply in nursing mothers. It has phytoestrogens, similar to estrogen, which is a hormone that also helps in producing more milk

Instructions

- ❖ You can use fennel seeds to make tea by infusing them in hot water for a few minutes. You can add honey for sweetness (optional). You may take this tea a couple of times a day. If you are not very enthusiastic about tea, you may chew a spoonful of Add- roasted seeds a few times a day.

2. Torbagun Leaves

This is a great herb for breastfeeding. Torbagun leaves are popularly used in Bataknese cuisine, but they have been in use for centuries for improving lactation in breastfeeding mothers.

Instructions

- ❖ You may use these miraculous leaves in any form. You may take half a teaspoon or so of the leaves and add them to a cup of boiling water to make some tea, add it to your soup, or your regular vegetable preparation and consume it regularly.

3. Fenugreek Seeds

Fenugreek seeds are one of the best herbs for breastfeeding mothers to increase milk production. It also contains diosgenin and phytoestrogen. These seeds are also loaded with galactagogue, which makes them great for mothers who wish to enhance their breast milk supply

How To Use

- ❖ You may take a teaspoon full of fenugreek seeds and boil them in water. Strain the seeds. You may add a teaspoonful of honey and a pinch of turmeric to this to enhance the taste. Drink this tea at least two to three times a day. Mix fenugreek sprouts with salad or veggies as well.

4. Shatavari

This Ayurvedic herb has been in use to overcome lactation problems in women. This herb has galactagogue properties that help increase the production of prolactin and corticoids, which help produce breast milk, which in turn improve lactation and the quality of breast milk too

How To Use

- ❖ You may take this herb by mixing it in water, or you may also buy Shatavari herbal supplements for increasing breast milk supply.

5. Cinnamon

Cinnamon is a fragrant herb that enriches the flavors of many culinary dishes. However, for a long time, many breastfeeding mothers who suffer from insufficient milk supply have been using this herb to increase their milk flow. It is also said to enhance the flavor of breast milk.

How To Use

- ❖ Lactating mothers may consume cinnamon by mixing a pinch of cinnamon powder in warm water, half a teaspoon of honey, or by adding it to milk. You may take cinnamon for a month or two to see the difference in your breast milk supply.

6. Anise

This herb has estrogenic properties; it contains anethole, which is a phytoestrogen. which helps unblocked clogged milk ducts and increases breast milk supply

How To Use

- You may make tea by infusing a few anise seeds in hot water. Add sugar or honey for taste. You may safely consume two to three cups in a day.

- The availability of these ayurvedic/natural herbs may make you pick some of them and begin consuming them right away. However, it's not as simple because you must consume what is healthy for your baby. Additionally, your body may not react the way it used to before after consuming the same ingredients. But you need not worry. Take these precautionary measures to ensure you gain the most health benefits from these ayurvedic herbs

7. Compresses

Cold Herbal Compresses

Materials:

- 2-4 cotton or linen washcloths
- Large glass bowl
- Plate/ lid for the glass bowl

Ingredients:

- Two herbal tea bags per each towel.
- Tea suggestions: Chamomile-Lavender, Green Tea Peppermint, and Peppermint.
- 1 cup of water per each towel used
- Essential oil suggestions:
- Lavender: calming and soothing
- Peppermint: energizing and cooling
- Eucalyptus: invigorating and awakening

Directions:

- **Make A Tea Concentrate:** Bring water to a boil. Place tea bags in a glass bowl, and cover with water. Cover and let steep for 15-20 minutes, until thoroughly cooled or place in the refrigerator to chill quickly.
- Soak a clean cotton or linen washcloth in the tea concentrate and allow it to become fully saturated. Then gently squeeze any excess tea out of the cloth. It should be heavy and wet, but not dripping.
- Lay towel flat, and apply two drops of desired essential oil. Be careful – we don't recommend applying undiluted essential oil directly onto your skin.
- Roll or fold the washcloth and apply it to the head, neck, chest, or feet.
- Relax and enjoy this restorative herbal practice.

8. Poultice

Ingredients

- 2-3 tablespoons (or more as needed) of fresh or dried herbs, healing clays, or activated charcoal as needed
- Enough hot water to form a thick paste
- Organic cheesecloth or cloth for covering
- Waterproof covering to keep poultice on

Instructions

- Make a thick paste with the desired herb, clay or charcoal, and water.
- Apply directly to the wound or place between two layers of cloth and apply the cloth to the wound (depending on the cloth and the wound). Leave for 20 minutes to 3 hours as needed and repeat as necessary.

Making A Soothing Yarrow Poultice

You Will Need:

- 25-50 g fresh yarrow herb (a good handful of the leaf)
- Water
- Pestle and mortar, muslin and scissors
- Pick leaves and brush off insects and dirt.
- Chop or tear the herb coarsely, and place in the mortar.
- Add a little water and crush and mash herbs into pulp or paste using the pestle.
- Cut a piece of muslin about twice the area of skin to be treated, and spread the herb paste onto the layer of muslin. Fold over the muslin onto the herb, like a sandwich.
- Apply the muslin with herb paste direct to the affected area, tie on with strips of muslin, leave on for 30 min, and repeat as needed.

What You'll Need:

- 1 teaspoon turmeric powder
- 1 ounce freshly chopped or grated ginger
- ¼ small raw sliced onion
- 1 chopped garlic clove
- 2 teaspoons coconut oil
- cheesecloth or cotton bandage

How To Do It:

- Add the coconut oil followed by the rest of the ingredients to a pan on low heat and allow it to heat until it's almost dry but not burnt.
- Turn off the stove and transfer ingredients to a bowl to cool so that it's warm to the touch.
- Lay the cloth flat and add the mixture to the center of the cloth.
- Fold the cloth over twice to create a pack or gather it and tie with some string or a rubber band to create a handle whatever you prefer as long as the ingredients stay inside the cloth.
- Place on the affected area for 20 minutes.

9. Tinctures

Ingredients

- For fresh herbs
- 1 oz fresh chopped herb to 2 oz of 95% alcohol
- For dried herbs
- 1 oz dried herb to 5 oz of 40% alcohol

Instructions

- Fill a glass jar with herbs without packing them down. Add alcohol to the jar and put the lid on the jar.
- Shake well and store the jar in a cool dark place, shaking the jar daily, for 4 to 6 weeks.
- Strain through a cheesecloth, squeezing the herbs to extract as much liquid as possible.
- Store the tincture in a glass jar in a dark place. Never leave your tincture in sunlight.

Ingredients

- dried herbs single or multiple
- vodka 80 proof or more (preferably 100 proof)

Instructions

- Put herbs in a quart-size Mason jar to about 1/2 full (not packed down).
- Pour a bit of boiling water over the herbs to help release nutrients (optional).
- Pour vodka overall to fill the jar to just below the bands.
- Cover the jar. Tip upside down a few times to wet all the herbs with the vodka.
- Put in a cool, dark location for 4 to 6 weeks. Each day during this time, tip the jar upside down a few times.
- After steeping for 4 to 6 weeks, strain. Discard herbs (compost) and put the extract in a jar(s) or 4-ounce dropper bottles.
- Store in a cool and dark location. Keeps a long time.
- Airtight, sterilized glass containers
- Enough chopped fresh herbs to fill each container halfway
- Dried herbs can be used instead to make more concentrated herbal tinctures
- High proof vodka. Everclear can also be used if it is legally available for purchase in your locale.
- Cheesecloth or a fine grade strainer

Instructions

- Chop your fresh herbs so that they naturally begin to release their aromatic oils.
- Place your herbs in each container using the measuring guidelines shown above.
- Fill with alcohol. Allow enough room at the top to ensure that there is room for the alcohol and herbs to mix well when shaken.
- Store in a cool, dry, dark area. Shake each container at least once per day for 30 days. Strain the tincture with layered cheesecloth or a fine grade strainer.

To Make An Herbal Infusion, You Will Need Three Things:

- 1 tablespoon dried herb of your choice
- 1 cup boiling water
- Glass jar with a tight lid (make sure it is very clean)
- The quantities of herbs and water can be increased proportionately to make a larger infusion if you wish. If you want to make 1 quart at a time, for example, this will require about 1 cup of dried herb and 1 quart of water. However, it's best to start with a small volume on your first infusion of any herb to avoid waste if you find you don't like it.
- While making the infusion, be sure to keep the jar covered at all times to contain the steam. The heat that's trapped inside is crucial to releasing those beneficial compounds in the herbs.
- Place the herbs in a glass container.
- Pour boiling water over the herbs so they are completely covered.
- Seal the jar with a tight-fitting lid to keep the steam and volatile oils from escaping.
- Allow the infusion to steep until the water cools to room temperature or for the time recommended by the infusion recipe. In general, roots and barks require the longest infusion (or a decoction) of about 8 hours. Leaves should be infused for a minimum of 4 hours, flowers for 2 hours, and seeds and fresh berries for at least 30 minutes.
- Strain the spent herbs out of the water using cheesecloth or a fine-mesh strainer (or both). Repeat if necessary to remove all of the herbs.
- The resulting liquid is called an infusion. Clean out the jar and pour the infusion back into it for storage. An infusion can be refrigerated for up to 48 hours. After this, it should be discarded.

ANTITUSSIVE

What Are Antitussives?

Antitussives are medicines that suppress coughing, also known as cough suppressants. Antitussives are thought to work by inhibiting a coordinating region for coughing located in the brain stem, disrupting the cough reflex arc; although the exact mechanism of action is unknown.

However, their use is not without controversy and they should only be considered for dry, irritating coughs that do not involve mucus production. Suppressing productive or mucus-producing coughs caused by some respiratory diseases with antitussives may be hazardous. Many viral coughs are best treated by increasing fluid intake and exposing the airways to humidity.

Many antitussives, including pholcodine, codeine, and dextromethorphan, are derived from opioids. Pholcodine and codeine may cause drowsiness and constipation and codeine may be addictive. Dextromethorphan can increase serotonin levels and may interact with other medicines that also increase serotonin. Benzonatate is a nonnarcotic antitussive that anesthetizes certain receptors located in the breathing passages, reducing the urge to cough.

Although antitussives are effective in adults, their effectiveness in children has not been established and their use in children should be discouraged.

Cough syrup

Ingredients

- ½ cup apple cider vinegar
- ⅓ cup raw honey
- ½ lemon, sliced
- ½ lime, sliced
- 2 teaspoons ground ginger
- 3 springs fresh rosemary

Instructions

- In a small saucepot over low heat, stir the vinegar and honey together until melted. Add lemon, lime, ginger, and rosemary and let steep for 1 hour until cooled.

- Pour into a glass jar and refrigerate until needed - lasts a couple of months in the fridge!

Soothing Cough And Cold Formula

Ingredients

- 1/2 cup water
- 1 cup evaporated cane juice or granulated sugar
- 1 tablespoon honey
- 1 tablespoon fresh lemon juice
- 1/4 to 1/2 teaspoon ground ginger add more for taste
- 1/8 to 1/4 teaspoon ground cloves
- Powdered sugar or cornstarch for coating

Instructions

- Gather your ingredients and prepare a baking sheet by lining it with parchment paper, or greasing it very well. A marble slab comes in handy and helps the drops cool quickly.
- Combine the ingredients, except for powdered sugar or cornstarch, in a heavy-bottomed pot or saucepan. Cook to the hard crack stage, about 300°F, whisking now and then to check the color and consistency. This may take between 15-20 minutes, or longer depending on the pan and stove. Test by dropping a little from a spoon into a bowl of ice water. If it cracks, it's ready. If it's chewy, cook for a few more minutes. Remove from the heat. Be careful not to let it burn - the temperature rises quickly at the end.
- Let the mixture cool slightly. Drop onto a baking sheet into rounds. Allow cooling completely.
- Once cool, dust with powdered sugar or cornstarch. Store in an airtight container in a cool, dry place away from any moisture. (Moisture will cause them to stick together.) Alternatively, they can be dusted and wrapped individually in small pieces of waxed or parchment paper.

Cough And Cold Formula

Ingredients

- 1 chunk of sliced ginger
- 1 cinnamon stick
- 4 cups of water
- Juice of half a lemon

- Raw honey to taste

Instructions

- Place ginger and cinnamon in a pot and cover with 4 cups of water.
- Bring to a boil and let simmer for 15 minutes.
- Strain and add the juice of half of the lemon.
- Add raw honey to taste.

Expectorating Cough And Cold Tea

Ingredients

- 4 cup boiling water (1 liter)
- 3 tea bags or 3 tbsp loose herbal leaves, such such as linden tea, rosehip, etc
- 3 tbsp ginger roots, peeled and thinly sliced, chopped or grated
- 1/3 cup honey
- 1 to 2 lemons, juice of a lemon
- Pinch chili flakes

Instructions

- Into a bowl or a large pot add peeled, sliced, or grated fresh ginger (3 tbsp), tea bags or loose tea (3 tea bags or 3 tbsp loses tea), chili flakes (pinch, only a few flakes, too much with the result is a tea that is too spicy).
- Pour boiling water over, cover, and let steep for 8-10 minutes. Strain the tea into a pot and flavor with honey (1/3 cup or use more as desired) and stir in freshly squeezed lemon juice (from 2 lemons).
- Pour the tea into the Thermos, close the lid, use as needed throughout the day.

Decongestant Tea

Ingredients

- 1/2 cup water
- 1/4 cup lemon juice
- 1/4 cup apple cider vinegar
- 1 teaspoon fresh minced ginger root or 1/4 teaspoon dried ground
- 1 teaspoon fresh minced turmeric or 1/4 teaspoon dried ground

- 1/4 teaspoon black pepper
- 1/4 teaspoon cayenne pepper
- Herbal tea bags such as Breath Easy or Throat Coat
- 1 drop oregano oil optional (make sure it's food-grade oil)

Instructions

- In a small pot over medium heat mix the water, lemon juice. apple cider vinegar, ginger root, turmeric, black pepper, and cayenne. Stir everything together and then add the teabag.
- Bring the mixture to a boil over medium-high heat and then reduce the heat to medium and allow the mixture to simmer for 10 minutes.
- Strain the mixture with a fine mesh colander and pour the tea into a mug. Add the drop of oregano oil, if using. Drink while the tea is still warm.

Mullein Cough Syrup

Ingredients For Mullein & Honey Cough Syrup:

- Mullein leaves and flowers (and please note that because mullein loves to live in disturbed areas, we have to be careful to check for pollution or other contaminants before harvesting; also, the seeds contain several compounds (glycosides, saponins, coumarin, rotenone) that are toxic to fish, and have been widely used as a piscicide, so just stick with the leaves and flowers which have little (if any) scientific study but as-yet little (if any) toxicity reports.
- Elderflowers from blue elderberry, de-stemmed and rinsed (all elder stems, leaves, and seeds contain cyanide-inducing glycosides, so absolutely remove all stems and leaves, and note that before preparing medicine, wine, jams, syrups, and other products, either strain the seeds, or heat (simmer) the berries to neutralize the glycosides)
- Organic honey

Cough Syrup Directions:

- First, make sure that the plant materials are clean and dry, and again, the elderflowers should be completely de-stemmed.
- Next, we need to make a hot infusion. In a medium pot, bring water to a boil and steep the mullein flowers, elderberry flowers, and the mullein leaves for 10 minutes.
- Alternatively, you can make a cold infusion: 1 oz of leaves and flowers in 1 quart of water for 4 hours.

- When ready, strain the infusion through a strainer bag, and place the infusion back on the stove.
- On a low simmer, stir in honey until dissolved. The affected person can also stand over the infusion and breathe in the steam for help with congestion and a croupy cough.
- Let cool before consuming. Don't forget to label with the name, date, and ingredients!
- Store in the fridge.

Elecampane Cough Syrup

Ingredients

- 1/2 cup Elecampane root (dried)
- 1/8 cup Horseradish root (dried)
- 1/4 cup Ginger root (dried)
- 2 cups water
- 4 cups honey
- 8 drops lemon essential oil (optional)
- 1 tablespoon powdered ascorbic acid

Procedure

- Pour the herbs into the cook pot and heat to boiling.
- Cover the pot with a lid and allow herbs to steep for a minimum of 20 minutes or until water darkens. If using a slow cooker, add a little more water to the recipe and keep the lid on.
- Pour herbs through the strainer and keep 2 cups of infused water for syrup.
- Using The Practical Herbalist's simple Syrup Making Instructions, heat honey and infused water to make syrup.
- More honey may be added for a sweeter syrup.
- Remove from heat and stir in ascorbic acid and lemon essential oil as flavoring and preservative value.
- Pour the finished product into the bottle and label it clearly.

Horehound Lozenges

Ingredients

- 1 cup dried horehound
- 3 cups boiling water
- 2 cups of brown sugar
- 1/2 cup of honey

Instructions

- To start make a strong decoction by steeping 1 cup of dried horehound leaves in 3 cups of boiling water.
- Cover and let steep for 15 minutes.
- Strain completely and squeeze leaves to get all the liquid out.
- You should have 2-3 cups of the decoction.
- Add all ingredients to a 3-quart pot.
- Stir in sugar to completely dissolve.
- Put a lid on the pot and begin to heat it over medium heat. When it boils rapidly, remove the lid and with a brush and water, dissolve any sugar crystals that may be adhering to the side of the pan.
- Do not stir the mixture or it will seize.
- Boil rapidly and insert a candy thermometer.
- Boil to the hard crack stage or 300 F.
- Remove from heat. Add flavoring if desired (eucalyptus, lemon, or vanilla) but stir as little as possible.
- Pour hot mixture out onto the greased baking sheet.
- Allow cooling for 2 minutes.
- Using two greased spatulas begin to fold the candy mixture over on itself and repeat until the mixture is cool enough to handle with gloves on.
- Then pull the candy as you would pull taffy. It's best to do this with two people, pulling a small amount of the recipe at a time.
- Once the candy begins to stiffen, cut into 1/2 inch pieces with buttered scissors. and drop onto a buttered pan.
- Allow cooling completely.
- Dust with icing sugar and wrap individually in parchment paper or wax paper.
- Store in a glass jar in air tight container.

BACK PAIN

Back pain is a common reason for absence from work and for seeking medical treatment. It can be uncomfortable and debilitating. Back pain is one of the most common reasons people go to the doctor or miss work, and it is a leading cause of disability worldwide.

Fortunately, you can take measures to prevent or relieve most back pain episodes. If prevention fails, simple home treatment and proper body mechanics often will heal your back within a few weeks and keep it functional. Surgery is rarely needed to treat back pain. It can result from injury, activity, and some medical conditions. Back pain can affect people of any age, for different reasons. As people get older, the chance of developing lower back pain increases, due to factors such as previous occupation and degenerative disk disease.

Lower back pain may be linked to the bony lumbar spine, discs between the vertebrae, ligaments around the spine and discs, spinal cord and nerves, lower back muscles, abdominal and pelvic internal organs, and the skin around the lumbar area. Pain in the upper back may be due to disorders of the aorta, tumors in the chest, and spine inflammation.

The Spine's Fine Tincture Herbal Tincture

Ingredients

- Dried Herbs Single Or Multiple
- Vodka 80 Proof or more (preferably 100 proof)

Instructions

- Put herbs in a quart-size Mason jar to about 1/2 full (not packed down).
- Pour a bit of boiling water over the herbs to help release nutrients (optional).
- Pour vodka overall to fill the jar to just below the bands.
- Cover the jar. Tip upside down a few times to wet all the herbs with the vodka.
- Put in a cool, dark location for 4 to 6 weeks. Each day during this time, tip the jar upside down a few times.
- After steeping for 4 to 6 weeks, strain. Discard herbs (compost) and put the extract in a jar(s) or 4-ounce dropper bottles.
- Store in a cool and dark location. Keeps a long time.

Warming Compress

Ingredients

- 3 Tablespoons organic Calendula flowers or organic Lavender flowers
- 3 Tablespoons organic Peppermint leaf
- 3 Tablespoons organic Sage leaf
- 3 Tablespoons organic Chamomile flowers
- 3 cups water
- Steep, strain, cool, soak, and wrap!

Instructions

- First make a strong tea with your desired herbs. I like to use about 3 Tablespoons per cup of water. I use a cotton muslin bag and a ceramic bowl for steeping, but you could do this in a saucepan or teapot too! Let your tea cool, or place it in the refrigerator to cool quickly.
- Soak a clean piece of fabric/cotton material in the tea and squeeze excess tea out of the cloth.
- Place soaked cloth on your skin and wrap it around the area in need. Let sit and enjoy the cooling herbal sensation!

Sciatic Pain Tea

Ingredients

- 2 tsp dried holy basil
- 1 tsp dried lemon balm
- 1 tsp dried chamomile
- 1/2 tsp dried lavender
- 1/2 tsp dried eleuthero root

Instructions

- Combine all ingredients in a mason jar or cup
- Top with hot water
- Place a plate or top onto a mason jar and let infuse for 20 minutes*
- Remove plate and filter tea through strainer or cheesecloth

- Add honey or sweetener if desired
- Sip and enjoy

Analgesic Daily Tea For Back Pain

Ingredients

- 1 cup water
- 1 cup freshly grated ginger root
- 1 cup freshly grated turmeric root
- 1 Tbsp. coconut oil
- Dash of black pepper
- A slice of lemon

Instruction

- Boil the water, then add the fresh roots and simmer for 15 minutes. Afterward, strain the debris and add the other ingredients. Feel free to top it off with honey if you'd like to sweeten the taste.

Soothing Back Pain Tea

Ingredients

- 1 ½ qt water
- ½ a lemon, sliced or rough chopped (or more to taste), rind included
- 1" ginger root, rough chopped (or more to taste)
- Big dash of turmeric
- Big dash cinnamon
- 2 tbsp maple syrup (more or less to taste)

Instructions

- Fill a 2-quart pot about ¾ full with water. Add in all other ingredients and bring to a boil on the stove. Reduce heat and simmer for 10 minutes. Then remove from heat and allow the drink to cool off. Strain into a glass jar.
- Chill overnight in the fridge for an iced tea (or enjoy hot straight away)!

BEDSORES

Bedsores also called pressure ulcers and decubitus ulcers are injuries to the skin and underlying tissue resulting from prolonged pressure on the skin. Bedsores most often develop on skin that covers bony areas of the body, such as the heels, ankles, hips, and tailbone.

What Are Bedsores?

Bedsores can happen when a person is bedridden or otherwise immobile, unconscious, or unable to sense pain. Bedsores are ulcers that happen on areas of the skin that are under pressure from lying in bed, sitting in a wheelchair, or wearing a cast for a prolonged time. Bedsores are also called pressure injuries, pressure sores, pressure ulcers, or decubitus ulcers. Bedsores can be a serious problem among frail older adults. They can be related to the quality of care the person receives. If an immobile or bedridden person is not turned, positioned correctly, and given good nutrition and skincare, bedsores can develop. People with diabetes, circulation problems and poor nutrition are at higher risk.

What Causes Bedsores?

Bedsore develops when blood supply to the skin is cut off for more than 2 to 3 hours. As the skin dries, bedsore first starts as a red, painful area, which eventually turns purple. Left untreated, the skin can break open and the area can become infected. Bedsore can become deep. It can extend into the muscle and bone. Once bedsore develops, it is often very slow to heal. Depending on the severity of bedsore, the person's physical condition, and the presence of other diseases (such as diabetes), bedsores can take days, months, or even years to heal. They may need surgery to help the healing process.

Bedsores Often Happen On The:

- Buttocks area (on the tailbone or hips)
- Heels of the feet
- Shoulder blades
- Back of the head
- Backs and sides of the knees

Bites And Stings

Formulas For Burns, Bites, Stings, Wounds, And Trauma

Traumatic injuries to the skin affect nearly everyone throughout a lifetime. Herbal therapies can promote healing and help alleviate pain and discomfort. Such herbs may be effective both topically and internally. Homeopathic medicines are often helpful for bites and stings and are specific for various presentations and qualities of pain. Home remedies can also be useful for minor kitchen burns and cuts, and many households have common remedies on hands such as onions (for poultices), an Aloe plant, or simple ice packs.

Following are homeopathic, topical, and internal remedies to help allay acute pain and itching due to venomous insects. While snakebites require expert medical care, and antivenom where available, Echinacea is a traditional North American herbal option, and several homeopathic details below may also help while en route to the hospital.

Field Poultices For Venomous Bites And Stings

The following herbs are classic remedies for bee stings and another insect venom. These herbs or mud and ashes are commonly available "in the field," where such stings typically occur. Herbalists may employ a so-called "spit poultice" where

Plantago or Stellaria leaves are simply chewed, and the masticated pulp is applied topically to the lesion. The pulp can be covered with a piece of torn leaf to help keep it moist and active for 15 to 30 minutes. Mud and clay can have natural drawing effects. Where available, vinegar or Epsom salt compresses may also be helpful.

- **Plantago Ovate Or P. Lanceolata:** Plantain leaves employed as a spit poultice
- **Stellaria Media:** Chickweed leaves employed as a spit poultice
- **Charcoal Or Ashes:** Activated charcoal is ideal, but in a pinch, can be prepared from campfire ash and moistened with water
- **Mud:** Obtained from a stream bank or made out of dirt and water

Any of the above may be applied topically and left in place for 15 to 30 minutes. A single application may suffice for minor stings, while wasp or other more painful stings may require repeat application as the poultice dries.

Essential Oils To Allay Itching

Mint, lavender, and tea tree essential oils can relieve stinging and itching sensations when topically applied. Small bottles of essential oils are light and easy to include in the first aid kit when camping or backpacking or to keep emergency supplies in the trunk of the car.

- Mentha piperita
- Lavandula augustifolia
- Melaleuca alternifolia

Simply apply a few drops of one of the above essential oils to mosquito bites, bee stings, and other insect stings, directly on the skin. Effects are typically immediate, and the essential oil can be reapplied as needed when the effects wear off over time.

Cooling Compress

Ingredients

- 1/3 cup fresh ginger (grated)
- 1 tablespoon turmeric powder
- 3-4 cloves
- 1 tablespoon cinnamon
- 1 tablespoon coriander
- 1/2 cup rice powder
- Yarn/thread
- Unbleached cloth or muslin
- Bowl for mixing

Steps:

- Place spices and rice powder in a bowl and mix well.
- Place herbal mixture into the center of your cloth, folding the edges up and over the herbs making a firm, round ball.
- Tie the top close to the mixture with yarn or thread to create a handle. Keep herbal compress ball tight so that it won't become loose when in use.
- Using a steamer, boil water and drop in the poultice until steamed about 30-to-45 minutes.
- Before application, check the temperature of the herbal compress ball on the inner forearm. Once the temperature is to your liking, firmly place the herbal compress ball on the affected area for up to 30 minutes.
- Use your Thai herbal compress up to four or five times each before making a new one.

Bug Bite Relief Spray

Materials And Ingredients For DIY Bug Spray

- 1/2 tsp Lemon Eucalyptus essential oil
- 1/4 tsp Rosemary essential oil

- 1/4 tsp Lavender essential oil
- Witch hazel
- Apple cider vinegar
- 1 tsp glycerine
- Glass spray bottle

Materials And Ingredients For DIY Citronella Luminary

- Citrus fruits
- Rosemary sprigs
- Lavender sprigs
- Thyme sprigs
- Flowers
- 1/2 tsp Citronella essential oil
- 1/2 tsp rosemary essential oil
- Water
- Floating candle
- Mason jar

Ingredients And Materials For Itchy Bite Relief

- Basil
- Blender (optional)

Materials And Ingredients For Soothing Chamomile Bite Relief

- Chamomile tea
- Ice cube trays

Directions For DIY Bug Spray

- Add Essential Oils to the bottle.
- Fill a little under half the bottle with Witch Hazel/Apple Cider Vinegar Mix.
- Put a cap on and shake the bottle.
- Take off the cap and fill it up with water, leaving a small space for glycerin.
- Add glycerin.

- Shake and use.

Directions For Luminary

- Add two/three citrus slices to the bottom of the mason jar.
- Add lavender, thyme, rosemary, and flowers.
- Pour in the Essential Oils.
- Fill up with water.
- Add a citrus slice to the top.
- Add a floating candle.

Directions For Bug Bite Relief

- Tear or blend basil to release juices and place on bites.

Directions For Chamomile Bite Relief

- Brew chamomile tea.
- Add to ice cube tray and freeze.
- Rub on bites to soothe.

Healing Ointment

Materials

- 1 oz. Beeswax
- 2 oz. organic coconut oil and
- 1 tsp. Vitamin E oil
- 1 oz. organic Jojoba oil
- 10 drops of German Blue Chamomile essential oil
- 20 drops Helichrysum essential oil

Instructions

- In a small saucepan on low heat. (can use a double boiler or glass mixing cup in the saucepan over water).
- Melt together the beeswax, coconut oil, and Jojoba oil. DO NOT BOIL!
- When it's all melted together, remove it from heat.

- Add the Vitamin E oil, German Blue Chamomile, and Helichrysum essential oils.
- Pour into containers and let cool.
- Label the containers.
- This ointment sets up beautifully at room temperature in about a half-hour. Store in closed containers.

Skin-Soothing Ointment

Ingredients

- 2 tablespoons beeswax
- 2 tablespoons coconut oil
- 1/4 cup extra virgin olive oil
- 1 tablespoon lanolin
- 5 drops tea tree essential oil
- 5 drops peppermint essential oil
- 5 drops calendula essential oil
- 5 drops chamomile oil or carrot seed oil

Instructions

- In a double boiler, melt the beeswax and coconut oil just until liquid. Stir in the extra virgin olive oil, the lanolin, and the essential oils. Pour into a small jar and allow to solidify as it cools. Rub onto skin to use.

BRONCHITIS

What Is Bronchitis?

The condition that falls in between the common cold and pneumonia in severity is called bronchitis. Symptoms include a frequent cough that produces mucus, fatigue, fever, and a wheezing sound when breathing. Find out how to treat, or better yet, prevent bronchitis. Bronchitis occurs when the bronchioles (air-carrying tubes in the lungs) are inflamed and make too much mucus. There are two basic types of bronchitis:

1. Chronic bronchitis is defined as cough productive of sputum that persists for three months out of the year for at least two consecutive years. The cough and inflammation may be caused by initial respiratory infection or illness, exposure to tobacco smoke, or other irritating substances in the air. Chronic bronchitis can cause airflow obstruction and then is grouped under the term chronic obstructive pulmonary disease (COPD).

2. Acute or short-term bronchitis is more common and usually is caused by a viral infection. Episodes of acute bronchitis can be related to and made worse by smoking. Acute bronchitis could last for 10 to 14 days, possibly causing symptoms for three weeks.

What Causes Bronchitis?

Usually, acute bronchitis is brought on by a viral infection, though it may also be caused by a bacterial infection. The flu and colds are examples of viral infections.

Chronic bronchitis is usually, but not always, caused by smoking tobacco. It can also be caused by exposure to secondhand cigarette smoke, air pollution, dust, or toxic gases. Your risk can be increased by a family history of bronchitis, having asthma and allergies, and having gastroesophageal reflux disease (GERD).

What Are The Symptoms of Bronchitis?

Symptoms Of Bronchitis Include:

- A cough that is frequent and produces mucus.
- A lack of energy.
- A wheezing sound when breathing (may or may not be present).
- A fever (may or may not be present).
- Shortness of breath.

Fire Cider

Ingredients

- 1 medium organic onion, chopped
- 10 cloves of organic garlic, crushed or chopped
- 2 organic jalapeno peppers, chopped
- Zest and juice from 1 organic lemon
- 1/2 cup fresh grated organic ginger root (or organic ginger root powder)
- 1/2 cup fresh grated organic horseradish root (or organic horseradish powder)
- 1 Tbsp. organic turmeric powder
- 1/4 tsp. organic cayenne powder
- 2 Tbsp. of dried rosemary leaves
- organic apple cider vinegar
- 1/4 cup of raw, local honey, or to taste

Directions

- Prepare your roots, fruits, and herbs and place them in a quart-sized glass jar. If you've never grated fresh horseradish, be prepared for a powerful sinus opening experience!
- Pour the apple cider vinegar in the jar until all of the ingredients are covered and the vinegar reaches the jar's top.
- Use a piece of natural parchment paper under the lid to keep the vinegar from touching the metal, or a plastic lid if you have one. Shake well.
- Store in a dark, cool place for a month, and remember to shake daily.
- After one month, use cheesecloth to strain out the pulp, pouring the vinegar into a clean jar. Be sure to squeeze as much of the liquidy goodness as you can from the pulp while straining.
- Next comes the honey. Add and stir until incorporated.
- Taste your cider and add more honey until you reach the desired sweetness.

Throat-Soothing Tea

Ingredients

- 2 TBSP marshmallow root
- 1 TBSP licorice root
- 2 TBSP fresh lemon juice

- 2-3 TBSP raw honey (to taste)
- 3¼ cups water

Instructions

- Place the marshmallow root in a jar with a lid (mason jars work well) and cover with 1 cup warm, filtered water. Be sure the water isn't hot! Put it in the fridge and let it steep for 4 hours or overnight.
- Put the licorice root into a pot along with 2 cups of water. Bring the mixture to a boil, then reduce and simmer with the lid on for 10 minutes. Strain the tea into a quart-sized jar.
- When the licorice decoction is very warm, but no longer hot, stir in the honey, lemon juice, and marshmallow infusion.
- Sip warm as needed for a sore, dry throat. This can be stored in the fridge for up to 6 days and reheated as necessary.

Notes

Be sure to check with your natural health care practitioner before use if you fall into any of the categories mentioned in the herbal info sections above. For adults, take about 1 cup three times a day. For children, adjust the dose to about 3/4 cup twice a day.

Sweet Soothing Tea

Ingredients

- 2 chamomile tea bags
- 1 inch thinly sliced fresh ginger
- Small pinch turmeric powder
- 1/2 teaspoon lemon juice
- 2 sprigs of fresh mint, plus more for garnish
- 1 teaspoon honey (or to taste)

Instructions

- To a teapot add the fresh mint sprigs.
- Add the infuser to the teapot and add the camomile tea bags, ginger, turmeric powder, lemon juice. Allow steeping for 5 minutes.
- Add a drizzle of honey (to taste) to each of the cups and pour over the tea. Stir to mix in the honey. Garnish with mint leaves.

Burns And Sunburns

Ingredients

- 1/4 cup raw honey, preferably Manuka honey
- 1/4 cup unrefined coconut oil
- 1 teaspoon beeswax
- 1 tablespoon Sea Buckthorn oil, optional
- 1/2 teaspoon aloe vera gel, aloe vera juice, or rosewater

Instructions

- In a small, heavy-bottomed saucepan or double boiler, heat the beeswax over the lowest heat possible.
- When the beeswax is nearly melted, add in the coconut oil and melt completely.
- Stir in the honey and Sea Buckthorn oil, if using, and whisk over the heat only until the whole mixture is one uniform liquid, about 30 seconds.
- Remove from the heat and either pour directly into tins or other containers OR stir in the aloe or rosewater briskly until the mixture is completely homogenous, then pour into your containers.
- Let sit until comfortable to touch before using. The mixture will fully harden in approximately 6-12 hours.

Burn-Healing Honey

Materials

- 1/4 cup extra virgin olive oil or coconut oil (for an added dose of healing, use calendula-infused oil following the methods outlined here)
- 1 heaping teaspoon beeswax pellets
- 1/4 cup raw honey (Manuka is best, see notes)
- 1 teaspoon Vitamin E oil
- 20 drops lavender essential oil

Instructions

- In a clean discarded tin can, add the oil and beeswax. Place the can in a pot filled with 1" of water. Bring water to a simmer over low heat and melt the mixture. Stir the mixture frequently with a wooden popsicle stick.
- When beeswax is completely melted, remove the can from heat and add in the honey, stirring vigorously until melted. Add in the Vitamin E oil and lavender essential oil. Stir well.
- Pour mixture into either the metal tins or plastic balm tubes. Let cool completely, about six hours, then cap, label, and store in a cool dark place for up to a year.
- To use: On minor burns, run the burn under cool water for at least 60 seconds, pat dry, and then spread the balm liberally on the burn site. Either cover in clean gauze or cotton dressing or let be exposed to air. Reapply the balm as needed to relieve pain and promote healing.

Healing Poultice

Ingredients:

- 1 ounce freshly grated or chopped turmeric
- 1 ounce chopped lemongrass
- 1/2 cup small raw sliced onion
- 2 chopped garlic cloves
- 1 ounce freshly grated or chopped ginger
- 1 teaspoon coconut oil
- 2 drops oregano essential oil
- 10 drops of eucalyptus
- White cloth, muslin, or a waterproof food wrap
- Thick string (optional)

Directions:

- In a pan on low heat, add the coconut oil and lightly sauté the ginger, turmeric, lemongrass, onion, and garlic. You can put a lid on it for a few seconds to let it steam. You want it to remain mostly dry or slightly moist from the coconut oil. You can use a tiny bit of water if needed as you do not want it to burn.
- Turn off and move the ingredients to a bowl to cool.
- Add the essential oils and stir to blend well.
- Next, layout your cloth. Take a big spoonful of the mixture and place it into the center of your cloth.

- Now, just fold or lay the outside pieces on top of each other so you have a pack. Some like to pull long pieces up into a "handle" at the top and tie it with yarn or thread. It doesn't matter as long as you keep the ingredients nestled tightly in the cloth so nothing falls out or becomes loose when in use.
- Next, place the poultice on the affected area for 20–30 minutes two or three times a day.
- You can place it in the fridge and reheat in a steamer or microwaves, using it four or fives times, before making a new one

Sunburn Relief Spray

Ingredients

- 1/4 cup apple cider vinegar
- 1/4 cup aloe vera gel
- 2 tbsp distilled water ((optional, to dilute if needed))
- 10 drops lavender essential oil
- 5 drops rosemary essential oil
- 1 4 oz spray bottle ((glass or PET plastic))

Instructions

- Add all ingredients to a small jar and shake to mix well.
- Transfer to a spray bottle.
- Shake well before use.
- Spray liberally on sunburned skin several times a day until healed.

Burn Poultice

Ingredients

- 2-3 tablespoons (or more as needed) of fresh or dried herbs, healing clays, or activated charcoal as needed
- Enough hot water to form a thick paste
- Organic cheesecloth or cloth for covering
- Waterproof covering to keep poultice on

Instructions

- Make a thick paste with the desired herb, clay, or charcoal and water.
- Apply directly to the wound or place between two layers of cloth and apply the cloth to the wound (depending on the cloth and the wound). Leave for 20 minutes to 3 hours as needed and repeat as necessary.

Immunity Strengthener

Ingredients

- 2 large raw beets, peeled
- 3-4 large Gala or Honeycrisp apples
- 2-inch piece of fresh ginger, peeled
- a large fistful of organic parsley
- 1 organic lemon, juiced

Instructions

- Place all of the ingredients in the juicer and juice.
- Stir and drink

Herbal Immune-Boosting Sore Throat Tea

Ingredients

- 1 tablespoon thyme
- 1 tablespoon dried elderberries
- 2 tablespoons licorice root
- 3 tablespoons nettles
- 3 tablespoons echinacea
- 1/4-1/2 teaspoon raw, local honey

Instructions

- Measure herbs and berries into a glass jar and seal. Shake well to mix.
- Steep 1 tablespoon of herbal tea mix in 12 ounces of boiling water.
- When steeped, stir in a drop or two (or three) of raw, local honey.
- Serve warm or chilled.

Notes: This recipe makes about a cup of herbal tea blend, which makes about 16 cups of herbal tea.

CANKER SORES

Canker sores also called aphthous ulcers, are small, shallow lesions that develop on the soft tissues in your mouth or at the base of your gums. Unlike cold sores, canker sores don't occur on the surface of your lips and they aren't contagious. They can be painful, however, and can make eating and talking difficult.

What Are Canker Sores?

Canker sores are small shallow ulcers that occur in the lining of the mouth. The medical term for canker sores is "aphthous ulcers." Canker sores start as white to yellowish ulcers that are surrounded by redness. They're usually very small (less than 1 mm) but may enlarge to ½ to 1 inch in diameter. Canker sores can be painful and often make eating and talking uncomfortable. There are two types of canker sores:

1. **Simple Canker Sores:** These may appear three or four times a year and last up to a week. Anyone can get canker sores but they typically occur in people between ages 10 and 20.

2. **Complex Canker Sores:** These are less common and occur more often in the people who have previously had them.

Anti-Inflammatory Mouthwash

Ingredients

- 10 drops Peppermint essential oil
- 6 drops Tea Tree essential oil
- 1 cup Purified or Distilled water
- 8 oz Mason Jar

Directions:

- Add all ingredients into a glass bottle, then shake well to mix.
- Take a small sip, swish the mixture around in your mouth, gargle for 30 seconds and spit out. Do not swallow.
- Shake well before each use. Use within 2 weeks for freshness, remember this is a natural mouthwash blend without preservatives.

Cold Sores

Ingredients

- Lemon Balm, dried, about 1/4 cup
- Peppermint, dried, about 1/4 cup
- Cloves, about 1 tbsp
- 1/2 cup coconut oil
- 1/4 cup jojoba oil (carrier oil)
- 1/4 cup Vitamin E oil (carrier oil)
- 10-20 drops Tea Tree Oil
- Beeswax, less than 1/4 cup

Recipe

- Infuse your oils. You can do this two ways - the long way OR the short way. I went with the short way. Here's how to do both. If you need some photo guidance, check back on my last salve-making post.
- Long Way. Fill a mason jar with your dried herbs. Pour your coconut oil, jojoba oil, and Vitamin E oil into the jar, cover the herbs, and give it a little stir. Seal tightly with a lid and let sit in a dark, cool place for about 2-3 weeks. This will get all of the goodness out of the herbs!
- Short Way. In a double boiler over medium heat, bring the water to a boil. Heat the coconut oil, jojoba oil, and Vitamin E oil. Stir in the dried herbs. You want the ratios to be 2:1. That would mean 1 cup of oil to 1/2 cup of dried herbs. Heat the herbs over medium/low heat for 30 minutes, stirring semi-constantly.
- You'll be using the lemon balm as it is filled with wonderful anti-viral properties and aids in stress and tension, which why most cold sores happen. The peppermint will aid in scent and is extremely therapeutic. The cloves will help to be a pain reliever - don't use too many!
- once your herbs have been infused, you'll want to strain them. Using a fine-mesh sieve or a cheesecloth, strain the herbs over a bowl to collect the oil. Toss the herbs or compost them!
- Heating your double boiler again, add the now-infused oil and beeswax. My beeswax was already melted in my crockpot. I used about 1/4 cup, and my salve set up a bit too thick. I would suggest using around 4 tbsp of melted beeswax. Stir them together for about 5-10 minutes to make sure they are melted well.
- Pour the melted beeswax + oil mixture into your desired container. I used two jam-size mason jars. Working quickly, drop in about 10-20 drops of tea tree oil and stir to incorporate. Make sure you use a wood stick or utensil to stir - beeswax is a pain to remove from metal.

- Place in the fridge for about 10-20 minutes or until set, mixing now and then. Finished!

Cold Sore Compress

Ingredients

- 1 tablespoon each dried chamomile, nettle, sage, peppermint, licorice root, AND echinacea
- 2 tablespoons elderberries

Instructions

- Bring water to a boil.
- Place herbs in a bowl and mix to combine. Add 1 heaping tablespoon of mixture to a large mug or liquid measuring cup.
- Pour 1 cup boiling water over herbs and let sit – covered – until cooled.
- Strain out herbs and stir in a teaspoon of honey, if desired.

Cold Sore Balm

Ingredients:

- 7 grams cocoa butter
- 4 grams shea butter
- 7 grams beeswax
- 2 grams argan oil
- 1 ml neem oil
- 10 drops tea tree oil
- 5 drops peppermint essential oil
- 5 drops lavender essential oil
- 3 drops vitamin E oil (optional)
- 3 drops rosemary extract (optional)

Instructions:

- Using a digital kitchen scale, weigh out the beeswax, cocoa butter, and shea butter. Melt in either a double boiler or in a glass Pyrex measuring cup in the microwave. Then weigh out and stir in the argan oil.

- Next, using a graduated plastic transfer pipette, measure out the neem oil and stir into the melted oil, butter, and wax. Now add the tea tree, lavender, and peppermint essential oils as well as the vitamin E and rosemary extract using a transfer pipette to measure out drops.
- Stir all the ingredients well then pour into lip balm pots or tins. This natural cold sore therapy lip balm recipe yields about 1 oz. and will fill three 10 grams or 1/3 oz. lip balm pots.
- To use, simply apply to the affected area several times per day until the affected area clears up completely.

Cold Sore Tea

Ingredients

- 2 cups boiling water
- 2 tsp cinnamon
- Juice of half a lemon
- 2 Tbs honey

Instructions

- Split cinnamon, lemon juice, and honey between two mugs.
- Pour boiling water over top and stir well.

Cold Sore Mouthwash

Ingredients

- 1 cup Peppermint tea
- 1 tsp fresh lemon juice
- 1 tsp raw honey
- 2 drops Bergamot
- 2 drops Lavender
- 1 drop Tea tree

Instructions

- Brew the tea, let cool, then add in everything else.
- Bottle it up and use it throughout the week. I recommend storing it in the refrigerator. If needed longer than a week, brew a new batch.

- Shake well before using.
- Swish vigorously and leave in the mouth for a minute or two before spitting out.
- Use several times a day. It's going to be most beneficial when used following oral care (brushing, flossing) after meals. You want to avoid drinking or eating within 20 minutes of using the mouthwash to allow the essential oils to be absorbed.

CONSTIPATION

What Is Constipation?

Having fewer than three bowel movements a week is, technically, the definition of constipation. However, how often you "go" varies widely from person to person. Some people have bowel movements several times a day while others have them only one to two times a week. Whatever your bowel movement pattern is, it's unique and normal for you – as long as you don't stray too far from your pattern.

Regardless of your bowel pattern, one fact is certain: the longer you go before you "go," the more difficult it becomes for stool/poop to pass. Other key features that usually define constipation include:

- Your stools are dry and hard.
- Your bowel movement is painful and stools are difficult to pass.
- You have a feeling that you have not fully emptied your bowels.

Constipation occurs when bowel movements become less frequent and stools become difficult to pass. It happens most often due to changes in diet or routine, or due to inadequate intake of fiber. You should call your doctor if you have severe pain, blood in your stools, or constipation that lasts longer than three weeks.

Bowel-Hydrating Infusion

Ingredients

- Lemon, Mint & Cucumber Detox Water
- 3 liters water
- 1/2 cucumber
- 2 lemons, sliced
- 10 - 12 mint leaves

How To Make Lemon, Mint & Cucumber Detox Water

- Add all ingredients to a large jug.
- Allow to steep overnight in the fridge to release all the flavors.

Bowel-Motivating Tincture

What You'll Need

- The plant parts you plan to tincture. To avoid diluting the alcohol with water, don't wash them. (Roots are the exception; you may need to rinse or even scrub them lightly before chopping.) If the plant parts are already wet, lay them out and blot gently with a clean towel to dry them off. Discard any diseased or damaged material.
- A bottle of 80-proof (or higher) ethyl alcohol. Many herbalists prefer vodka because it's relatively colorless, tasteless, and odorless.
- A glass jar with a tight lid. You don't need large bottles for making an alcohol tincture; a tincture is a potent plant medicine administered only a few drops at a time. Start with small containers such as pint canning jars or empty peanut-butter or jam jars.
- Some small, dark bottles for storing the decanted tincture(s). Storing them in the dark helps protect their potency.

How To Make An Herbal Tincture

- Chop large leaves, flowers, or roots; leave delicate leaves and flowers whole. Then fill the glass jar loosely with the plant material, and add enough alcohol to cover the plant materials. Seal the jar tightly.
- Label and date the jar. Include the plant parts tinctured and the type of alcohol used. Set the jar in a cool, dark place for a month or longer, shaking or stirring occasionally and adding more alcohol if needed to keep the plant materials covered.
- Strain the tincture over a clean cheesecloth into a glass or ceramic container twisting the cloth to remove as much of the tincture as possible. Funnel the tincture into dark glass bottles and cap (or cork) tightly. Label and date each tincture and store it in a cool, dark place. You can increase the concentration of a tincture by straining out the original plant materials and adding fresh material.

Bowel-Soothing Tea Purifying Digestive Tea Couch And Cold

Ingredients

- 1 chunk of sliced ginger
- 1 cinnamon stick
- 4 cups of water
- Juice of half a lemon
- Raw honey to taste

Instructions

- Place ginger and cinnamon in a pot and cover with 4 cups of water.

- Bring to a boil and let simmer for 15 minutes.
- Strain and add the juice of half of the lemon.
- Add raw honey to taste.

Lung-Lubricating Tea

Ingredients

- Organic Ginger Root: Ginger root can be effective in relieving congestion and increasing circulation to the lungs. Ginger is also known to help reduce inflammation.
- Organic Licorice Root: Licorice root is used to help soothe the respiratory system, relieve irritation, and expel sticky mucus. Licorice root can help the body produce new, clean mucus which helps the respiratory system function smoothly.
- Organic Ginkgo Biloba: Ginkgo biloba may help to reduce asthma symptoms. It can help reduce inflammation which can make breathing easier.
- Organic Lemongrass: Lemongrass may help to provide relief from coughs and colds. It strengthens the immune system and has a calming effect on the body.
- Organic Sage: Sage is a member of the mint family and is a great source of antioxidants. It can also help reduce inflammation and provide relief from congestion caused by the build-up of mucus.
- Organic Oregano: Oregano is an immune booster that can help remove toxins from the body. It may also provide relief from allergy symptoms.
- Organic Slippery Elm: Slippery elm provides stress relief, but is mainly known for its ability to coat the throat providing relief from sore throats, coughing, and other respiratory ailments.

Ingredients

- Add all the ingredients
- Add 1-2 teaspoons of tea to 8 oz of boiling temperature water
- Let the tea steep for 5-7 minutes
- For best results, use filtered water (water can affect the taste of the tea if it is not filtered).

FEVER

A fever is a temporary increase in your body temperature, often due to an illness. Having a fever is a sign that something out of the ordinary is going on in your body. For an adult, a fever may be uncomfortable, but usually isn't a cause for concern unless it reaches 103 F (39.4 C) or higher. For infants and toddlers, a slightly elevated temperature may indicate a serious infection. Fevers generally go away within a few days. Several over-the-counter medications lower a fever, but sometimes it's better left untreated. Fever seems to play a key role in helping your body fight off several infections.

Fever-Inducing Tea

Ingredients:

- 1teaspoonyarrow
- 1/2teaspooncatnip
- 1/2teaspoonpeppermint(or spearmint)
- 2cupswater
- Try using a 1/2 cup of each herb instead to prepare an infusion and pour it into a warm bath for the child. This is a great solution for babies too young to drink this tea.

Instructions:

- Boil 2 cups of water.
- Place the herbs into a tea ball or fine strainer.
- Once boiling, pour the water over the herbs and steep for 10 to 15 minutes.
- Remove the herbs and discard them.
- Sweeten the tea lightly, if desired, and serve. This tea will keep 2 to 3 days in the fridge.

Fever-Breaking Tea

Ingredients

- ½ tsp fresh ginger (minced)
- ½ tsp catnip leaf (dried)

- ½ tsp yarrow flowers (dried)
- 1 tsp peppermint leaf (dried)
- 1 tsp chamomile flowers (dried)
- 1 pinch cinnamon (optional)

Instructions

- Place herbs in a cup or a tea ball or strainer.
- Boil water and pour into the cup.
- Cover the cup with a plate to keep the steam and important oils in.
- Steep for 10 minutes.
- Strain the tea through a fine-mesh strainer or remove the teabag.

Notes: Sweeten with 1 teaspoon honey, if desired.

Fever relief tea

Ingredients

- 2tablespoons dried stinging nettle
- 1-1/2tablespoon fresh ginger finely diced
- 1tablespoon dried peppermint leaves
- 1-1/2teaspoon ground cinnamon
- 1/2teaspoon ground turmeric
- 1/4teaspoon ground black pepper
- 32ounces just-boiled water

Instructions

- Add the nettle, fresh ginger, peppermint leaves, cinnamon, turmeric, and black pepper to a French press or loose-leaf teapot.
- Fill the French press or loose-leaf teapot with just-boiled water. I LOVE my electric ceramic tea kettle!
- Steep at least 5 minutes and up to 10 minutes.
- Pour into teacups or mugs. Add a slice of lemon, raw honey, or stevia, if desired.
- Drink liberally during illness, especially the cold or flu.

Quick-Acting Fever Tea

Ingredients

- 1 medium yellow or white onion
- 4-5 cloves garlic, peeled and chopped
- 3-4 tbsp fresh horseradish, grated
- 3-4 tbsp fresh ginger, grated
- Raw apple cider vinegar (enough to pour over other ingredients and fill the jar)
- Raw honey, added later – after weeks of infusion
- Cayenne pepper powder also added later (if other hot peppers aren't added during infusion)
- Optional: citrus, 3-4 tbsp freshly grated turmeric, black pepper, hot chili peppers (instead of cayenne later), and fresh herbs such as oregano, lemongrass, thyme, rosemary, sage, or calendula blooms

Instructions

- Chop or use a food processor to prepare the above-listed onion, garlic, horseradish, and ginger – per quart jar. Scale-up as needed for larger batches.
- Slice the optional citrus into slices or quarters, e.g. one lemon and/or orange per quart jar.
- Pack your container of choice with the prepared ingredients until it is about ¾ of the way full.
- Pour the ACV over the prepared ingredients until the container is full.
- Place a lid on the container, and store at room temperature for 3 to 4 weeks minimum.
- Shake the jar daily to help the ingredients steep and infuse.
- After a minimum of 3 to 4 weeks, strain the contents of the jar using a cheesecloth and/or fine mesh strainer, separating the solids from the liquid. Retain the liquid! Squeeze solids to extract as much liquid as possible.
- Add honey into the reserved liquid to taste – we usually do just a couple tablespoons per infused and drained quart jar, Also add chili or cayenne powder to taste, and thoroughly stir to combine. *As a vegan variation, either skip the sweeter or use agave syrup – though it doesn't have the same healing properties as local raw honey.
- Bottle the liquid and store it in your refrigerator or a cool dark place. Fire cider should last up to a year or longer. As long as it is doesn't develop mold or a sudden change in flavor or odor, it's still good.

- It is now ready to drink! Enjoy often to stay healthy during the winter months. It is recommended to take 1-2 tablespoons of fire cider per day throughout the fall and winter as a preventative measure. If you are feeling some crud coming on, up to your dose to a full 1 oz "shot"! You can repeat it a few times a day. You can also use fire cider as a zesty salad dressing! Remember to shake the bottle before pouring to ensure you're getting all the good stuff that may have settled.

FOOD INTOLERANCES

Food intolerance is a detrimental reaction, often delayed, to a food, beverage, food additive, or compound found in foods that produce symptoms in one or more body organs and systems, but generally refers to reactions other than food allergy. Food hypersensitivity is used to refer broadly to both food intolerances and food allergies. Food allergies are immune reactions, typically an IgE reaction caused by the release of histamine but also encompassing non-IgE immune responses. This mechanism causes allergies to typically give immediate reaction (a few minutes to a few hours) to foods. Food intolerances can be classified according to their mechanism. Intolerance can result from the absence of specific chemicals or enzymes needed to digest a food substance, as in hereditary fructose intolerance. It may be a result of an abnormality in the body's ability to absorb nutrients, as occurs in fructose malabsorption.

Gut-Heal Tea

Ingredients

- 2 teaspoons marshmallow root
- 2 teaspoons plantain
- 1 teaspoon cinnamon chips or 2 cinnamon sticks
- 1 teaspoon rose petals
- 6 cloves
- 2-star anise pods, whole or crushed
- ½ to 1 teaspoon licorice root (optional)
- Pinch of freshly grated nutmeg (optional)

Directions

- **Method 1:** Combine the herbs in a quart-size French press or jar and cover with hot water. Let it steep on the counter, or in the refrigerator overnight or all day. Strain well, squeezing out as much liquid as you can, and drink throughout the day, hot or cold.
- **Method 2:** Combine the herbs in a small pot. Add water, bring to a boil, then reduce the heat and let simmer, covered, for 20 minutes. Remove from the heat and let sit overnight. Strain. Reheat as desired before serving.

- **Method 3:** Prepare the tea as a basic decoction or, though weaker in action, an infusion (steep for 60 minutes or longer, preferably in an insulated thermos).

Build-Up Broth

Ingredients

- 1-gallon water (or whatever quantity your crockpot will carry)
- 4-6 fresh sprigs of parsley (Petroselinum crispum)
- 4-6 sprigs of fresh thyme (Thymus vulgaris) (or 1 tablespoon dried thyme)
- 2 sprigs of fresh rosemary (Rosmarinus officinalis) (or 1 tablespoon dried)
- 2 sprigs of fresh sage (Salvia officinalis) (or 1 tablespoon dried)
- 1 bay laurel (Laurus nobilis) leaf
- ¼ cup apple cider vinegar
- 2 pounds of animal bones (ex: lamb, beef, fish)

Directions

- Add the animal bones and vinegar to a crockpot then cover with water until there is 1 inch of water above the bones. Turn on the crockpot to the high setting until the broth is simmering. Reduce the heat to low and cook for 48-72 hours. The water will reduce while the broth is cooking, check on the broth periodically, and add hot water as needed to maintain the original water level. If the bones float to the top of the liquid, simply keep the crockpot relatively full with water.
- Add the parsley, thyme, rosemary, sage, and bay laurel leaf when the broth is 2-3 hours away from completion.
- Turn off the heat and let the broth cool slightly once it is done cooking. Strain the broth into a soup pot then discard the bones and herbs.
- Allow the broth to cool completely before pouring it into a container to store in the refrigerator or freezer. In the refrigerator, the broth will keep for up to 1 week and in the freezer, the broth will keep for up to 6 months.

Stop-Flatulence Tea

Ingredients

- ½ tsp whole dried fennel seeds
- ½ tsp whole dried coriander seeds

- ¼-½ tsp whole dried cumin seeds (to taste- using the smaller amount provides less of the cumin flavor that many people have trouble with)
- 3 cups water

Instructions

- Optional prep step: For the best flavor, I like to roast the seeds on a baking sheet at 350 for about 5-8 minutes until fragrant and golden. This is optional but I find it improves the flavor.
- Grind the seeds- place the fennel, coriander, and cumin seeds in a coffee grinder or use a mortar and pestle to create a fine powder.
- Place this powder and the water in a small saucepan and bring to a boil. Simmer for 5 minutes until fragrant and remove from heat. Add cinnamon or ginger if using and stir. Let cool to warm before adding raw honey (if using). Note: some sources recommend letting the spices soak in the water for up to an hour before simmering, though I haven't noticed any extra benefit when I've done this personally.
- Strain through a fine-mesh metal strainer and drink immediately or pour over ice for a cool drink. Can also be made in big batches, cooled, and kept in the refrigerator until ready to consume.

Colon-Soothing Tea

Ingredients:

- ½ cup 100 percent pure organic apple juice
- 2 tablespoons fresh lemon juice
- 1 teaspoon ginger juice
- ½ teaspoon sea salt
- ½ cup warm purified water

Directions:

- Start with a tall glass and a spoon.
- Place 3.5 ounces of purified water in a pan. You want to warm the water, not boil it so that you can drink the water at a safe temperature.
- Once it is warm, pour it into your glass. Then add the sea salt and stir.
- Add the apple juice, ginger juice, and fresh lemon juice. Stir.
- Drink first thing in the morning on an empty stomach. Then have this mixture again just before a light lunch, and again mid-afternoon.

Quick-Acting Flatulence Tea

Ingredients

- Tablespoons fresh chamomile flowers
- Cups boiling water
- Slices apples (thin slices)
- Honey

Directions

- Rinse the flowers with cool water.
- Warm your teapot with boiling water.
- Add the apple slices to the pot and mash them with a wooden spoon.
- Add the chamomile flowers and pour in the 2 cups boiling water.
- Cover and steep for 3-5 minutes.
- Strain the tea into two cups.
- Add honey to taste.
- Drink and enjoy!

Gut-Clearing Tea

Ingredients

- 1 Cup Filtered Water
- 1-Inch Fresh Ginger Root (Thinly Sliced)
- 1 Tbsp Fresh Lemon Juice
- Dash Cayenne Pepper
- Optional Fresh Parsley

Instructions

- Heat water just below boiling.
- Add sliced ginger and lemon juice to a mug.
- Pour hot water into a mug and allow to steep for 5 minutes.

- Add a dash of cayenne, and parsley, if using.

Daily Digestive Tea

Ingredients: 1 part each

- Chamomile Flowers
- Dandelion Root
- Marshmallow Root
- Spearmint Leaf
- ½ part Ginger
- (Part can be any unit of measurement, 1 teaspoon, tablespoon, etc.)

Method: How To Prepare 1 Cup Of Tea

- Add 2 teaspoons (up to 1 Tablespoon) of tea to a mesh tea infuser, muslin bag, or tea filter, and place in a pretty mug.
- Pour boiling water over the herbs and steep for 15 minutes.
- Remove herbs and enjoy with a bit of raw local honey.

Note: Avoid giving honey to children under age 2. This tea is delicious as is, unsweetened for children, or substitute maple syrup instead of honey.

Peppery Indigestion Tea

Ingredients

- 2 heaped teaspoons fennel seeds
- 1 teaspoon freshly grated ginger
- 1 teaspoon dried lemon verbena
- 500ml water

Instructions

- It is essential to crushing the fennel seeds to release their volatile oils. Crush by using a pestle and mortar or the back of a large chef's knife.
- Grate a teaspoon of fresh ginger (without the skin).

- Boil 500ml of water in a saucepan along with the crushed fennel seeds, grated ginger, and dried lemon verbena.
- Once it has started to bubble then allow it to simmer on low heat for 10 minutes.
- Serve immediately by pouring through a tea strainer. Alternatively, turn off the heat and leave it in the saucepan to enjoy when you are ready.

HANGOVER

A hangover is a group of unpleasant signs and symptoms that can develop after drinking too much alcohol. As if feeling awful weren't bad enough, frequent hangovers are also associated with poor performance and conflict at work. As a general rule, the more alcohol you drink, the more likely you are to have a hangover the next day. But there's no magic formula to tell you how much you can safely drink and still avoid a hangover. However unpleasant, most hangovers go away on their own, though they can last up to 24 hours. If you choose to drink alcohol, doing so responsibly can help you avoid future hangovers.

Typical symptoms of a hangover may include headache, drowsiness, concentration problems, dry mouth, dizziness, fatigue, gastrointestinal distress (e.g., vomiting, diarrhea), absence of hunger, light sensitivity, depression, sweating, nausea, hyper-excitability, irritability, and anxiety.

Take-It-Easy Next Day Infusion

Ingredients

The Herbal Beauty Infusion

- 2 part nettle leaf
- 2 part raspberry leaf
- 1 part goji berries (optional)

The Herbal Immune Boosting Infusion

- 2 part echinacea purpurea
- A few slices of fresh ginger
- A few drops of lemon juice

The Herbal Stress Relief Infusion

- 2 part oat straw
- 2 part nettle leaf

- Or 1 part hibiscus
- With fresh lemon juice to taste

The Herbal Women Support Infusion

- 2 part raspberry leaf
- 2 part nettle leaf

Instructions

- For example for The Herbal Beauty Infusion, for about 10-ounce cups (300 ml), add 4 tablespoons of nettle leaf, 4 tablespoons of raspberry leaf, and 2 tablespoons of goji berries.
- Simply adjust these measurements for a stronger brew or a larger/smaller serving. For a stronger brew, I use the same measurements but then for 8 ounces. Bring water to a boil and pour over the herbs in the jar.
- I always use a French coffee press for this, since this makes the process extremely easy and effective.
- Cover the jar with a lid and let steep for a few hours or overnight. Slowly push the lid of the French press down to strain the herbs and serve.
- You can safely enjoy 2-3 cups a day.
- Drink before the day is over and make a new one for the next morning.

Tip: Once you finished the jar you will be left with a French press with herbs on the bottom of the jar. I simply add more boiling water and enjoy a diluted herbal infusion, more like a tea. As such, nothing is wasted and you are sure to get all the nourishment from the herbs.

Notes: The infusion will (of course) be cold once it has been steeping for several hours. I don't mind drinking room temperature tea, but if you prefer a warm drink add a little splash of boiling water to your cup before serving or reheat it on the stove so that your tea is hot.

If you have a celiac or severe gluten intolerance, please take caution with oat straw as there is the possibility of gluten contamination.

If you have a medical condition or if you are pregnant, please check with your physician if you can use any of these herbs.

No-Fuss Hangover Tea

Ingredients

- 2 tablespoons extra virgin olive oil
- 10-15 medium-sized shiitake (Lentinula edodes) mushrooms (dried or fresh), chopped
- 5 garlic cloves, minced
- 1-inch piece of fresh ginger (Zingiber officinale), minced
- 1 teaspoon of dried chopped angelica (Angelica Sinensis) root (optional)
- 2 teaspoons of dried chopped astragalus (Astragalus membranaceous) root (or two 2-inch slices of dried astragalus root)
- 1 tablespoon dried chopped lemongrass (Cymbopogon citratus)
- 2 quarts water
- A handful of fresh parsley (Petroselinum crispum) leaves (or 2 teaspoons dried parsley leaves)
- Sea salt and ground black pepper, to taste
- 2 teaspoons lemon or lime juice per serving

Directions

- Add the olive oil to a large pot and warm over medium heat. Add the mushrooms, garlic, ginger, angelica (if using), astragalus, and lemongrass to the pot. Cook for about 5 minutes, stirring frequently.
- Add the water and increase the heat to high until the mixture has reached a boil. Reduce the heat to low. Simmer the broth for 15 to 20 minutes, or until the roots have softened.
- At the very end, add the parsley and salt and pepper to taste.
- Strain the broth. Add the lemon or lime juice to each serving and enjoy hot.

Quick-Acting Hangover Tea

Ingredients

- 6 ounces chopped cantaloupe (about 1 cup)
- 5 ounces spinach (about 3 packed cups)
- 5 ounces red grapes (about 3/4 cup)
- 3 ounces celery (2 small stalks)

Instruction

- Step 1: Juice in an electric juicer. Serve immediately for the best quality, or within 24 hours.

- Step 2: Pulp Fix: Jazz up your plain 1/3-less-fat cream cheese with the pulp from this juice for a sweet-and-savory blend that's deliciously schmeared over whole-grain bagels, pizza crust, or in place of mayo on a sandwich.

Spicy Hangover Tea

Ingredients

- 1 clove garlic, peeled
- Juice of 1 lemon
- 1/8 tsp. cayenne pepper
- 1 Tbs. apple cider vinegar
- 1 knob fresh ginger root, peeled and sliced

Preparation

- Combine all ingredients in a high-speed blender.
- Blend on high for 1–2 minutes, until smooth. If your blender is too large to effectively blend this small volume of ingredients, double the recipe or add 1/2 cup water to dilute.
- Pour into a shot glass, and drink immediately. It will be sour, strong, and spicy! Follow with plenty of water.

HEADACHE

Headache is a pain in any region of the head. Headaches may occur on one or both sides of the head, be isolated to a certain location, radiate across the head from one point, or have a viselike quality. A headache may appear as a sharp pain, a throbbing sensation, or a dull ache. Headaches can develop gradually or suddenly and may last from less than an hour to several days. Headaches are a common health problem most people experience at some time. Headaches can be more complicated than most people realize. Different kinds can have their own set of symptoms, happen for unique reasons, and need different treatments. Once you know the type of headache you have, you and your doctor can find the treatment that's most likely to help and even try to prevent them.

Factors That Lead To Headaches May Be:

- Emotional, such as stress, depression, or anxiety
- Medical, such as migraine or high blood pressure
- Physical, such as an injury
- Environmental, such as the weather

Frequent or severe headaches can affect a person's quality of life. Knowing how to recognize the cause of a headache can help a person take appropriate action.

Cooling Headache Tea

Ingredients

- Dried catnip
- Dried feverfew
- Dried valerian root
- Dried white willow bark (chopped, not powdered)

Instructions

- Mix equal parts, by volume, of the four dried herbs. Store in a glass container with an airtight lid. Keep in a dark place, for up to a year or longer.
- **To Brew Headache Tea:** In a medium-sized saucepan, combine 4 cups (1 liter) filtered water with 1 tablespoon of the Headache Tea herb mixture. Bring to a boil, then reduce the heat to medium-low. Cover the pot with a lid, and simmer the tea for 10 minutes. Strain through a tea strainer into a mug. Add honey to taste, if desired.

- Keep the remaining tea, covered, on the lowest heat – just low enough to keep it hot until you drink the last of it. You can also pour it into a thermos or thermal carafe to keep hot until you finish it. Leave the herbs in the tea to continue steeping and strain them out for each cupful as you pour it.
- Sip all the tea over several hours, starting as soon as you feel the first symptoms of a headache coming on.

Notes: Do not use Headache Tea when pregnant or nursing, or if using blood thinners, and do not give it to children. As with all herbal and natural remedies, use with caution and seek the advice of a medical expert if you have any pre-existing medical conditions, are on any prescription drugs, or develop symptoms from using the herbal remedies.

Warming Headache Tea

Ingredients

- 2 cups water
- inch piece ginger peeled and sliced into rounds
- 1-2 slices lemon optional--for a more lemony drink
- 2 teaspoons Lemon or Lemon Raspberry Natural Calm

Instructions

- Combine water, ginger, and lemon slices in a small saucepan; bring to boil over high heat. Once the mixture has come to boil, reduce heat to low and simmer for 10 minutes. Remove from heat and cool slightly. Place Natural Calm in a large mug; pour tea into a mug, discarding lemon and ginger. Add sweetener if desired.

Peppery Headache Tea

Ingredients

- 1 frozen banana
- 1 cup fresh pineapple
- 1/2 cup 2% or nonfat plain Greek yogurt
- 1/4 cup unsweetened almond milk, plus more if necessary
- 1/2 teaspoons fresh grated ginger or 1/4 tsp ground ginger
- 1/2 teaspoons ground turmeric
- 2 teaspoons of chia seeds

- Optional: A few fresh mint leaves

Instructions

- Place all ingredients in a blender and mix until smooth. Pour into 2 glasses and enjoy immediately. Makes 2 smoothies.

Soothing Headache Tea

Ingredients

- 1 Cup Plant-based Milk (unsweetened)
- 1 Cup Water1 Tbsp. Dried Chamomile (or 1 teabag)
- 2 tsp. Honey (or maple syrup to be vegan)
- 2 tsp. MCT oil or Coconut Oil
- 1/4 tsp. Cinnamon
- Pinch Ginger
- 12 Drops Anxiety Ally tincture (optional but amazing!)

Instructions

- Bring the milk and water to a boil, add chamomile and remove the tea from the heat.
- Let steep for five minutes.
- Strain the tea into a blender with honey (or maple syrup), oil, tincture, cinnamon, and ginger.
- Puree until frothy with a whisk or in a blender. Divide among 2 mugs and garnish with a pinch more cinnamon.

Heartburn/Reflux/GERD Marshmallow Infusion

Ingredients

- 1 TBSP Marshmallow Root
- 1 tsp Peppermint Leaf optional- for taste
- 1 cup warm not boiling water

Instructions

- Combine the herbs and water in a pint-size mason jar and put on the lid.

- Shake gently and put in the refrigerator for a few hours or overnight.
- Strain and drink cool.

Preventive Bitter Tincture

What You'll Need:

- High-proof alcohol (at least 80 proof). If you're in the United States and have access to Everclear, use that. Otherwise, vodka or brandy works well.
- An alternative to alcohol if necessary: high-quality apple cider vinegar. Organic, if you can find it.
- An herb of your choice: fresh or dried
- A pint jar (16oz) with a tight-fitting lid
- Small, dark glass bottles for storing the tinctures. Cobalt or amber glass is great and should have tight-fitting screw-on or snap-down lids.
- A fine strainer
- Fine cheesecloth or muslin
- A bowl or glass measuring cup with a spout
- A small funnel

How To Make A Tincture

- It's incredibly easy to make your tinctures: you just need to soak plant matter in a menstruum (solvent) for a few weeks so all of its "good stuff" can be absorbed into the liquid. While vodka is usually the best choice, you can use brandy instead. Remember that regardless of that alcohol is chosen, it has to be at least 80-proof (namely, 40 percent alcohol) to prevent any mildewing of the plant material in the bottle. 100-proof (50 percent alcohol) is better if you can get your hands on it. This high-proof alcohol acts as a preservative, and if you store your tinctures in a cool, dark place, they can have a shelf life of 7-10 years.
- If you're using fresh herbs, chop them up a bit or bruise them with a mortar and pestle. You'll be putting enough of the fresh herb to fill your jar about 3/4 full, but don't pack it in too tightly: it should fill the jar well, but be loose enough to move around. The reason you should leave a bit of headroom in the jar is that you need to cover the plant matter completely with the alcohol—no part of the plants should be exposed to the air. You'll fill the jar with alcohol to the spot where the lid ring begins, and then screw the lid on tightly.
- For dried herbs, you'll fill your pint jar halfway, and then fill it with alcohol the same way you did with fresh plants. The reason you have to use less dry root than fresh is that the vodka/brandy/etc. will partially re-constitute the plant matter, causing it to swell up: you

need to leave some room for this to happen. Be sure to stir the dried root well to ensure that it absorbs the liquid.

- Generally, the ratio of fresh herbs to alcohol is 1:2 (so 1 part plant to 2 parts alcohol), and the ratio of dried herbs to alcohol is 1:4 or 1: 5, but there will always be exceptions to this: be sure to do thorough research on the herb you'll be tincturing before you begin so you have a good idea of what the required ratio is.

- Label your jars and date them, and then let them steep in a cool, dark, dry place. During the first week, give the jar a little shake every day to swish the alcohol around the plant matter and move it around a little bit. You'll then let it just sit in that cupboard (or another appropriate place of your choosing) for another 5 weeks, so it'll steep for 6 weeks in total.

- After it has steeped for several weeks, line a fine-mesh strainer with a layer or two of muslin or cheesecloth, and then hold that over your bowl or measuring cup. Pour the tincture over the cloth so that it strains well, pressing gently on the herbs to squeeze out the liquid. You can even gather the sides of the cloth and twist it to squish out every last drop. Compost the used plant matter, and wash out the cloth to be used again another time.

- Now, you'll use the funnel to decant the tincture into your little glass bottles (preferably the kind with droppers), filling them close to the top. Label each bottle with the herb used, as well as the date decanted, and then store them away from direct sunlight.

Soothing Heartburn Tea

Ingredients

- 2 quarter-sized slices of ginger root
- 4 Tablespoons chamomile flowers or a chamomile tea bag
- 1-2 Tablespoons Honey
- 12 oz water

Instructions

- Slice up 3 quarter sized pieces of ginger root. Simmer gently in 12 oz of water for 30 minutes. Keep the pot covered.

- Remove the ginger pieces. Pour into a large mug with chamomile and let steep for 5 minutes. Add the honey or Maty's Acid Indigestion Relief.

- For best results, drink the tea 15 minutes before eating a meal. The tea can also be used after a meal if you feel indigestion coming on.

HYPERTENSION

High blood pressure (hypertension) is a common condition in which the long-term force of the blood against your artery walls is high enough that it may eventually cause health problems, such as heart disease. Hypertension is another name for high blood pressure. It can lead to severe health complications and increase the risk of heart disease, stroke, and sometimes death.

Blood pressure is the force that a person's blood exerts against the walls of their blood vessels. This pressure depends on the resistance of the blood vessels and how hard the heart has to work.

Blood pressure is determined both by the amount of blood your heart pumps and the amount of resistance to blood flow in your arteries. The more blood your heart pumps and the narrower your arteries, the higher your blood pressure. A blood pressure reading is given in millimeters of mercury (mm Hg). It has two numbers.

- The top number (systolic pressure). The first, or upper, number measures the pressure in your arteries when your heartbeats.
- The bottom number (diastolic pressure). The second, or lower, number measures the pressure in your arteries between beats.

You can have high blood pressure for years without any symptoms. Uncontrolled high blood pressure increases your risk of serious health problems, including heart attack and stroke. Fortunately, high blood pressure can be easily detected. And once you know you have high blood pressure, you can work with your doctor to control it.

Softhearted Tea

Ingredients

- 1 cup Hawthorn berries, dried
- ½ cup Linden leaves and flowers, dried
- ½ cup Yarrow flowers and leaves, dried
- ½ cup Cramp bark, black haw bark, or black hawthorn bark, dried and chopped
- ½ cup German chamomile flowers

Instructions

- Add the herbs to a 1 quart/liter mason jar. The jar will be 3/4s full. The contents will sift together to fill the jar about ½ full. Fill the jar with vodka or another 100 proof or higher mild-tasting liquor.

- Overnight the dried herbs will absorb the alcohol and swell filling the jar almost to the top. Top up with more alcohol to keep the herbs completely covered.
- Allow the menstruum to macerate in the jar for 6 to 8 weeks, shaking the jar daily or as often as you think of it.
- After 6 to 8 weeks strain out the plant material and reserve the liquid. Press the spent herbs to obtain as much tincture as possible. The liquid is the medicinal tincture. The spent plant material can be composted.

Free-Flowing Circulation Tea

Ingredients

- 1 Fuji apple, cored and sliced
- 1 lemon, peeled
- 1 orange, with peel
- 2 carrots, whole
- 6 kale leaves, rinsed
- 1 inch of ginger root

Directions

- Slice up the apple, orange, and lemon.
- Remove the peel from the lemon and add all of the ingredients to your electric juicer.

Anti-Congestive Tea

Ingredients

- 1 bag good quality organic echinacea tea (optional)
- 3 or 4 thin slices of fresh organic ginger root
- 3 tablespoons organic lemon juice, fresh squeezed
- 2 tablespoons raw organic honey
- 1/2 teaspoon organic ground cinnamon
- 1/4 teaspoon organic ground clove
- Cayenne pepper to taste

Instructions

- In a large cup of hot filtered water, steep the teabag and the sliced ginger (you may omit the tea bag if you'd like).
- Add the lemon juice, honey, and spices and stir well. The tea will be cloudy.
- If you'd like, you may strain the tea through a cheesecloth to remove the ground spices and ginger. At our house, we just drink it as is.

Soothing Marshmallow Rose Tea

Ingredients

- 3 parts organic marshmallow root
- 2 parts organic rosebuds
- 1 part organic sweet cinnamon chips, or 1 organic sweet cinnamon stick, or 1/2 part organic sweet cinnamon powder
- Distilled, spring, or filtered water
- Raw, local honey, optional

Directions

- Measure out herbs in proportions above to fill a pint-size jar one-third of the way—if desired, bundle the herbs in cheesecloth first.
- Fill the jar with cool water and put it on the lid.
- Refrigerate overnight.
- Add honey to taste if you'd like a little more sweetness. Drink and enjoy!

Indigestion tea

Ingredients

- 6 cups apples chopped pieces, cores, or peels from (preferably) a variety of apples
- 6 to 7 tablespoons sugar or honey 1 tablespoon for every 1 cup of water used
- 6 to 7 cups pure water warm, but not hot

Instructions

- Fill Mason jar(s) 3/4 of the way with apples or apple scraps.
- Stir the sugar or honey into the warm water. Stir to dissolve.
- Pour sweetened water over the apples. Leave 2 to 3 inches of room at the top of the jar.
- Cover with cheesecloth, thin fabric or coffee filter, and a rubber band or mason jar screw-top lid.
- Set in a warm dark place for 2 weeks. (Place on a warm surface, and cover with a tea towel. The smell is wonderful during this process.)
- After 2 weeks, strain out the solids, pressing on them gently to extract extra liquid. (Taste the vinegar at this point. It is super delicious!! It's a fermented apple cider!)
- With the solids removed, you will be able to ferment in a smaller jar. Cover with fresh cheesecloth. Set the fermenting cider in a warm dark place for about 4 weeks.
- The apple cider vinegar is complete when it has a strong apple cider vinegar smell and taste. Allow fermenting longer, if not.

Pre-Emptive Bitter Tincture

Ingredients

- 4 parts organic maple or coconut sugar
- 2 parts organic cardamom powder
- 1 part organic ginger root powder
- 1 part organic licorice root powder
- 1 part organic acacia powder
- Distilled water or organic fennel extract

Directions

- Thoroughly combine maple or coconut sugar with herbs in a bowl.
- Use a glass dropper to add one dropper-full of distilled water or fennel extract at a time to the mixture, incorporating as you go.
- Keep adding one dropper-full at a time until the mixture just holds together in a clump, similar to the consistency of cookie dough. Be careful not to add too much liquid! Form into small lozenges about the size of a pencil eraser.
- Coat the outsides with additional licorice root powder if desired.
- Allow drying on a screen or plate for a few days.

- Store in a glass jar or tin.

Carminative Tincture

Ingredients

- 1 part organic dried orange peel
- 1 part organic dried dandelion root
- 1 part organic cacao nibs
- 1/4 part organic gentian root
- Unflavored vodka

Directions

- Measure out herbs in proportions above to fill a 4 oz. jar one-third of the way.
- Pour unflavored vodka over the herbs until the jar is full.
- Allow herb mixture to extract for 2 weeks before straining.
- Label jar and store in your liquor or apothecary cabinet.
- Use several dropper-fulls in a pint of bubbly water with a squeeze of fresh grapefruit juice, or take a few drops straight on the tongue.

Digestive Tea

Ingredients

- 1 tbsp. chamomile flowers
- 1 tbsp. rose petals and buds
- Boiling water

Instructions

- Put chamomile and rose into a tea ball and place into a large mug.
- Top with 6-8 oz. boiling water.
- Steep 7-10 minutes.

Strong Digestive Tea

Ingredients

- 2 heaped teaspoons fennel seeds
- 1 teaspoon freshly grated ginger
- 1 teaspoon dried lemon verbena
- 500ml water

Instructions

- It is essential to crushing the fennel seeds to release their volatile oils. Crush by using a pestle and mortar or the back of a large chef's knife.
- Grate a teaspoon of fresh ginger (without the skin).
- Boil 500ml of water in a saucepan along with the crushed fennel seeds, grated ginger, and dried lemon verbena.
- Once it has started to bubble then allow it to simmer on low heat for 10 minutes.
- Serve immediately by pouring through a tea strainer. Alternatively, turn off the heat and leave it in the saucepan to enjoy when you are ready.

Quick-Acting Digestive Tea

Ingredients

- 2 tbsp edible aloe vera cubes or edible aloe vera gel
- 2 medium cucumbers
- 1 medium lemon, peeled
- 1-inch fresh ginger, peeled
- ¼ cup fresh mint and 1 cup cold water

Instructions

- Place all the ingredients in a blender and blend until smooth.
- Pour in glasses. Add a few ice cubes (optional) and serve.
- If you want, you can strain the drink through a fine-mesh sieve or nut bag and then serve.

INSOMNIA

Insomnia is a sleep disorder in which you have trouble falling and/or staying asleep. The condition can be short-term (acute) or can last a long time (chronic). It may also come and go. Insomnia is a sleep disorder that regularly affects millions of people worldwide. Someone with insomnia finds it difficult to fall asleep or stay asleep. Acute insomnia lasts from 1 night to a few weeks. Insomnia is chronic when it happens at least 3 nights a week for 3 months or more

The Elixir

Ingredients

- 750ml – 1L mason jar
- 375ml flask of whiskey
- 175glocal, organic clear runny honey
- 20g damiana (loves to grow in temperate climates, but also easily found in health food stores)
- 20g rose dried (or if using fresh, 50g)
- 20g angelica root (if unable to find you can replace with: 1 grated nutmeg, 1 whole vanilla pod (split), and a pinch of saffron – all aphrodisiac spices in their own right)
- 15g whole cardamom
- 2 cinnamon sticks

Method

- Sterilize your jar by pouring in boiled water and swishing around, including the lid. Drain dry on a clean cloth.
- Pour in the whiskey and slowly drizzle the honey in, swirling the mixture around and imagining all the elements you want to capture. You may need to give the mix a shake to make sure the honey has fully dissolved. It should look like golden nectar.
- In a mortar and pestle, add the angelica root, cardamom, and cinnamon. Grind down to a coarse texture. You don't want it too fine, or else it will form a sludge that will be difficult to press out. Close your eyes and take three deep breaths of all the aromas that have been released. Ooh, la la!
- Spoonful by spoonful, add the mixture into the jar with the whiskey and honey mixture (if you're using the other spice combination instead of angelica root, you can add it in now).

- Sprinkle in the rose petals and tell them what part of your heart needs soothing. Be specific and honest. A touch of vulnerability will make this elixir all the more effective.
- Allow your imagination to get a bit wild, picturing the part of your creativity or sensuality you're wanting to harness....Whatever that means for you. With that in mind, add in the damiana and stir to mix in.
- Put the lid on and give a good shake to make sure the whole mixture is covered. You'll have quite a dense mix.
- For a month, shake every day to move that nectar around all the plant parts.
- At the month's end, have a couple of clean bottles at the ready (enough to allow for 400ml), sterilize them as you did the jar. Fix a funnel into the mouth of the bottle, add a double layer of cheesecloth, and spoon in a large portion of the mix. Squeeze out everything your can. Have a taste whilst you're at it and you'll be happy you waited the month. Repeat until you have very dry plant material on one side and a bottle full of elixir on the other.
- Cap, label, and consume.
- Enjoy 1/4 – 1/2 teaspoon of this elixir at the end of the day. Have as is, add to hot cacao, or mix with cream and enjoy with berries whilst telling stories to your lover. If they haven't arrived yet, tell stories to yourself. The secret, creative, soulful kind.
- Plant medicines work in subtle ways. You're welcoming their energy into your body and allowing them to work through you. Don't expect a lightning bolt surge of passion. Just nurture the opening and be delighted by what it brings. Just as the plants do

Sleep! Formula

Ingredients

- 1 cup + 2 tablespoons water
- 2 heaped tablespoons raw macadamia nuts
- 1 Medjool date or a teaspoon of raw Manuka honey
- ¼ - ½ teaspoon cinnamon powder
- 2 pinches of nutmeg powder
- 2 pinches of clove powder
- Pinch of fine sea salt
- 1/3 – ½ vanilla bean
- 1 teaspoon ashwagandha root powder equivalent to 1g

Instructions

- Add all ingredients (even the vanilla bean – no need to scrape the seeds out) in a blender and whizz till smooth and creamy. Transfer to a pot and heat gently.
- To serve, add a sprinkle of cinnamon powder. In my photos, I used cinnamon, freeze-dried plums, dried rose petals, and cornflowers.

Insomnia Relief Tea

Ingredients

- 1 tablespoon dried lemon balm
- 2 teaspoons dried peppermint
- 1 teaspoon fennel seeds
- 1 teaspoon dried rose petals
- 1 teaspoon dried lavender flowers
- 2 slices dried licorice root
- Honey (as needed)
- Heavy cream (as needed)

Instructions

- Place a kettle of filtered water onto the stove and bring it to a boil.
- While the water comes to a boil, place herbs and spices into a mortar and crushes with a pestle until roughly combined. Transfer to a teapot, pour boiling water over the herbs, and steep for three to five minutes.
- Strain and serve with honey and cream, as you like it.

Sweet Dreams Tea

Ingredients

- 1 tsp chamomile & catnip blend (or passionflower & lavender blend)
- Grass-fed gelatin (i use about 1 tbsp per cup, both the regular gelatin which dissolves in hot liquids & hydrolysate which dissolves in cold liquids will work)
- Raw honey
- Pinch sea salt (i use a scant 1/8 teaspoon)
- 1 cup water

Instructions

- Boil water and pour it into your mug. Add 1 teaspoon of your tea blend to a tea ball and place it in the mug. Allow to steep for 5-7 minutes, then add the other ingredients and enjoy.

Herbal Tea For Relaxation

Ingredients

- 1 teaspoon Dried Oatstraw
- 1 teaspoon Dried Lavender
- 1 teaspoon Dried Chamomile
- Maple Syrup or Honey to sweeten, if desired
- 8 ounces Boiling Water

Instructions

- Combine the herbs in a tea ball.
- Place tea ball in the cup.
- Add sweetener to cup, if using.
- Pour boiling water overall. Let steep 10 minutes.
- Strain herbs. Enjoy.

MENSTRUAL CYCLE IRREGULARITIES

Menstrual irregularities are problems with a girl's normal monthly period. For example, girls may miss periods, have them too frequently, have painful periods, or have an excessively heavy flow. Menstrual irregularities can sometimes be a sign of an underlying health issue.

What's The Menstrual Cycle?

The menstrual cycle is the monthly series of changes a woman's body goes through in preparation for the possibility of pregnancy. Each month, one of the ovaries releases an egg a process called ovulation. At the same time, hormonal changes prepare the uterus for pregnancy. If ovulation takes place and the egg isn't fertilized, the lining of the uterus sheds through the vagina. This is a menstrual period.

What's Normal?

The menstrual cycle, which is counted from the first day of one period to the first day of the next, isn't the same for every woman. Menstrual flow might occur every 21 to 35 days and last two to seven days. For the first few years after menstruation begins, long cycles are common. However, menstrual cycles tend to shorten and become more regular as you age.

Your menstrual cycle might be regular about the same length every month or somewhat irregular, and your period might be light or heavy, painful or pain-free, long or short, and still be considered normal. Within a broad range, "normal" is what's normal for you.

Keep in mind that the use of certain types of contraception, such as extended-cycle birth control pills and intrauterine devices (IUDs), will alter your menstrual cycle. Talk to your health care provider about what to expect.

When you get close to menopause, your cycle might become irregular again. However, because the risk of uterine cancer increases as you age, discuss any irregular bleeding around menopause with your health care provider.

How Can I Track My Menstrual Cycle?

To find out what's normal for you, start keeping a record of your menstrual cycle on a calendar. Begin by tracking your start date every month for several months in a row to identify the regularity of your periods.

If you're concerned about your periods, then also make note of the following every month:

- **End Date:** How long does your period typically last? Is it longer or shorter than usual?
- **Flow:** Record the heaviness of your flow. Does it seem lighter or heavier than usual? How often do you need to change your sanitary protection? Have you passed any blood clots?

- **Abnormal Bleeding:** Are you bleeding in between periods?
- **Pain:** Describe any pain associated with your period. Does the pain feel worse than usual?
- **Other Changes:** Have you experienced any changes in mood or behavior? Did anything new happen around the time of change in your periods?

Causes

Possible Causes Include:

- Pregnancy
- Eating disorders
- Extreme weight loss
- Excessive exercise
- Polycystic ovary syndrome (PCOS)
- Premature ovarian insufficiency (POI)
- Endometriosis
- Pelvic inflammatory disease (PID)
- Uterine fibroids

Symptoms

Menstrual Irregularities Include:

- Periods that are too far apart instead of once a month
- Periods that are too close together occurring every two or three weeks
- The period doesn't start by age 16 (amenorrhea)
- Periods stop occurring (amenorrhea) for at least 3 months and the woman is not pregnant
- Periods that don't come regularly (oligomenorrhea) occurring infrequently
- Heavy periods, or prolonged bleeding
- Painful periods (dysmenorrhea) severe menstrual cramps

Steady Cycle Tea

Ingredients

- 2 cups red raspberry leaf

- 1 cup dried stinging nettle leaf
- 1 cup dried peppermint
- 1 cup red clover
- 1/2 cup green tea leaves optional

Instructions

- Combine all herbs and optional green tea into a bowl.
- Stir to combine and store in an airtight container away from direct sunlight.

To Drink As A Tea:

- Add 1/4 cup herb blend to a coffee or tea press.
- Add boiling water, cover, and allow to steep for 10 minutes.
- Discard used herbs, then enjoy tea in a mug with a touch of honey or a lemon slice.

To Drink As An Infusion:

- Add 1/2 cup herb blend to a quart-sized Mason jar.
- Fill with tepid water to the top. Close the jar and leave it at room temperature overnight.
- In the morning, pour infusion through a strainer into another quart-sized Mason jar.
- Discard herbs and drink infusion as desired!
- Store in the refrigerator if it will not be consumed within 12 hours.

Bleed On! Tea

Ingredients

- 1 cup dairy-free milk
- 1/2 tsp turmeric
- 1 tsp cinnamon
- 1/4 tsp ginger
- 1 scoop stevia (or another low-carb sweetener)

Instructions

- Heat milk on the stovetop until hot.
- Stir in the spices and stevia.

- Enjoy.

Daily Soothing Menstrual Tea

Ingredients:

- 1 part Raspberry Leaf, crumbled
- 1 part Chamomile flowers, dried
- 1 part Peppermint leaves, crumbled
- 1/2 part Calendula blossoms, crumbled
- ½ part Motherwort leaves, crumbled
- ½ part Cramp Bark or Black Hawthorn Bark, shredded
- ¼ part Marshmallow Root, shredded
- 1/8 part Ginger powder

Method:

- Mix the dried herbs and store them in a glass jar, in a cool, dark cupboard. This will last a year or more without loss in potency.
- To use place 1 tsp of the dried herb mixture in a tea ball. Pour boiling water over the tea ball, in a teapot with a tight-fitting lid. Allow steeping for 5 minutes.
- Drink hot for period cramps, as often as necessary.

Tincture For Painful Periods

Ingredients

Mix the ingredients as listed using a ½ cup as the part. It will look like this:

- ½ cup Raspberry Leaf
- ½ cup Chamomile
- ½ cup Peppermint
- ¼ cup Motherwort
- ¼ cup Cramp Bark or Black Hawthorn Bark, shredded
- 2 tbsp. Marshmallow Root
- 1 tbsp. Ginger powder or 2 tbsp. freshly grated ginger

Instructions

- Place the ingredients in a 1 quart, wide-mouth mason jar. Pour vodka over the herbs, filling up the jar. Place a tight-fitting lid on the jar. Place the jar in a cool, dark cupboard. Shake the jar once a day or as often as you think of it.
- After 5 to 6 weeks, strain the herb, reserving the liquid. You can compost the herb. Put the tincture in a dark, glass, bottle with a drop reducer to prevent spills.
- To use take 1 tsp. 3 times a day, or as often as needed for painful periods.
- Herbal tinctures last for years without loss of potency.

Dysmenorrhea Tea

Ingredients

- 1/2 cup baby kale
- 1/2 cup baby spinach
- 1 cup mango fresh or frozen
- 1/2 avocado
- 1-1/2 cups almond milk or cashew milk, or raw milk if you tolerate dairy
- 2 tablespoons walnuts preferably soaked and dehydrated
- 2 teaspoons flaxseed meal
- 1 teaspoon coconut oil
- 1-inch knob fresh ginger minced
- 1/4 teaspoon ground turmeric
- 1 pinch ground black pepper

Instructions

- Combine all ingredients in a blender.
- Blend until smooth and enjoy right away.
- If you want a smoother consistency, feel free to add more almond milk.

Cramp Relief Tea

Ingredients

- 1-inch chunk of fresh ginger (no need to peel), sliced into pieces no wider than ¼-inch
- 1 cup water
- Optional flavorings (choose just one): 1 cinnamon stick, 1″ piece of fresh turmeric (cut into thin slices, same as the ginger), or several sprigs of fresh mint

Instructions

- Combine the ginger slices and water in a saucepan over high heat. If you're adding a cinnamon stick, fresh turmeric, or fresh mint, add it now. Bring the mixture to a simmer, then reduce the heat as necessary to maintain a gentle simmer for 5 minutes (for extra-strong ginger flavor, simmer for up to 10 minutes).
- Remove the pot from the heat. Carefully pour the mixture through a mesh sieve into a heat-safe liquid measuring cup, or directly into a mug.
- If desired, serve with a lemon round and/or a drizzle of honey or maple syrup, to taste. Serve hot.

NAUSEA AND VOMITING

What Are Nausea And Vomiting?

Nausea and vomiting are not diseases, but rather are symptoms of many different conditions, such as infection ("stomach flu"), food poisoning, motion sickness, overeating, blocked intestine, illness, concussion or brain injury, appendicitis, and migraines. Nausea and vomiting can sometimes be symptoms of more serious diseases such as heart attacks, kidney or liver disorders, central nervous system disorders, brain tumors, and some forms of cancer.

What Is The Difference Between Nausea And Vomiting?

Nausea is an uneasiness of the stomach that often accompanies the urge to vomit, but doesn't always lead to vomiting. Vomiting is the forcible voluntary or involuntary emptying ("throwing up") of stomach contents through the mouth. Some triggers that may result in vomiting can come from the stomach and intestines (infection, injury, and food irritation), the inner ear (dizziness and motion sickness), and the brain (head injury, brain infections, tumors, and migraine headaches).

Calming Tea

Ingredients

- 2 parts lemon balm (Melissa officinalis) leaf
- 1 part chamomile (Matricaria chamomilla) flowers
- 1 part linden (Tilia spp.) bract and flower
- 1 part rose (Rosa spp.) petal
- ½ part spearmint (Mentha spicata) leaf

Directions

- Blend the herbs in a bowl and store tea blend in a glass jar until ready for use. Note: each part can be any measure you'd like—1 teaspoon, 1 tablespoon, or 1 cup, etc. depending on the batch size you'd like to make.
- To brew a cup of tea, use 1-2 tablespoons of the tea blend per cup of water.
- Place the herbs in a heat-proof glass vessel with a tight-fitting lid, and cover with boiling water.
- Cover and let steep for 10-15 minutes, strain, and enjoy 3-4 cups per day while encouraging your stress to melt away.

Ginger Emergency Formula

Ingredients

- 1-inch ginger peeled and cut into thin slices
- Honey to taste or sweetener of choice

Instructions

- Place ginger and water in a pot and place on high heat. Bring to a boil then reduce the heat to medium and let it boil for 5 minutes.
- Strain and add honey or sweetener of choice and stir. Serve hot or let it cool completely then place in the fridge to chill before serving.

Recipe Notes

- Use more or less ginger depending on how much ginger flavor you want in your tea.
- This recipe makes 1 serving. Feel free to double, triple, quadruple, or multiply the recipe as needed if you are making a ginger drink for several people.
- I find that organic ginger is best for a ginger drink because it is more fragrant so use organic ginger if you can. Health food stores like Whole Foods or Sprouts sell organic ginger.
- For Cold Ginger Drink: follow all the steps for making the ginger drink as stated above. Let the drink cool completely then pour it into a bottle or container with a tight-fitting lid and place it in the fridge to chill before drinking.
- For Variation in Flavor: boil the ginger with some fresh lemongrass (if you can find it), mint leaves, or squeeze some lemon or lime juice into the ginger drink before drinking.
- Nutritional information is based on the assumption that the ginger drink is sweetened with 2 teaspoons of strained honey.

RASH

Rashes are abnormal changes in skin color or texture. They usually result from skin inflammation, which can have many causes. A rash is defined as a widespread eruption of skin lesions. It is a very broad medical term. Rashes can vary in appearance greatly, and there are many potential causes. Because of the variety, there is also a wide range of treatments. A rash can be local to just one small part of the body, or it can cover a large area.

Rashes come in many forms, and common causes include contact dermatitis, bodily infections, and allergic reactions to taking medication. They can be dry, moist, bumpy, smooth, cracked, or blistered; they can be painful, itch, and even change color. There are many types of rashes, including eczema, granuloma annulare, lichen planus, and pityriasis rosea.

Dry Rash Salve

Ingredients

- 8 oz. Infused herbal oil
- 1 oz. Beeswax, either grated or pellets
- A double boiler
- Clean glass jars or metal tins
- Essential oils, if desired

Directions:

- Warm oil in a double boiler. Add beeswax and stir until melted. Test the consistency of your salve by dipping a clean spoon into the mixture, and putting it in the freezer for a few minutes. If it's softer than you'd like, add more beeswax.
- Pour the still-warm salve into containers (old jam jars or small metal tins work well). If adding essential oils, do so now (only a few drops are needed) and stir with a chopstick or other clean implement.
- Put the cap on the containers, and store it in a dark, cool place. Salves will last up to a year.

Weepy Rash Poultice

Ingredients

- 1 handful of fresh calendula flowers (Calendula officinalis)

- 1 heaping handful of fresh violet leaves (Viola sororia and V. odorata)
- 1 heaping handful of fresh plantain leaves (Plantago spp.)
- 4 to 6 ounces very hot water (not boiling)
- 2 Tablespoons powdered clay
- 10 drops lavender essential oil (Lavandula angustifolia), optional

Instructions

- Using a food processor or a blender, combine four ounces of hot water with all other ingredients until the poultice is smooth, with the consistency of pesto. You may need to add more herbs, clay, or water to achieve the desired consistency. Refrigerate for up to three days, and apply as needed. If using dried herbs, substitute ¼ cup (60 ml) of the dried herb for one handful of the fresh herb.

Skin-Soothing Tea

Ingredients

- 1 part lavender
- 1 part calendula
- 1 part chamomile
- 1 part lemon balm
- 1 part oats

Instructions

- Combine all ingredients in a mixing bowl.
- Store in a mason jar until ready to use.
- When ready to take a bath, fill an empty unbleached paper or muslin tea bag and place it in the bathwater.
- Let steep until you and the tea are done!

RASH WASH

A rash is defined as a widespread eruption of skin lesions. It is a very broad medical term. Rashes can vary in appearance greatly, and there are many potential causes. Because of the variety, there is also a wide range of treatments.

A rash can be local to just one small part of the body, or it can cover a large area. Rashes come in many forms, and common causes include contact dermatitis, bodily infections, and allergic reactions to taking medication. They can be dry, moist, bumpy, smooth, cracked, or blistered; they can be painful, itch, and even change color. Rashes affect millions of people across the world; some rashes may need no treatment and will clear up on their own, some can be treated at home; others might be a sign of something more serious.

The word "rash" means a change in the color and texture of skin that usually causes an outbreak of red patches or bumps on the skin. In common usage of the term, a "rash" can refer to many different skin conditions. A rash can be caused, directly or indirectly, by a bacterial, viral, or fungal infection. Alternatively, a rash may be unrelated to an infectious organism, such as from an underlying medical illness. Medications, chronic medical conditions, and allergic reactions (hives) are among the multiple different causes of rash. Doctors use specific terms to describe rashes. A macular rash refers to flat, small red patches on the skin, while a papular rash refers to small raised red bumps. If both rash symptoms and signs are present, a rash is called maculopapular. Scaling, blister formation, or ulceration of the skin may be present with a rash. A rash with accompanying blisters is termed a vesicular rash. Itching (pruritus) may or may not accompany a rash.

Sinusitis Herbal Tea

Ingredients

- 1/2 cup water
- 1/4 cup lemon juice
- 1/4 cup apple cider vinegar
- 1 teaspoon fresh minced ginger root or 1/4 teaspoon dried ground
- 1 teaspoon fresh minced turmeric or 1/4 teaspoon dried ground
- 1/4 teaspoon black pepper
- 1/4 teaspoon cayenne pepper
- Herbal tea bags such as Breath Easy or Throat Coat

- 1 drop oregano oil optional (make sure it's food-grade oil)

Instructions

- In a small pot over medium heat mix the water, lemon juice. apple cider vinegar, ginger root, turmeric, black pepper, and cayenne. Stir everything together and then add the teabag.
- Bring the mixture to a boil over medium-high heat and then reduce the heat to medium and allow the mixture to simmer for 10 minutes.
- Strain the mixture with a fine mesh colander and pour the tea into a mug. Add the drop of oregano oil, if using. Drink while the tea is still warm.

Sinus-Clearing Steam Bath

Ingredients

- ¼ cup Eucalyptus leaves
- 2 Tbsp. peppermint leaf
- 2 Tbsp. rosemary leaf
- 3 Tbsp. thyme
- 1 Tbsp. lavender buds
- ¼ cup the Dead Sea salt
- 2 drops Eucalyptus essential oil, optional (Not for children under 10.)
- 2 drops peppermint essential oil, optional (Not for children under 6.)
- 2 drops lavender essential oil (optional)

Directions

- If using essential oils, mix into Dead Sea salt until completely distributed evenly.
- Mix in all of the herbs and stir until well combined. Store in a Mason jar in a cool dark location, when not in use.
- Bring 4-6 cups of water to a boil. To a large bowl, add 1 Tbsp. of the herbal salt mixture.
- Pour boiling water over the herbs and cover the bowl. Let steep for 5-10 minutes.
- Cover your head with a towel and position your face over the bowl, using the towel as a tent to hold the steam in.
- With your eyes closed and face 5-10 inches away from the hot water, breathe in the herbal goodness for no more than 10 minutes at a time.

- You can also use ½ cup of this in a foot bath!

Sinus-Relieving Tea

Ingredients

- 1 knob fresh ginger
- 4 fresh lemon
- 1 tbsp apple cider
- 1 tbsp honey

Instructions

- Peel ginger (a spoon works great for this!), slice it, and bring to a boil in about 1.5 cups water. Simmer for 5 minutes.
- Meanwhile, squeeze a lemon into a mug. Add apple cider and honey.
- After ginger tea is done boiling, add it to the mug. I let the ginger pieces fall in too - they keep steeping as the tea cools.
- Drink this up to 3x a day as soon as you feel the first sign of a cold coming on!
- Enjoy!

Mucus-Freeing Tea

Ingredients

- Mullein leaf
- Red clover
- Plantain leaf
- Fenugreek seed
- Stevia leaf
- Licorice root
- Calendula flower

How To Use

- Place tea bag into a cup and add boiled water. Allow the tea bag to steep for 2 minutes. Cool to suitable drinking temperature. Add sweetener of choice (e.g. 100% grade B maple syrup, agave nectar (from sap), or raw honey) and a little lemon juice if you desire. Drink and enjoy warm or cold.

Sore Throat Tea

Ingredients

- 1 ½ cups boiling water
- 1 teaspoon ground ginger (or feel free to use fresh-see notes)
- 1–2 teaspoons honey
- Squeeze lemon

Instructions

- Pour hot water into a mug.
- Stir in ginger, honey, and a squeeze of lemon.
- Adjust honey and lemon to your liking. Sip slowly and repeat as needed.

Herbal Gargle

Ingredient

- Sage
- 1/4 teaspoon of Cayenne (powder)
- 1 teaspoon of Salt
- 1/2 cup of water (boiling)
- 1/2 cup of Apple Cider Vinegar (preferably unpasteurized)
- 1 1/2 tablespoons of Sage (dried leaves)

Directions

- Sage has anti-inflammatory properties that make it a useful herb for healing sores. Regular use of this gargle will soothingly reduce swelling and pain in the throat.

- Pour the boiling water over the dried sage in a cup. Cover, and leave to steep for 30 - 45 minutes. (45 minutes)
- Strain the leaves from the liquid and discard. Add salt, cayenne, and apple cider vinegar while the tea is still warm. Stir to dissolve the ingredients. (2 minutes)
- Gargle a teaspoon of the mixture every 30 minutes. The rinse will be more effective the longer you gargle for; do not swallow, as the taste will be unpleasant.

Throat-Soothing Tea

Ingredients

- 1 cup milk use your favorite dairy or plant-based
- ½ teaspoon ground cinnamon
- ½ teaspoon powdered ginger
- 1 tablespoon mild-tasting honey

Instructions

- Place milk in a small saucepan and scald (heat) on low until hot but not boiling. Stir in the cinnamon, ginger, and honey until well mixed. Sip to soothe.
- Or, place all ingredients in a microwave-safe cup and microwave on high for 1-1 ½ minutes (microwave times will vary), or until hot. Stir, and sip.

Fruity Gargle

Ingredient

- 2 cups water
- ½ teaspoon ground turmeric
- ½ teaspoon chopped fresh ginger
- ½ teaspoon ground cinnamon (optional)
- 1 tablespoon honey

- 1 lemon wedge

Instructions

- Bring water to a boil in a small saucepan; add turmeric, ginger, and cinnamon. Reduce heat to medium-low and simmer for 10 minutes. Strain tea into a large glass; add honey and lemon wedge.

Sweet Cough Drops

Ingredients

- 1-1/2" segment fresh ginger
- 1 cinnamon stick
- 1-1/2 cups water
- 1-1/2 cups sugar
- 1/2 cup honey
- 2 tablespoons lemon juice
- 1 teaspoon lemon zest
- 1/2 cup superfine sugar, for dusting

Ingredients

Step 1:

- Gather Ingredients
- Natural cough drops are prepared in the same way hard candy is made, but with a few added cough-busting ingredients commonly found in the kitchen to help calm a cough and soothe a sore throat.

Step 2:

- Chop Ginger
- Peel a 1-1/2" piece of ginger root and cut it into slices.

Step 3:

- Boil Ginger and Cinnamon Water
- Place ginger slices and a cinnamon stick in 1-1/2 cups of water in a heavy saucepan and bring to a boil over high heat. Reduce heat and simmer for 10 minutes.

Step 4:

- Remove Ginger and Cinnamon
- Remove the ginger root and cinnamon stick from the saucepan and discard.

Step 5:

- Add Sweeteners
- Add 1-1/2 cups of sugar and 1/2 cup of honey to the infused water in the saucepan and return to boil over high heat.

Step 6:

- Dissolve Sugar
- Stir until sugar has dissolved and placed a candy thermometer in the pot to monitor heat.

Step 7:

- Turn Up The Heat
- Once the sugar has dissolved, stop stirring and keep an eye on the pot as temperatures rise. As the temperature rises, the boil will be volatile but will calm as the sugar approaches the 300 degrees F necessary for the candy to harden when it cools (this is known as the "hard crack" stage).

Step 8:

- Water Evaporates
- As it nears "hard crack", the water will have cooked away, the color will darken and the consistency is molten.

Step 9:

- Watch Temperature
- Watch closely. When the candy thermometer reads between 300 and 305 degrees, remove it from heat.

Step 10:

- Add Citrus
- Stir in 2 tablespoons lemon juice and 1 teaspoon lemon zest. Take caution when adding the juice, which will sputter and splash as it comes in contact with the sugar.

Step 11:

- Pour Into Molds
- Immediately pour into candy molds. The number of lozenges will vary depending on the size of the molds. We got about 50 pieces, some shaped like traditional lozenges and others as hearts, Christmas trees, and candy canes.

Step 12:

- Remove From Molds
- Once cooled completely (at least an hour), remove from molds and place in a lidded container with 1/2 – 1 cup of superfine sugar to keep the lozenges from sticking together when they are stored. Shake to coat.

Step 13:

- Store
- Brush excess sugar off cough drops and store in an airtight container in a cool, dark location. Use anytime to soothe a sore throat or cough. Your movie date will thank you.

SPRAINS AND STRAINS

Sprains and strains both refer to damage to the soft tissues in the body, including ligaments, tendons, and muscles. They are common injuries that share some symptoms but affect different body parts. People can often treat sprains and strains at home.

A sprain is an overstretched, torn or twisted ligament. A ligament is a tough band of fibrous tissue that connects bones to other bones or cartilage. Ligaments are usually located around joints. Commonly sprained areas include the wrists, ankles, thumbs, and knees. A sprain is a stretch or tears in a ligament. Ligaments are bands of fibrous tissue that connect bones to bones at your joints.

A strain is an overstretched, torn, or twisted tendon or muscle. A tendon is a tough cord of fibrous tissue that connects muscles to bones. Commonly strained areas include the legs, knees, feet, and back. A strain is also a stretch or tear, but it happens in a muscle or a tendon. Tendons link muscles to bones.

Soft Tissue Injury Liniment

Ingredients

- 1 cup Witch Hazel or Rubbing Alcohol
- 1 tsp menthol crystals
- 2 Tbsp dried meadowsweet
- 2 Tbsp dried willow bark
- 2 Tbsp dried yarrow
- 2 Tbsp dried comfrey
- 2 Tbsp dried calendula
- 2 Tbsp dried arnica flower
- ½ tsp cayenne pepper
- 1 oz St. John's Wort Tincture
- 25 drops peppermint essential oil

Instructions

- Coarsely grind all dried herbs with your mortar and pestle. Put all the ground herbs in a pint-sized mason jar. Pour witch hazel or alcohol over the top. Steep for 4-6 weeks, shaking daily. Strain and compost herbs. Add St. John's Wort tincture and essential oil. Bottle and label.

Topical Pain Relief

Ingredients

- 1/2 cup olive oil
- 3 tablespoons cayenne powder
- 1 cup coconut oil
- 1 coffee filter or cheesecloth
- 1 heat-proof glass jar or bowl
- 1 glass jar with a tightly fitting lid for storage

Directions

- Add olive oil and cayenne powder into a heatproof glass jar.
- Place that glass jar into a saucepan that contains about an inch of water to create a double boiler.
- Stir the mixture in the glass jar while the water simmers for 15 minutes over medium heat.
- Remove the jar to cool for 30 minutes.
- Strain the newly infused oil through a coffee filter or cheesecloth into a storage jar.
- In a separate bowl, microwave the coconut oil for 20 seconds.
- Add the coconut oil to the storage jar and mix it with the infused oil.
- Chill the mixture in the refrigerator for 30 minutes.
- Apply daily as needed for pain.
- Store mixture in the refrigerator when not in use.

Quick-Acting Pain Relief

Ingredients

- 1 quart of water
- ¼ cup fresh or 1/8 cup dry rosemary leaves

- 3 lemons, sliced
- ¼ cup honey
- 1 cup raspberries
- ice cubes

Instruction

- Boil the water, then steep the leaves for 10-15 minutes. Strain the leaves, add the honey, and stir. Lastly, add the other ingredients and enjoy.

Tea Sweet Relief Tea

Ingredients

- Elderberry
- Nettles
- Cinnamon
- Sarsaparilla
- Honeybush
- Rosemary
- Licorice

How To Brew:

For Sweet Relief:

- Use 1 teaspoon per 8 ounces of water. Bring water to a boil and immediately pour over herbs. Allow to steep 5-7 minutes, remove herb. Enjoy hot, warm, or cold.

For Cold Tea:

- **Method 1:** Brew in half the water, then add ice.
- **Method 2:** Brew full strength, then allow to cool to at least 100 degrees. Put in fridge overnight and enjoy the next day.
- There you go! Perfect iced herbal tea!

For Hot Tea:

- Add herb to hot water. For a stronger tea, steep longer – be careful brewing longer, as some herbs will become bitter the longer they steep. It is suggested to cover all tea while brewing to save the volatile oils.

STRESS

What Is Stress?

Stress is a normal human reaction that happens to everyone. The human body is designed to experience stress and react to it. When you experience changes or challenges (stressors), your body produces physical and mental responses. That's stress.

Stress responses help your body adjust to new situations. Stress can be positive, keeping us alert, motivated, and ready to avoid danger. For example, if you have an important test coming up, a stress response might help your body work harder and stay awake longer. But stress becomes a problem when stressors continue without relief or periods of relaxation.

What Happens To The Body During Stress?

The body's autonomic nervous system controls your heart rate, breathing, vision changes, and more. Its built-in stress response, the "fight-or-flight response," helps the body face stressful situations. When a person has long-term (chronic) stress, continued activation of the stress response causes wear and tear on the body. Physical, emotional, and behavioral symptoms develop.

Physical Symptoms Of Stress Include:

- Aches and pains
- Chest pain or a feeling like your heart is racing
- Exhaustion or trouble sleeping
- Headaches, dizziness, or shaking
- High blood pressure
- Muscle tension or jaw clenching
- Stomach or digestive problems
- Trouble having sex
- Weak immune system

Stress Can Lead To Emotional And Mental Symptoms Like:

- Anxiety or irritability
- Depression
- Panic attacks
- Sadness

Often, People With Chronic Stress Try To Manage It With Unhealthy Behaviors, Including:

- Drinking too much or too often
- Gambling
- Overeating or developing an eating disorder
- Participating compulsively in sex, shopping, or internet browsing
- Smoking
- Using drugs

Rescue Elixir

Ingredients

- ½ cup organic Krishna holy basil
- ¼ cup organic ashwagandha root
- ¼ cup organic astragalus root
- ½ cup raw, local honey
- 2 ½ cups alcohol of choice

Directions

- Combine holy basil, ashwagandha, and astragalus in quart size jar.
- Add honey and stir well to combine.
- Pour in alcohol until completely covered.
- Cover the jar and shake well.
- Infuse for at least 2 weeks, storing in a cool dark place.
- Shake the blend every few days.
- Strain the elixir and transfer it to clean glass bottles.
- Label and date the elixir.
- Enjoy about one teaspoon to support you during stressful times.

Pro Tips

- Store in a cool, dark place where it can last for several years.

- As with any herbal preparation, the dosage should be determined based on the status of your health and guidance from a qualified herbal practitioner. A teaspoon seems to do well for most people, but this should not be taken as a dosage recommendation.

Soothe Up! Tea

Ingredients

- 2 chamomile tea bags
- 1 inch thinly sliced fresh ginger
- Small pinch turmeric powder
- 1/2 teaspoon lemon juice
- 2 sprigs of fresh mint, plus more for garnish
- 1 teaspoon honey (or to taste)

Instructions

- To a teapot add the fresh mint sprigs.
- Add the infuser to the teapot and add the camomile tea bags, ginger, turmeric powder, lemon juice. Allow steeping for 5 minutes.
- Add a drizzle of honey (to taste) to each of the cups and pour over the tea. Stir to mix in the honey. Garnish with mint leaves.

Nerve-Soothing Tea

Ingredients

- 2 tablespoons dried lemon balm
- 2 tablespoons dried rose hips, cut & sifted
- 1 tablespoon dried oat straw
- 1 tablespoon dried chamomile
- 1/2 teaspoon dried lavender

Directions

- Combine all ingredients & mix thoroughly. Store in a sealed container in a cool place out of direct sunlight.

For A Hot Cup Of Tea:

For a single serving hot cup of tea, place 1 tablespoon of the tea blend into a tea ball or bag. In a mug, add the filled tea ball or bag and fill with 1 cup (8 fl oz) hot water. Cover & let steep for 8-10 minutes, then enjoy! (Sweeten if desired!)

For A Cold Infusion:

In a 1 quart jar, add 1/4 cup of the tea blend & fill the rest of the jar with water. Cover and let sit 8-10 hours, or overnight. Then strain out herbs. Enjoy as-is, add ice for extra refreshment, & sweeten with honey or another sweetener of choice if desired. (Drink tea within ~3 days.)

Calming Tea Recipe

Ingredients

- 2 parts lemon balm (Melissa officinalis) leaf
- 1 part chamomile (Matricaria chamomilla) flowers
- 1 part linden (Tilia spp.) bract and flower
- 1 part rose (Rosa spp.) petal
- ½ part spearmint (Mentha spicata) leaf

Directions

- Blend the herbs in a bowl and store tea blend in a glass jar until ready for use. Note: each part can be any measure you'd like—1 teaspoon, 1 tablespoon, or 1 cup, etc. depending on the batch size you'd like to make.
- To brew a cup of tea, use 1-2 tablespoons of the tea blend per cup of water.
- Place the herbs in a heat-proof glass vessel with a tight-fitting lid, and cover with boiling water.
- Cover and let steep for 10-15 minutes, strain, and enjoy 3-4 cups per day while encouraging your stress to melt away.

Calm Down Tea

Ingredients

- 1 tablespoon chamomile
- 1 tablespoon catnip
- 1 tablespoon fennel seed
- 1 tablespoon rose hips

- 1 teaspoon lavender
- 1 teaspoon spearmint
- 4 cups filtered water

Instructions

- Combine all herbs in a medium mixing bowl. Stir to evenly distribute herbs. Store in an airtight glass container {like a mason jar} if you're not making the tea right away.

To Make The Tea:

- In a medium-size saucepan or tea kettle, bring filtered water to a boil. Remove from heat and allow to cool for 5 minutes.
- Add 2 tablespoons of the herbal tea to the hot water. COVER and steep for 5-7 minutes {a maximum of 10 minutes}.
- When the tea is done steeping, strain tea with a fine-mesh strainer into a heatproof bowl or glass jar/container.
- Serve hot with a generous spoonful of honey - if desired.

Shake-It-Off Tea

Ingredients

- 1 cup warm water
- 1–2 tablespoons raw honey
- 2 tablespoons fresh lemon juice
- 2 tablespoons raw apple cider vinegar
- 2 tablespoons fresh ginger, grated
- Dash of cinnamon
- Dash of cayenne pepper

Instructions

- Combine warm water with raw honey.
- Add in fresh lemon juice and apple cider vinegar.
- Grate fresh ginger and add it into a mason jar.
- Add a dash of fresh cinnamon and cayenne pepper.
- Combine well with a whisk or adding a lid and shaking up.

WOUNDS

A wound is a type of injury that happens relatively quickly in which skin is torn, cut, or punctured (an open wound), or where blunt force trauma causes a contusion (a closed wound). In pathology, it specifically refers to a sharp injury that damages the epidermis of the skin.

Classification

According to the level of contamination, a wound can be classified as:

- **Clean Wound:** Made under sterile conditions where there are no organisms present and the skin is likely to heal without complications.
- **Contaminated Wound:** Usually resulting from accidental injury; there are pathogenic organisms and foreign bodies in the wound.
- **Infected Wound:** The wound has pathogenic organisms present and multiplying, exhibiting clinical signs of infection (yellow appearance, soreness, redness, oozing pus).
- **Colonized Wound:** A chronic situation, containing pathogenic organisms, difficult to heal (e.g. bedsore).

Wound Wash

Ingredients:

- 4 ounces aloe vera gel
- 2 ounces witch hazel infused with calendula flowers, sage leaves, thyme leaves and flowers, yarrow, and/or goldenseal root
- 2 ounces lavender hydrosol (flower water)
- 1 teaspoon castile soap, liquid
- 5 drops grapefruit seed extract
- 20 drops lavender essential oil
- 15 drops tea tree oil
- 5 drops thyme essential oil
- 5 drops myrrh essential oil

Directions:

- Gather the plant material you will be using based on affordability and availability – either dried or fresh, or a mix of both...I use garden-fresh as often as possible. Place herbs and flowers into a glass jar. Pour enough liquid witch hazel extract over the plant material to cover it completely.
- **Note:** Proceed using these basic tincturing methods for making an herb-infused witch hazel.
- Once the witch hazel is tinctured, gather the remaining ingredients. In a glass jar, combine all ingredients. Shake the jar vigorously to mix. Pour mixture into a dark or colored mister/spray bottle. Label with name, contents, and date. The spray is shelf-stable for 1-2 years depending on the quality of raw materials used. Keep away from heat and direct sunlight.

Pine Resin Salve

Ingredients

- ¼ cup pine resin
- ½ cup oil (olive, almond, etc.)
- ½ – 1-ounce beeswax, grated

Directions

- Add pine resin to oil in a simmering double boiler. Heat together on low heat until pine resin melts.
- Strain mixture through a coffee filter or strainer.
- Return to double boiler and add grated beeswax. Gently heat until the mixture is melted. Pour into tins or jars and store in a cool, dark place.
- This is the basic pine resin salve recipe, but note that you could substitute herb-infused oils such as plantain, Calendula, comfrey, or yarrow for the plain oil to incorporate more vulnerable and antimicrobial herbs to support the body's wound healing process. There is certainly room to tweak this formula to your own needs!

Calendula Succus Simple For Lacerations And Abrasions

Calendula officinalis (calendula) is a first aid kit staple. A succus has lower alcohol content than a tincture and is made from fresh juice. Calendula officinalis succus is unlikely to sting very much when topically applied. Use a dropperful of succus on a sterile gauze pad and apply topically, repeating each hour until the wound has scabbed over.

Calendula-Comfrey Poultice For Lacerations And Abrasions

Calendula officinalis (pot marigold or calendula) and Symphytum officinale (comfrey) are the classic duos for trauma and wounds. Calendula enhances circulation and connective tissue regeneration in the dermis, and comfrey contains the cell-proliferating agent allantoin.

- Calendula officinalis succus
- Symphytum officinale roots

When fresh comfrey roots are available, thoroughly wash several inches of a supple root, then mince or grate, and cover in a small amount of water. Add Calendula officinalis succus and allow it to stand for 10 minutes to yield a gummy mass for topical application. Dry comfrey roots can be macerated in hot water until mucilaginous. Symphytum officinale root tincture would also do in a pinch, but fresh roots or long-macerated dry root preparations are superior. If using fresh root pulp, place the gummy mass on a thin gauze pad, place the fabric side against the skin, saturate with Calendula officinalis succus, and cover with plastic or more gauze and tape to hold in place. Apply 3 to 5 times daily for acute injuries, allowing the injury to air-dry between applications.

You can also make this poultice by combining equal parts of Calendula and Symphytum tinctures, applying to a sterile gauze pad, and using topically, or by making a paste out of the combined dry powders and water.

Antimicrobial Black Drawing Salve For Tick Bites And Splinters

Ingredients

For The Oil

- 1 part dried Andrographis
- 1 part dried or fresh calendula flowers (if fresh, see notes)
- 1 part fresh chickweed (see notes)
- 1 part fresh plantain (see notes)
- Organic extra virgin olive oil

For The Salve

- 1/2 cup infused oil
- 1 tablespoon beeswax pellets
- 2 tablespoons activated charcoal
- 2 tablespoons bentonite clay
- 1/2 teaspoon vitamin E, optional, works as a preservative

- 20 drops lavender essential oil, optional, works as a skin soother
- 10 drops tea tree essential oil, optional, works as an antimicrobial and anti-inflammatory

Instructions

1. To Infuse The Oil Using The Solar Method: Place the herbs in a wide mouth pint-sized mason jar, filling the jar about 2/3 full. Using a marker or piece of tape, mark the top level of the herbs on the outside of the jar. Then cover the herbs with 1" of the oil. The herbs may float, but just fill the jar until the oil reaches 1" above the marking. Set in a sunny spot for 4-6 weeks, shaking daily (or as often as you remember). Strain through a cheesecloth-lined sieve before using.

2. To Infuse The Oil Using A Double Boiler: Fill a saucepan with 1" of water, then place a glass bowl over top. Bring the water to a gentle simmer, and then add in about 1 cup of olive oil to about 1/2 cup of mixed herbs. Let infuse over a very low burner for 2-3 hours, or until the oil takes on the color and scent of the herbs. Do not let the oil get hot enough to cook the herbs. It's best to err on the side of too cool here. I prefer to use the smallest burner on my stove at its lowest setting. Strain through a cheesecloth-lined sieve before using.

3. To Make The Salve: Fill a saucepan with 1" of water, then place a glass bowl over top. Bring the water to a gentle simmer. Add in the beeswax and 1/2 cup of the infused oil. Stir constantly until the wax is completely melted. Remove from heat, and then add in the charcoal, clay, vitamin E, and essential oils, and stir until completely smooth. Pour into a glass container and let cool completely. Label and store.

4. To Use On Tick And Other Insect Bites: Place a heaping glob on the clean bite site, then cover with a large bandage (the salve will stain). Remove after 24 hours.

5. To Use On Splinters, Embedded Glass, And Other Foreign Objects: Place a heaping glob on the clean site and cover with a large bandage. Check after 12 hours to see if the foreign object has moved enough to be grabbed with tweezers. If not, apply more of the salve and check again in another 12 hours. Deep splinters might take a few days. If the site becomes inflamed, red, warm, has pus, or shows any other signs of being infected, immediately contact your healthcare professional.

Notes: When using fresh herbs, it's important to "fresh wilt" the herbs to get a little bit of the moisture out of them before adding them to the oil. Oil and water don't mix! To fresh wilt, just place the herbs in a warm, dry spot (sun works, too) until they are floppy and a bit shriveled, it shouldn't take more than a few hours.

NATIVE AMERICAN REMEDIES FOR YOUR CHILD

Natural Herbal Remedies, Sacred Medicinal Plants, and Recipes to Heal Common Ailments in Children

Taahira Maskwa

HERBAL REMEDIES FOR YOUR CHILD

0-2 Months

1. Newborn Dill [Anethum Graveolens]

Baby Dill is an aromatic herb, botanically classified as Anethum graveolens. The herb is a member of the Umbelliferae family, also known as the celery, carrot, or parsley family, and is cultivated for its delicate fresh leaves. Baby Dill is harvested at the very early stages of growth when the plant is still small and tender, and the flavor is milder. Though the herb is most often associated with pickling, Baby Dill is also popular in Scandinavian, Eastern European, Indian and Mediterranean cuisines.

Nutritional Value

Baby Dill is a great source of vitamins A and C and a good source of manganese, iron, and folate. The herb also contains calcium, riboflavin, niacin, and potassium and trace amounts of vitamin B6, dietary fiber, magnesium, phosphorus, zinc, and copper. Its medicinal properties are due to the presence of monoterpene compounds, flavonoids, volatile oils, and amino acids. Dill has also demonstrated antibacterial properties.

Applications

Baby Dill is most often used fresh, but it is also used in its dried, or dehydrated, form. It may be used in fresh or cooked preparations, or as a garnish. It is often paired with fish, especially salmon, and in cream or wine-based sauces. Pair Baby Dill with yogurt, soft cheeses or cream, cucumbers, lentils, tomatoes, dried fruit, seafood, poultry, and beans. Use it as a salad herb or in pasta dishes with smoked fish or caviar, or in barley, quinoa, couscous, or bulgur wheat dishes. In Greek, Turkish and Slavic cuisine the herb is paired with chicken, spinach, mushrooms, and lamb. In Germany, it is paired with eggs, cheese, and potatoes. Keep Baby Dill dry until ready to use. If it becomes wilted, you can put the stems in a glass of water and cover it with a plastic bag. Baby Dill will keep refrigerated for up to a week and it can be frozen and kept for up to 2 months.

Recipe For Dill For Newborns Is As Follows:

- Pour a teaspoon of shredded fennel blooms over a glass (200ml) of hot water and put in a water bath to cook for 40 minutes.
- Pour the finished brew into a bottle.
- Leave to cool at room temperature.
- Fennel has similar properties, but they are more marked. If you like, prepare a remedy for fennel colic. This can be done as follows:
- Take a teaspoon of fennel seeds and a glass (200ml) of water for a daily dose.
- Pour the seeds with boiling water.
- After 1-1.5 hours, drain the infusion through the gauze and leave it to cool.

2. Lavender (Lavandula angustifolia)

You want the absolute best for your little one. You want to help them sleep well; feel better quickly if they get sick, and stop any pain or discomfort. Most of all, you want them to be happy and content. And you want to do it using a safe natural remedy.

Enter lavender essential oil. Just one whiff of lavender can immediately make your kid (and you) feel calm and more relaxed. It's the most widely used essential oil to ensure a good night's sleep for your baby or child. But its aromatherapy benefits don't stop there. It's also a great pain reliever, can help with colic and skin rashes, ease a fever and congestion, and naturally boost your child's mood and emotions. Most importantly, it's kid-safe.

One study found that mothers that bathed their infants in lavender-scented water experienced multiple benefits for both mom and baby. Mothers became more relaxed and touched and smiled at their babies more often. Their babies, in turn, looked at their mothers more, cried less often, and spent more time in deep sleep after bath-time.

It's also been found that a lavender oil massage can also help relax a fussy baby and encourage longer and deeper sleep. After introducing a bedtime massage routine with mothers and their babies, a study found that bedtime becomes easier, and the babies experienced less night-time waking.

As lavender essential oil quickly and safely relaxes the body and calms the mind, it can also be a life savior if your little one is anxious, insecure, or in any form of emotional distress - helping to soothe that incessant crying that can be so stressful for any mother.

Lavender is soothing and non-toxic, making it a favorite for babies not less than 2 months of age. In addition to being a natural antiseptic, lavender is also naturally sedative and its calming effects can alleviate muscle pains. To use, dilute lavender at a ratio of up to .5 percent and massage the blend along the baby's jawline.

3. Roman Chamomile

Roman Chamomile is one of the safest essential oils, and you can use it with very young babies (as young as zero to two months). At birth, the baby's digestive system is not fully developed yet. It is therefore common that during his first months of life, your baby experience digestive disorders such as colic, gas, bloating, or constipation. Chamomile is effective to relieve these issues and promote digestion in children thanks to its antispasmodic, anti-inflammatory, and soothing properties.

Benefits

Soothe Skin Irritation

Chamomile helps soothe irritated skin, redness, itching, and common skin conditions in infants. It has soothing and anti-inflammatory properties thanks to its rich concentration of flavonoids and is perfectly suited to the sensitive skin of babies. To soothe the baby's skin, you can use chamomile in different forms: hydrosol, floral water, essential oil, or herbal tea.

To Calm The Itching:

Pour 2 to 3 tablespoons of chamomile hydrosol into the baby's bathwater. If you do not have a hydrosol, you can make a cup of chamomile tea and mix it with the baby bathwater.

To Relieve Irritation And Redness:

Apply chamomile hydrosol or floral water to a sterilized compress. Apply it on the irritated area (previously cleaned and dried) 2 to 3 times a day. You can also put chamomile hydrosol and floral water in a spray bottle and apply it to the irritated skin.

Promote Sleep And Reduce Anxiety

All parents know it well: from your baby's birth, you are very unlikely to have an uninterrupted night. Although babies' sleep cycles evolve over the months, sleep disorders are common among infants and can have various causes: anxiety, toothache, fear of darkness, nightmares, etc. ... Chamomile helps calm the nervous agitation in baby, relax and improve sleep quality.

Before Putting Baby To Bed:

Give her a few teaspoons of chamomile tea diluted with a little water before bedtime.

You can also give her/him a relaxing massage with 1 drop of the essential oil of noble chamomile (Chamaemelum Nobile) diluted in a teaspoon of sweet almond oil. Not only will it help your little one relax and fall asleep serenely, but it will also strengthen your bond.

Calm Eye Irritation

Chamomile can be used in infants with conjunctivitis and eye irritation. It is effective in decongesting the eyes and calming the inflammation of conjunctivitis that causes itchy eyes. Its use is very simple and safe for babies. Just clean the eyes several times a day with chamomile tea, and after a few days, conjunctival symptoms and eye irritation will fade.

To Soothe Conjunctivitis:

Apply cooled chamomile tea on a compress. Clean the baby's eyes with the soaked compress by emphasizing the corners of the eyes and eyelashes. Soak a new compress of chamomile tea and apply it gently on the eyelids for 1 to 2 minutes. Repeat 4 to 5 times a day (or more) to help fight off the infection.

4. Astragalus

Like many safe herbs for infants, astragalus is known to boost the function of the immune system, thereby strengthening an infant's resistance to catching diseases. It is known to prevent children from contracting any illness or disease and also strengthening the immune system of a child after a disease.

How To Use

Add a slice of the root to a cup of water to make tea, or add it to stews, soups, or even to your pot of rice. The root itself should not be consumed, but it will release its beneficial properties in the boiling process.

2-12 Months

1. Geranium

Geranium essential oil is derived from steam distillation of the leaves of Pelargonium graveolens, a plant species native to South Africa. The geranium essential oil can be diluted with a carrier oil, such as sesame oil, and used topically on the skin. You can use it as a spot treatment for acne or itchy skin, or as a massage oil.

Some carrier oils may cause an allergic reaction when applied to the skin. Before using, do a patch test on a small area to make sure it doesn't cause a reaction. When diluting essential oils with a carrier oil, it's important to follow these dilution guidelines for one-two months to the one-year-old baby; 3 to 6 drops of essential oil per 6 teaspoons of carrier oil is a safe amount.

How To Make Geranium Oil At Home

If you have several weeks to spare, you can make geranium oil at home:

- Snip about 12 ounces of rose geranium leaves off the plant.
- Fill a small, clear glass jar around halfway up with olive or sesame oil and submerge the leaves, covering them completely.
- Seal the jar tightly and place it on a sunny windowsill for a week.
- Strain the oil through a cheesecloth into a different glass jar. Leave the geranium leaves behind.
- Add a supply of fresh geranium leaves into the oil.
- Seal the new jar and again leave it on a sunny windowsill for one week.
- Continue these steps each week for an additional three weeks (total of five weeks).
- Pour the essential oil into a bottle that can be kept tightly closed. Keep it in a cool, dry place, and use it within one year.

2. Mandarin (Citrus Reticulata) –Promoting Sleep.

Mandarin has calming effects similar to lavender, making it a great nighttime alternative for babies who are allergic to the scent of lavender. The sweet scent of mandarin is favorable to other orange varieties because it's not phototoxic. This means that even when diluted and applied directly to the skin, it shouldn't cause skin irritation.

3. Eucalyptus globulus

Eucalyptus oil is an extract from the leaves of the eucalyptus tree. The oil has a composition of more than 100 different compounds. Single distilled eucalyptus oil, which is crude oil, may contain more compounds in different quantities than the double-distilled eucalyptus oil, which is rectified. For instance, eucalyptus globulus oil has nearly 60% cineole and 40% other compounds. Following rectification, the oil contains 80% cineole and 20% other compounds.

Eucalyptus oil, one such essential oil, is said to have antibacterial and antiseptic action. The oil is used for these healing properties and has been in use as a popular home remedy for thousands of years. It is used as a therapy to treat respiratory problems such as cold, bronchitis, cough, and pneumonia in some cultures.

Eucalyptus is a natural expectorant that can help unclog respiratory congestion as it possesses antiseptic and antibacterial properties, making it a favorite during the cold winter months. Eucalyptus oil is used as a natural therapy to treat pneumonia, bronchitis, coughs, colds, and other respiratory ailments. It helps strengthen the immune system as well by improving respiratory circulation and providing antioxidant benefits. Cineole – more commonly known as camphor – is an organic compound present in eucalyptus oil that can help reduce pain and inflammation.

The type of eucalyptus species you buy for your baby is critical. When using Eucalyptus essential oil to treat congestion, parents should only use Eucalyptus Radiata for their children and infants. Eucalyptus Radiata contains a lower content of cineole than the widely available Eucalyptus Globulus and can, therefore, when diffused, be used with babies. While Eucalyptus globulus is safe for adults, it should not be used on children under the age of two. Eucalyptus Globulus contains a high content of cineole which is too harsh for the babies and can cause central nervous system and breathing problems. Eucalyptus Globulus should not be "applied to or near the faces of" or "otherwise inhaled by" children under one year of age.

4. Tea Tree (Melaleuca Alternifolia) –Reducing Germs

The botanical name of the tea tree, which is native to Australia, is 'Melaleuca alternifolia'. It is the source of tea tree oil. The leaves and twigs of it are treated with a steam and distillation process to obtain the medicinal oil. The oil has medicinal and disinfectant properties. Tea tree is a natural antimicrobial, antifungal, and disinfectant. Adding a few drops of tea tree oil to an unscented oil can help with diaper rash and fungal infections. Tea tree is a stronger oil that can be harsh on the skin, so it should be avoided on babies younger than six months old and carefully patch-tested on older infants.

Benefits Of Tea Tree Oil For Infants

The tea tree oil has several health benefits, which makes it a herbal remedy you need to have at your disposal. Mentioned below are some of the benefits of this oil.

1. Cures Skin Infections.

This oil is a natural antibacterial and antiseptic. It can be used to treat topical skin infections in babies and children. It is highly effective against wounds, insect bites, diaper rashes, and more.

2. It Helps Heal Wounds Faster.

When applied to injuries, the oil's antibacterial nature kills bacteria that are present on wounds and helps them recover more quickly. The oil can also reduce scarring of skin after a wound heals or in cases such as chickenpox blisters.

3. Treats Fungal Infections.

The tea tree oil for baby skin is highly effective in treating fungal infections such as ringworm in babies as it has a powerful anti-fungal effect. It also kills several harmful microbes in the protozoan family that can cause skin infections, rashes, and disease.

4. Strengthens The Immune System.

When you apply tea tree oil to the skin, it strengthens your immune system and helps build resistance to diseases. It does so by having a stimulating effect on hormone secretion and blood circulation. Due to this, your baby will be less prone to infections.

5. Cures Cough And Cold.

The tea tree oil for baby cold and cough is an excellent remedy to ease your baby's respiratory congestion. Since the oil has expectorant properties, it has been used for a long time to treat cold and cough. The treatment is as simple as rubbing oil on the baby's chest and throat to provide relief from a cough.

6. Improves Blood Circulation.

The anti-inflammatory properties of this oil help ease the pain in the body. Rub this oil on the muscles of your baby and he will feel better. The oil also reduces inflammation and improves blood circulation when applied over sore muscles. This promotes faster recovery.

7. Keeps The Skin Healthy.

The oil enables sweating which in turn helps your baby's skin to expel waste and other toxic substances that may have accumulated over time. This helps in keeping the baby's skin healthy.

8. Promotes Good Health.

Adding a few drops of tea tree oil to your baby's bathwater can promote good health. Its balsamic properties boost a baby's overall health.

How To Use Tea Tree Oil On Baby

Tea tree oil is available in the concentrated form as an essential oil. It should never be applied directly to the baby's skin. Mix it with a carrier oil such as olive oil, sweet almond, or coconut oils to dilute it, and then use it on your baby.

12 Months-5 Years

1. Palmarosa [Cymnopogon martinii]

Naturally balancing for the skin and emotions, palmarosa blends well with bergamot, cedarwood, and geranium. With a beautiful fresh, green, and floral scent, this soothing organic oil is steam distilled from the wild-growing grass near Tororo, in eastern Uganda. We've worked with a young farmer, Joel, to set up the distillery for aromatic crops grown on local farms, creating valuable employment.

Key Action: Cleansing

Latin Name: Cymbopogon martini

Country Of Origin: Uganda

Blends Beautifully With: bergamot, cedarwood, and geranium

Ingredients: Cymbopogon Martini Oil

Range: Essential Oils

Directions

1. Bath & Shower

Inhale the aromatic stream while your skin absorbs all the benefits of the oil. For adults, add up to 5 drops in 2 tbsp bath oil, shower gel, full-fat milk, or carrier oil. For children over 2 years old or adults with sensitive skin, reduce the amount to up to 2 drops per 2 tbsp.

2. Inhalation

This technique helps to clear your head and nose. For adults, add 4–6 drops to a bowl of steaming water, place a towel over your head and breathe. Children over 2 years old, adults with sensitive skin, and asthmatics should not inhale directly. Instead, place the bowl of hot water with added oils in the room nearby.

3. Massages

Balances your body and mind while helping to ease aching muscles. For adults, use up to 7 drops in 1 tbsp of base oil. For children over 2 years old or adults with sensitive skin, use up to 3 drops in 1 tbsp of base oil.

4. Diffusers & Burners

A natural air freshener, this technique creates a balancing ambiance and sets a mood. For adults, add 1–3 drops in a diffuser or burner. For children over 2 years old, add 1–3 drops in a diffuser.

Warning: Do not use undiluted on the skin. For external use only. Avoid contact with the eyes. Keep out of the reach of children. Flammable. Use within 12 months of opening.

5 years-12 years

1. Clary Sage [Salvia sclarea]

Clary sage (Salvia sclarea) is a flowering herb that's native to the Mediterranean Basin. The essential oil that's extracted from the leaves and buds of the plant has a clean, refreshing scent that you can use as a skin balm or gently inhale as part of an aromatherapy treatment

Clary sage is easy to grow in high-temperature areas. It's usually cultivated for its use as a flavoring in tea. It's also known by the names "clear eye" and "eyebright" because of its traditional use as a treatment for eye health. But it's now being studied for a variety of other health benefits.

Clary sage (Salvia sclarea) is traditionally used to boost confidence and self-esteem, as well as to improve mood. Studies show that clary sage has powerful antidepressant effects, and it seems to work by modulating dopamine and serotonin, brain chemicals linked with feelings of pleasure, happiness, and well-being. It may be even more effective when combined with ylang-ylang oil studies show that ylang-ylang can improve mood and boost self-esteem. Mix clary sage and ylang ylang essential oils in a diffuser in your child's room or combine in a spray bottle of water and spritz throughout your house. Sprinkle a few drops of clary sage on a cotton ball and inhale or sniff it right from the bottle. Or stir a few drops into a tub of warm water for a mood-lifting bath.

Ingredients

10 drops clary sage oil

Directions

Add 10 drops to an air diffuser or inhale directly from the bottle

2. Nutmeg [Myristica fragrans]

Nutmeg is the seed or ground spice of several species of the genus Myristica. Myristica fragrans (fragrant nutmeg or true nutmeg) is a dark-leaved evergreen tree cultivated for two spices derived from its fruit: nutmeg, from its seed, and mace, from the seed covering. It is also a commercial source of an essential oil and nutmeg butter. The California nutmeg, Torreya californica, has a seed of similar appearance, but is not closely related to Myristica fragans, and is not used as a spice.

Possible Benefits Of Nutmeg For Babies

Nutmeg contains several bioactive compounds possessing therapeutic properties. Its use is common in folk and alternative medicine to treat ailments and offer overall health benefits.

1. Relieve Indigestion: The use of nutmeg to treat digestive disorders is prevalent in traditional medicine. A freshly prepared decoction of nutmeg with honey is known to relieve gastrointestinal issues, such as indigestion. This decoction may be useful for babies older than 12 months who can consume honey.

2. Improve Appetite: Nutmeg has carminative effects, helping relieve flatulence, gas, and bloating . These effects may also help promote appetite in babies.

3. Support Immunity: Nutmeg has several bioactive compounds, such as eugenol, isoeugenol, and methoxyeugenol, with antioxidant properties. Besides, it has anti-inflammatory and immunomodulatory properties that may boost an infant's immunity in the long run

How To Use Nutmeg Or Jaifal In Babies

Take a grinding stone and wash it properly. Then pour some milk or water on it and rub the whole Nutmeg or Jaifal on the grinding stone in a circular motion and alternatively to and fro until you get some paste around 0.5 ml. Collect this paste in a spoon and pour some more milk or water to dilute it. Then give it to your baby directly post that feed her immediately to change the taste of the baby.

Dose: You can give around 0.5 ml of it one time during summers and two times during winters.

Precautions To Take While Feeding Nutmeg To Babies

- Before grating the whole nutmeg for use, wash it thoroughly under cold running water to remove dust and dirt that might be present on its surface.
- Grate the whole nutmeg to make its smooth paste, ensure no lumps or chunks are left.
- Every time you use ground nutmeg, rub a small amount of powder between your fingers and smell. If there is a faint aroma or no aroma, it usually signifies that the powder has become stale.
- Mix only a pinch or two of nutmeg paste or powder to a serving of baby food. Feeding nutmeg in excess can increase the risk of nutmeg intoxication (3).
- Preferably feed nutmeg with a food item that your baby is already consuming comfortably. It will help identify intolerance, sensitivity, or allergy towards nutmeg easily.
- If your baby looks uncomfortable after ingesting nutmeg, discontinue feeding and try again later.
- Nutmeg allergy is rare but possible . Consult a pediatrician before feeding nutmeg to the baby, especially if they have a family history of food and seed allergies.

- Keep the ground nutmeg away from your child's reach to avoid accidental ingestion.
- Nutmeg is a fragrant and flavorful spice with potential health benefits. You can use whole or ground nutmeg in minimal amounts to add flavor to your baby and toddler's foods. Purees, soups, stews, porridges, cereals, drinks, and baked goods are some recipes where nutmeg can go with other complementary herbs and spices.

NATIVE AMERICAN HERBAL DISPENSATORY

Discover The Secrets of Native Americans. Learn to Source Powerful Herbs, and Create The Best Herbal Remedies to Naturally Improve Your Wellness

Taahira Maskwa

CHAPTER 1 : HERBS FOR WEALTH AND POWER

1. Fenugreek

Description

Fenugreek is an herb native to southeastern Europe, northern Africa, and western Asia, but is widely cultivated in other parts of the world. Its botanical name is Trigonella foenum-graecum; its English name comes from two Latin words meaning Greek hay. Fenugreek is an annual plant that grows 2–3 ft (0.6–0.9 m) tall, with a strong odor and small pale yellow flowers. The seed of the fenugreek plant contains many active compounds with pharmaceutical applications. The seeds are collected in the autumn. The chemical components of fenugreek seed include iron, vitamin A, vitamin B1, vitamin C, phosphates, flavonoids, saponins, trigonelline, and other alkaloids. The seed is also high in fiber and protein.

General Use

Quite apart from its therapeutic value, fenugreek is used as a seasoning and flavoring agent in foods, particularly in Egypt, India, and the Middle East. The maple smell and flavor of fenugreek have led to its use as a spice in foods, beverages, confections, tobacco, and imitation maple syrup. In some countries, the seeds are eaten raw or boiled, or the greens are enjoyed as a fresh salad. Extracts of fenugreek are used in some cosmetic products as well.

The best-documented medical use of fenugreek is to control blood sugar in both insulin-dependent (type 1) and noninsulin-dependent (type 2) diabetics. Some studies also show that serum cholesterol levels in diabetics, and perhaps in others, are reduced by fenugreek. Doses as low as 15 mg per day may produce beneficial effects on fasting blood sugar, the elevation of blood sugar after a meal, and overall glycemic control.

The use of fenugreek is likely to alter the diabetic patient's need for insulin or other medications used to control blood sugar. This treatment should be supervised by a health care provider familiar with the use of herbal therapies for diabetes. The recommended doses of fenugreek can vary rather widely.

The seeds of fenugreek can also act as a bulk laxative as a result of their fiber and mucilage content. These portions of the seed swell up from being in contact with water, filling the bowel, and stimulating peristaltic activity. For laxative purposes, 0.5–1 tsp of freshly powdered herb per cup of water, followed by an additional 8 oz water, can be taken one to three times daily. Patients should begin with the lowest effective dose of fenugreek; they should also avoid taking oral medications or vitamins at the same time as the herb.

Fenugreek may encourage a flagging appetite and is sometimes given during convalescence from illnesses to improve food intake, weight gain, and speed of recuperation.

Cancer researchers are also studying fenugreek for its potential effectiveness as a cancer chemopreventive. It is thought that fenugreek may help to prevent cancer by raising the levels of vitamin C, vitamin E, and other antioxidants in the bloodstream.

Historically, fenugreek has been used as a topical treatment for abscesses, boils, burns, eczema, gout, and ulceration of the skin as it has an anti-inflammatory effect. It is also reputedly useful for some digestive complaints, including gastritis and gastric ulcers.

Fenugreek reportedly can be helpful in the induction of childbirth, as it is known to stimulate uterine contractions. For this reason, it should not be taken during pregnancy. As a gargle, fenugreek may relieve sore throats and coughing. Arthritis, bronchitis, fevers, and male reproductive conditions are other traditional but unsubstantiated indications for this herb.

Preparations

Fenugreek may be purchased as bulk seeds, capsules, tinctures, or in teas. Due to the strong, bitter taste, capsules are used most often. The dose is variable, depending on the form of the herb that is used. The seeds may also be soaked to make tea. For topical use, powdered fenugreek seed is mixed with water to form a paste. Herbal supplements should be stored in a cool, dry place, away from direct light and out of the reach of children.

Precautions

Fenugreek may when taken in larger amounts than are used to season foods, cause contractions of the uterus. For this reason, women who are pregnant should avoid therapeutic doses. Frequent topical use of fenugreek preparations may cause skin irritation and sensitization. Symptoms of an allergic reaction include swelling, numbness, and wheezing. This herb should not be used by anyone with sensitivity to fenugreek. Large doses (over 100 g per day) may cause intestinal symptoms, including diarrhea, nausea, and gas. Blood sugar can also drop to abnormally low levels. Fenugreek is generally recognized as safe, but its safety is not well-documented for use in small children, lactating women, or persons with liver or kidney disease.

Side Effects

Depending on the dose used, fenugreek may cause a maple syrup odor in the patient's sweat and urine.

Interactions

Fenugreek can enhance anticoagulant activity, and should not be used with other herbs or medications (heparin, warfarin, ticlopidine) that have this effect due to increased risk of bleeding. It can lower blood sugar to a marked degree; blood sugar levels should be monitored closely, particularly in people who are taking insulin, glipizide, or other hypoglycemic agents.

Medications that are being taken to control diabetes may need to have dosages adjusted, which should be done under medical supervision. In theory, since fenugreek is high in mucilage, it can alter the absorption of any oral medication. Corticosteroid and other hormone treatments may be less effective. Monoamine oxidase inhibitors (MAOIs) may have increased activity when used in conjunction with fenugreek.

2. Bergamot Oil

Bergamot essential oil, extracted from the peel of the bergamot orange (Citrus bergamia), has a light citrus scent with floral notes that are said to have healing properties. Commonly used in aromatherapy to elevate mood and alleviate stress, bergamot oil is also said to have characteristics similar to grapefruit essential oil in that it is antiseptic, antispasmodic, and analgesic (pain-relieving), possibly offering some benefit for health issues like skin infections. It may also have some utility for high cholesterol.

Some practitioners add bergamot oil to the water for use as a health tonic, while others recommend using it topically or orally. However, it's worth noting that bergamot oil is known to cause side effects and interactions, particularly when used in excess.

Health Benefits

Practitioners of aromatherapy believe that inhaling essential oils or absorbing them through the skin transmits signals to the limbic system, the region of the brain that regulates emotions and memories. Doing so can induce physiological effects, including a reduction in blood pressure, heart rate, and respiration, and an increase in the "feel-good" hormone serotonin and the neurotransmitter dopamine.

Bergamot oil can also be used as a nasal decongestant when inhaled and an antibacterial agent when applied to the skin. In alternative medicine, bergamot oil is believed to treat or prevent a range of unrelated health conditions, including:

- Acne
- Anxiety
- Chronic fatigue syndrome
- Depression
- Eczema
- Food poisoning
- Headache
- High cholesterol
- Insomnia
- Non-allergic rhinitis
- Non-arthritic joint pain
- Psoriasis
- Ringworm
- Side Effects

Bergamot essential oil should never be applied to the skin at full strength. Doing so can cause extreme skin inflammation, stinging, and photosensitivity. It should instead be diluted with a neutral carrier oil (such as sweet almond or jojoba oil) before applying it to the skin.

Bergamot contains a substance known as bergapten which is highly phototoxic. If skin exposed to bergamot oil is then exposed to UV radiation from the sun (or a tanning bed), a potentially serious skin condition called photodermatitis may occur. Symptoms include redness, pain, swelling, blistering, and rash. Bergamot oil has the highest concentration of bergapten of any essential oil. So phototoxic is the oil that even soaking in a bath with a few drops can trigger photosensitivity.

Interactions

Bergamot oil is known to intensify the effects of photosensitizing drugs, further increasing the risk of skin inflammation, rash, and blistering. Here are just some of the possible drug-drug interactions:

Alpha-hydroxy acids in cosmetics

Antibiotics like Avelox (moxifloxacin), Cipro (ciprofloxacin), Floxin (ofloxacin), Levaquin (levofloxacin), and tetracycline

Antifungals like Ancoben (flucytosine), griseofulvin, and Vfend (voriconazole)

Antidepressants like Elavil (amitriptyline)

Phototherapy-enhancing drugs like Oxsoralen (methoxsalen) and Trisoralen (trioxsalen)

Vitamin A derivatives (a.k.a. retinoids) like Soriatane (acitretin) and isotretinoin

Bergamot oil also contains significant amounts of a substance known as bergamottin, which is associated with a wide range of grapefruit drug interactions. Though the impact of these interactions is unknown, it is important to advise your doctor if you use bergamot oil and take chronic medications of any sort.

Dosage And Preparation

Bergamot essential oil is typically sold in dark amber or cobalt blue bottles with a dropper cap. The colored glass reduces oxidative damage caused by UV radiation. If used topically, bergamot oil used should be diluted with a cold-pressed carrier oil. The proportion of essential oil to a carrier oil can vary based on your skin type, but some organizations.

Bergamot oil also can be inhaled by sprinkling a few drops onto a cloth or tissue, or by using an aromatherapy diffuser or vaporizer. You can also add three to four drops to bathwater.

There are no guidelines for the appropriate use of bergamot oil when taken internally. Many alternative practitioners will tell you that one drop of bergamot oil diluted in four ounces (15 ml) of water can safely be consumed on an occasional basis. Even so, you should use bergamot oil with extreme caution and ideally under the supervision of a qualified physician who can monitor for side effects and interactions.

Storage Tips

Essential oils should be stored in a cool, dry room away from direct sunlight, ideally in their original light-resistant bottles. They also keep well in the refrigerator. If an essential oil accidentally freezes, let it come to room temperature gradually. Do not try to heat it. Essential oils are flammable and have different flash points at which they can ignite. Even though essential oils have a long shelf life, you should discard any that have become cloudy, smell funny, or have thickened in consistency. Always keep the cap screwed on tightly to prevent oxidation and evaporation.

3. Cinnamon Bark

Description

Cinnamon bark (Cinnamomum Verum, C. zeylanicum, C. cassica) is harvested from a variety of evergreen tree that is native to Sri Lanka and India. The tree has thick, reddish-brown bark, small yellow flowers, and its leathery leaves have a spicy smell. It grows to a height of approximately 20-60 ft (8-18 m) and is found primarily in tropical forests. Cinnamon bark belongs to the Lauraceae family. Related species are Cinnamomum cassia and Cinnamomum saigonicum (Saigon Cinnamon).

Cinnamon bark is cultivated in such tropical regions as the Philippines and the West Indies. It is not grown in the United States. Every two years the trees are cut to just above ground level. The bark is harvested from the new shoots, then dried.

The outer bark is stripped away, leaving the inner bark, which is the main medicinal part of the herb. Moses included cinnamon in an anointing oil that he used. By the seventeenth century, cinnamon was considered a culinary spice by Europeans. American nineteenth-century physicians prescribed cinnamon as a treatment for stomach cramps, nausea, vomiting, diarrhea, colic, and uterine problems.

General Use

Cinnamon bark is a common ingredient in many products such as toothpaste, mouthwash, perfume, soap, lipstick, chewing gum, cough syrup, nasal sprays, and cola drinks. A popular food flavoring, it is valued as one of the world's most important spices. It is also valuable in the treatment of various ailments. Modern herbalists prescribe cinnamon bark as a remedy for nausea, vomiting, diarrhea, and indigestion. Chinese herbalists recommend it for asthma brought on by cold, some digestive problems, backache, and menstrual problems.

The medicinal value of the herb is attributed to the oil extracted from the inner bark and leaves. The cinnamon bark harvested from the young branches is primarily used for culinary purposes. The cinnamon sticks commonly used in cooking are pieces of rolled outer bark.

The active ingredients of the bark contain antibacterial, antiseptic, antiviral, antispasmodic, and antifungal properties. A study published in 2002 indicates that oil from cinnamon bark inhibits the production of listeriolysin, a protein released by Listeria bacteria that destroys healthy cells. Japanese research has shown cinnamaldehyde, one of the constituents of cinnamon bark, to be sedative and analgesic. Eugenol, another component, contains pain-relieving qualities.

Cinnamon bark helps strengthen and support a weak digestive system. Research reports that cinnamon bark breaks down fats in the digestive system, making it a valuable digestive aid. It is used to treat nausea, vomiting, diarrhea, stomach ulcers, acid indigestion, heartburn, lack of appetite, and abdominal disorders.

A traditional stimulant in Chinese medicine, cinnamon bark has a warming effect on the body and is used for conditions caused by coldness. The twigs of cinnamon enhance circulation, especially to the fingers and toes. Cinnamon bark contains antiseptic properties that help to prevent infection by killing decay-causing bacteria, fungi, and viruses. One German study showed that the use of cinnamon bark suppressed the cause of most urinary tract infections and the fungus responsible for vaginal yeast infections. It is also helpful in relieving an athlete's foot.

Cinnamon bark is a frequent ingredient in toothpaste, mouthwash, and other oral hygiene products because it helps kill the bacteria that cause tooth decay and gum disease. Inflammations of the throat and pharynx may be relieved through its use.

Cinnamon bark is also known to control blood sugar levels in diabetics. United States Department of Agriculture (USDA) researchers have found that cinnamon bark may reduce the amount of insulin required for glucose metabolism. A dose of 1/8 to 1/4 tsp of ground cinnamon

Preparations

Cinnamon bark is available in several forms from Chinese pharmacists, Asian grocery stores, and health food stores: fresh or dried bulk, pill, tincture, and as an essential oil.

Dosage

In Chinese medicine, cinnamon is usually taken in combination with other herbs. Below are some typical dosages for cinnamon alone.

Tincture: Take up to 4 ml with water three times daily.

Tea: Take 1 cup 2–3 times daily at mealtimes.

Crushed: Take 1/2 tsp (2–4 g) daily.

Precautions

Cinnamon bark may cause an allergic reaction in some individuals.

Cinnamon bark is not recommended for pregnant or nursing women.

Do not take essential oil of cinnamon bark internally unless under professional supervision. Internal ingestion may cause nausea, vomiting, and possible kidney damage.

The essential oil of cinnamon bark is one of the most hazardous essential oils and should not be used on the skin. External application of the oil may cause redness and burning of the skin.

Cinnamon bark should not be given to children under two years of age.

Cinnamon bark is considered toxic if taken in excess.

Cinnamon bark should not be given to persons with inflammatory liver disease; in large quantities, it can irritate the liver.

Side Effects

Mild side effects include stomach upset, sweating, and diarrhea. Large doses can cause changes in breathing, dilation of blood vessels, sleepiness, depression, or convulsions. Excessive use of cinnamon bark may cause red, tender gums; mouth ulcers; inflamed taste buds; and a severe burning sensation in the mouth.

Interactions

Some interactions with other medications have been reported. Cinnamon oil may cause skin irritation if applied to the skin together with acne medications that contain retinoic acid.

Cinnamon bark has also been reported to intensify the effects of medications given to lower blood pressure. Persons taking cinnamon bark should discontinue its use two weeks before any surgery requiring general anesthesia because the herb tends to lower blood pressure.

4. Marjoram

Marjoram is a plant. You probably recognize it as a common cooking spice. But it also has an interesting place in early Greek mythology. As the story goes, the goddess of love, Aphrodite, grew marjoram, and, as a result, marjoram has been used ever since in various love potions.

People make medicine from marjoram's flowers, leaves, and oil. Tea made from the leaves or flowers is used for runny nose and colds in infants and toddlers, dry and irritating coughs, swollen nose and throat, and ear pain. Marjoram tea is also used for various digestion problems including poor appetite, liver disease, gallstones, intestinal gas, and stomach cramps.

Some women use marjoram tea for relieving symptoms of menopause, treating mood swings related to menstrual periods, starting menstruation, and promoting the flow of breast milk.

Other uses include treating diabetes, sleep problems, muscle spasms, headaches, sprains, bruises, and back pain. It is also used as a “nerve tonic” and a “heart tonic,” and to promote better blood circulation.

Marjoram oil is used for coughs, gall bladder complaints, stomach cramps, and digestive disorders, depression, dizziness, migraines, nervous headaches, nerve pain, paralysis, coughs, runny nose; and as a “water pill.”

Insufficient Evidence To Rate Effectiveness For

- Asthma
- Coughs
- Colds
- Runny nose
- Stomach cramps
- Colic
- Liver problems
- Gallstones
- Headache
- Diabetes
- Menopause symptoms
- Menstrual problems

- Nerve pain
- Muscle pain
- Sprains
- Promoting breast milk
- Improving appetite and digestion
- Improving sleep

How Does Marjoram Work?

There isn't enough information to know how marjoram might work.

Are There Safety Concerns?

Marjoram is likely safe in food amounts and possibly safe for most adults when taken by mouth in medicinal amounts for short periods. Marjoram is possibly unsafe when used long-term or when applied to the eye or skin as fresh marjoram. There is some evidence that marjoram could cause cancer if used long-term. Applying fresh marjoram might cause eye or skin irritation.

- Special Precautions & Warnings:
- Pregnancy and breast-feeding
- Children
- Bleeding disorders
- Slow heart rate (bradycardia)
- Allergy to basil, hyssop, lavender, mint, oregano, and sage
- Diabetes
- Gastrointestinal tract blockage
- Ulcers
- Lung conditions:
- Seizures
- Surgery
- Urinary tract obstruction

5. Vervain

Vervain (Verbena Officinalis) is a flowering plant in the verbena family of herbs. While there are well over 250 species of verbena, vervain refers specifically to the types used for medicinal purposes. In addition to V. Officinalis, less common varietals include blue vervain (V. hastata) and white vervain (V. urticifolia).

Verbena Officinalis is a perennial plant with delicate, jagged leaves and small, five-petaled blossoms. Although vervain has no scent, alternative practitioners believe that vervain has anti-inflammatory, antibacterial, antispasmodic, and analgesic (pain-relieving) properties beneficial to one's health.

Vervain is also referred to as American blue verbena, simpler's joy, holy herb, mosquito plant, and wild hyssop. In traditional Chinese medicine, it is known as mǎ biān cǎo. Verbena Officinalis should not be confused with lemon verbena, a garden herb used for cooking that also has medicinal properties.

Health Benefits

The medicinal use of vervain can be traced back to the 18th-century book "Sauer's Herbal Cure," where it was said to aid in the treatment of kidney stones. The name "verbena" is believed derived from the Celtic word ferfaen meaning "to drive away stones." Vervain regained popularly in the 1930s as one of the 38 flowering plants used in a homeopathic tincture called Bach Flower Remedy, variations of which are still sold today. Among its purported benefits, vervain may help treat:

- Headaches
- General aches and pain
- Insomnia
- Digestive dysfunction
- Upper respiratory tract symptoms
- Urinary tract infections
- Depression and anxiety

As with many homeopathic remedies, some of the health claims are better supported by research than others.

Possible Side Effects

As an herb, V. Officinalis is considered safe for consumption with a few side effects, namely indigestion, and gas.

The herb also produces an oily substance that may cause contact dermatitis, but a generally mild form with localized rash and redness. Before using a vervain tincture, always apply a little to the skin and wait an hour to see if a rash develops. Severe anaphylactic reactions are rare. It is not known if vervain interacts with other drugs. Advise your doctor about any supplements you are taking to avoid possible interactions.

Vervain should be avoided in people with kidney disease. The verbenalin found in the plant can irritate the kidneys if overused, causing inflammation and a potential worsening of the condition. Little is known about the long-term safety of vervain supplements. For this reason, they should not be used in children, people who are pregnant or breastfeeding, or for the treatment of any serious medical condition. Self-treating any medical condition without input from a qualified doctor or avoiding the standard care of treatment is unadvised and may put you in harm's ways.

Selection and Preparation

There are no guidelines for the appropriate use of vervain in treating medical conditions. Supplements are typically sold in capsule form but are also available as tinctures, extracts, astringents, teas, powders, and dried herbs. Capsules are available in doses ranging from 150 milligrams to 1,000 milligrams. When taken within this range, they are generally considered safe. Vervain supplements are intended for short-term use only. Dietary supplements in the United States are not regulated in the same way as pharmaceutical drugs. They are not required to undergo rigorous testing or research and, as such, can vary in quality.

6. Mints

The mint family (Labiatae or Lamiaceae) is a large group of dicotyledonous plants occurring worldwide in all types of climates except in extreme arctic and antarctic conditions. There are about 3,000 species in the mint family and 200 genera. The most diverse groups are the genus Salvia with 500 species, Hyptis with 350 species, and Scutellaria, Coleus, Plectranthus, and Stachys, each with 200 species. Some species in the mint family are economically important and are grown as herbs used to flavor foods and beverages or for the production of essential oils that are used as fragrances in perfumery. Some species are also grown as showy or fragrant ornamentals in gardens.

Biology of Mints

Most species in the mint family are annuals or herb-like perennials, and a few species are shrubs. Most species of mints have aromatic glands and hairs on their stems and foliage, and when the leaves are crushed strongly scented vapors are released. The stems of mints are commonly four-sided in cross-section, and most species have oppositely arranged leaves.

The flowers of mints are bilaterally symmetric. Because they are mostly pollinated by insects, mints have relatively brightly colored, nectar-rich flowers usually grouped into a larger inflorescence The lower, fused petals of the flower provide a platform for pollinators to land on called a lip (or in Latin, labia, from which the family name Labiatae is derived). Most species in the mint family have bisexual flowers, containing both male (staminate) and female (pistillate) organs. The fruits are small, one-seeded nutlets.

Native Mints Of North America

Many species in the mint family are native to natural plant communities of North America. Many additional species have been introduced from Eurasia and elsewhere, especially species that are grown in agriculture or horticulture, and some of these have escaped from gardens and become naturalized in appropriate habitats in North America.

Some of the more interesting and attractive groups of native species include the skullcaps (Scutellaria) spp., physostegias (Physostegia) spp., hemp-nettles (Stachys) spp., sages (Salvia) spp., horse-mints or bergamots (Monarda) spp., bugle-weeds (Lycopus) spp., and true mints (Mentha) spp.

Economic Products Obtained From Mints

Several herbs are derived from aromatic species in the mint family, sometimes as cultivars that have been selectively bred to enhance the aromatic qualities of the plants. The most commonly known of these herbs are derived from several herbaceous, perennial species in the genus Mentha, originally native to Eurasia but now cultivated widely in suitable, usually temperate climates. The common mint (Mentha arvensis), spearmint (M. spicata), and peppermint (M. Piperita) are all used to flavor candies, chewing gum, toothpaste, and tea, and are sometimes used to prepare condiments to serve with meats and other foods.

The hoarhound (Marrubium vulgare) of Europe and Asia is another species used to flavor candies. Common sage (Salvia officinalis) is used to flavor foods, toothpaste, and mouthwash. Sweet marjoram (Origanum majorana) is used to flavor some types of cooked meats, stews, and other foods, as are basil (Ocimum basilicum), rosemary (Rosmarinus officinalis), summer savory (Satureja hortensis), thyme (Thymus vulgaris), hyssop (Hyssopus officinalis), clary (Salvia sclarea), and balm (Melissa officinalis).

Various species in the mint family contain aromatic essential oils that can be extracted and used to scent potpourri and other decorations or as fragrances in the mixing of perfumes. Lavender (Lavandula officinalis) is a Mediterranean shrub that is commonly used for these purposes. Lavender is an important ingredient of eau de cologne and lavender water, and it is commonly dried and put into small bags called sachets and used to scent clothing cupboards and drawers. Other species of the mint family from which

Key Terms

Bilateral Symmetry: About flower shape, this means that vertical sectioning of the flower will produce two halves with symmetric features.

Cultivar: A distinct variety of a plant that has been bred for particular, agricultural or culinary attributes. Cultivars are not sufficiently distinct in the genetic sense to be considered to be subspecies.

Essential Oil: These are various types of volatile organic oils that occur in plants and can be extracted for use in perfumery and flavoring.

Inflorescence: A grouping or arrangement of florets or flowers into a composite structure, often to make the flowers more attractive to animal pollinators.

Nutlet: A diminutive nut, or a small, dry, one-seeded fruit with a hard coat.

Mints As Ornamental Plants

Some species in the mint family are commonly grown indoors or in gardens as leafy ornamentals. One of the more popular groups of foliage plants is the various species and varieties of coleus (Coleus spp.,) bee-balm (Monarda fistulosa), bergamot (Monarda didyma), gardens (Salvia splendens), and common sage (Salvia officinalis).

Mints As Weeds

Many species in the mint family are grown in gardens and agriculture, and these have been transported around the world for cultivation in suitable climates. In some cases, these species have escaped from cultivation and have become minor weeds of agriculture, lawns, and disturbed areas. Examples of such weeds in North America include catnip, ground-ivy (Glechoma hederacea), heal-all (Prunella vulgaris), hemp-nettle (Galeopsis tetrahit), henbit (Lamium amplexicaule), and motherwort (Leonurus cardiaca).

7. What Is Dill?

Dill is a plant that has a long history as a culinary spice. But it has also been used as a magic weapon and a medicine. During the Middle Ages, people used dill to defend against witchcraft and enchantments. More recently, people have used dill seeds and the parts of the plant that grow above the ground as medicine. Dill is used for digestion problems including loss of appetite, intestinal gas (flatulence), liver problems, and gallbladder complaints. It is also used for urinary tract disorders including kidney disease and painful or difficult urination.

Other uses for dill include treatment of fever and colds, cough, bronchitis, hemorrhoids, infections, spasms, nerve pain, genital ulcers, menstrual cramps, and sleep disorders. Dill seed is sometimes applied to the mouth and throat for pain and swelling (inflammation).

- Insufficient Evidence To Rate Effectiveness For
- Loss of appetite
- Infections
- Digestive tract problems
- Urinary tract problems
- Spasms
- Intestinal gas (flatulence)
- Sleep disorders
- Fever
- Colds
- Cough
- Bronchitis
- Liver problems
- Gallbladder problems
- Sore mouth and throat

How Does Dill Work?

Some chemicals contained in dill seed might help relax muscles. Other chemicals might be able to fight bacteria and increase urine production like a "water pill."

Are There Safety Concerns?

Dill is likely safe when consumed as a food. Dill is possibly safe for most people when taken by mouth as a medicine. When applied to the skin, dill can sometimes cause skin irritation. Fresh dill juice can also cause the skin to become extra sensitive to the sun. This might put you at greater risk for sunburns and skin cancer. Avoid sunlight. Wear sunblock and protective clothing outside, especially if you are light-skinned.

- Special Precautions & Warnings:
- Pregnancy and breast-feeding
- Allergy to plants in the carrot family
- Diabetes
- Surgery

8. Myrrh

Myrrh is a sap-like substance (resin) that comes out of cuts in the bark of trees that are members of the Commiphora species. Commiphora Mukul, a related species, is not a source of myrrh. Myrrh is used to make medicine. Myrrh is used for indigestion, ulcers, colds, cough, asthma, lung congestion, arthritis pain, cancer, leprosy, spasms, and syphilis. It is also used as a stimulant and to increase menstrual flow. Myrrh is applied directly to the mouth for soreness and swelling, inflamed gums (gingivitis), loose teeth, canker sores, bad breath, and chapped lips. It is also used topically for hemorrhoids, bedsores, wounds, abrasions, and boils.

Insufficient Evidence to Rate Effectiveness For

- Indigestion
- Ulcers
- Colds
- Cough
- Asthma
- Congestion
- Joint pain
- Hemorrhoids
- Bad breath
- Sore mouth or throat
- How Does Myrrh Work?
- Myrrh can help decrease swelling (inflammation) and kill bacteria.

Are There Safety Concerns?

Myrrh seems safe for most people when used in small amounts. It can cause some side effects such as skin rash if applied directly to the skin, and diarrhea if taken by mouth. Large doses may be unsafe. Amounts greater than 2-4 grams can cause kidney irritation and heart rate changes.

- Special Precautions & Warnings:
- Pregnancy and breast-feeding
- Diabetes
- Fever
- Heart problems
- Surgery
- Systemic inflammation
- Uterine bleeding

9. Dragon Blood

Blood of the dragon (Croton lechleri) is a flowering tree found throughout South America. It gets its name from its dark red, latex-containing sap, which has long been used to treat traveler's diarrhea and help heal wounds. Among practitioners of alternative and traditional herbal medicine, the sap is also believed to offer antioxidant and anti-inflammatory properties that may prevent or treat peptic ulcers, indigestion, and certain forms of cancer. Some of these claims are better supported by research than others.

Also Known As

- Dragon's blood
- Sangre de drago (Ecuadorian Spanish)
- Sangre de Grado (Peruvian Spanish)
- Sangue do dragão (Portuguese)

Health Benefits

Blood of the dragon has both proven and unproven medical benefits. Current research supports its use in treating certain forms of diarrhea. Claims that it can treat ulcers, reduce fever, swelling, and redness, or promote wound healing are more loosely supported. There is currently no evidence that the blood of the dragon can aid in the treatment or prevention of cancer, although there are some promising findings.

Possible Side Effects

Little is known about the long-term safety of the blood of the dragon. When taken by mouth, common side effects may include:

- Flatulence
- Cough
- Nausea
- Bronchitis

When applied topically, the blood of the dragon may cause a burning or stinging sensation. Blood of the dragon may also increase bilirubin levels in the blood, indicating liver inflammation. As such, liver function should be checked before beginning blood of the dragon supplements, as well as periodically during use. People with liver impairment should use these supplements with caution, ideally under the care of a qualified physician.

Because the blood of the dragon affects calcium channels, it may amplify the action of calcium channel blockers and increase the risk of side effects, including headaches, dizziness, flushing, and palpitations. The safety of blood of the dragon supplements in pregnant women, nursing mothers, and children has not been established. It is always best to advise your doctor if you are using or planning to use the blood of the dragon so that your condition can be monitored.

Selection, Preparation, And Storage

In the United States, the blood of the dragon is mainly sold in liquid extract or tincture forms. Dried C. lechleri sap is also available, as are oral capsules or tablets and topical soaps or creams. You may also notice the blood of the dragon listed as an ingredient in certain higher-end skincare products. There are no guidelines for the appropriate use of the blood of the dragon. Some manufacturers endorse the use of the blood of the dragon tincture for both topical and oral use; the safety of this practice is unknown. Others offer their tinctures purely for skincare purposes, which is generally safer. Blood of the dragon capsules or tablets offers consistent dosing. Per manufacturers, they are generally dosed at 100 to 500 milligrams (mg) per day.

Because few manufacturers of the blood of the dragon products voluntarily submit their products for quality testing, and such testing is not required by the FDA, it is up to you to make an informed choice when choosing brands. Here are some tips that can help:

1. Always Read The Product Label: It should say "Croton lechleri," not just "blood of the dragon." It should also state the percentage of C. lechleri in the formulation as well as any inactive ingredients (such as carrier oils or preservatives). If you don't know what an ingredient is, ask your pharmacist.

2. Buy Organic: Organic goods are less likely to expose you to pesticides and other unwanted chemicals. For a product to be labeled organic, it must be certified by the U.S. Department of Agriculture (USDA).

3. Avoid Wildcrafted Products: These include powders, resins, and dried bark that are marketed as blood in the dragon in its "most natural form." There is no way of knowing if these products are contaminated or even authentic.

4. Don't Assume That Higher Prices Mean Higher Quality: Instead, follow the above guidelines and omit from consideration any product that doesn't meet these minimum requirements. If you're not 100% sure about a product, it is best not to use it. Most blood of the dragon products can be stored safely at room temperature.

10. Frankincense Essential Oil

An essential oil commonly used in aromatherapy, frankincense oil is typically sourced from the resin of the Boswellia carterii or Boswellia sacra tree. Also called olibanum, frankincense oil has a sweet, woody scent and is sometimes used to ease stress. People use it to make medicine. Frankincense is used for pain and swelling in people with various diseases. Also used for gas (flatulence), wound healing, and many other conditions, but there is no good scientific evidence to support any use. Frankincense is also used as a flavoring agent in foods and as a fragrance in soaps, lotions, and perfumes.

- Commonly Known As
- Frankincense
- Boswellia carterii
- Boswellia sacra
- Olibanum

In aromatherapy, inhaling the scent of essential oil (or absorbing it through the skin) is thought to send messages to the limbic system, a brain region that influences our emotions and nervous systems. Proponents suggest that essential oils may affect several biological factors, such as heart rate, stress levels, blood pressure, breathing, and immune function. Frankincense essential oil is also used as an ingredient in perfume, incense, and skin care products.

Uses

In aromatherapy, frankincense oil is typically used for the following conditions:

- Anxiety
- Colds
- Coughs
- Indigestion
- Ulcers

Frankincense essential oil is also used to alleviate stress and relieve pain. When used as an ingredient in skin care products, frankincense essential oil is said to treat dry skin and reduce the appearance of wrinkles, age spots, scars, and stretch marks.

Health Benefits

While preliminary research suggests that frankincense essential oil may offer certain health benefits, there is currently a lack of research testing the health effects of frankincense oil. A component in frankincense, boswellic acid, has been studied for its anti-inflammatory and anti-tumor properties. Here's a look at the science.

Possible Side Effects

In addition, some individuals may experience irritation or an allergic reaction when applying frankincense essential oil to the skin. A skin patch test should be done before using any new essential oil. Additionally, essential oils shouldn't be applied to the skin undiluted.

Pregnant or nursing women and children should consult their healthcare providers before using essential oils. It's also important to note that self-treating a condition with frankincense essential oil and avoiding or delaying standard care may have serious consequences.

Dosage And Preparation

There is no standard or recommended dose for frankincense essential oil. When a drop or two is combined with a carrier oil (such as jojoba, sweet almond, or avocado oil), frankincense essential oil can be applied to the skin or added to baths in small amounts. Frankincense essential oil can also be inhaled after sprinkling a drop or two of the oil onto a cloth or tissue, or by using an aromatherapy diffuser or vaporizer. In aromatherapy, several other essential oils are often used in combination with frankincense.

What To Look For

Essential oils are not regulated by the FDA and do not have to meet any purity standards. When purchasing essential oils, look for a supplier who either distills their material or deals directly with reputable distillers and uses gas chromatography and mass spectrometry (GC/MS) to analyze the quality of the product. When buying pure frankincense essential oil, check the label for its Latin name, Boswellia carterii or Boswellia sacra. No other oil ingredients should be listed. If you see another oil, such as fractionated coconut oil, jojoba oil, or sweet almond oil, the frankincense is diluted and should not be used in a diffuser. Essential oils should be packaged in a dark amber or cobalt bottle and stored out of sunlight.

Is It Safe To Ingest Frankincense Essential Oil?

While some essential oil companies recommend ingesting frankincense essential oil for a wide variety of health ailments, there is no evidence to support its safety or efficacy. If you choose to ingest essential oils, be sure you are using pure oils and follow the manufacturer's directions carefully and discuss it further with your doctor.

Can Frankincense Essential Oil Be Applied Directly To The Skin?

Frankincense is a mild oil and most people can apply it directly to the skin, or neat, without any issues. However, if you experience any burning, tingling, or irritation, dilute the oil by rubbing a carrier oil, such as fractionated coconut oil, jojoba oil, or grapeseed oil, over the irritated area. Do not apply frankincense oil close to your eyes as its vapors may irritate your eyes.

11. Thyme

Thyme is an herb. The flowers, leaves, and oil are used as medicine. Thyme is sometimes used in combination with other herbs. Thyme is taken by mouth for bronchitis, whooping cough, sore throat, colic, arthritis, upset stomach, stomach pain (gastritis), diarrhea, bedwetting, a movement disorder in children (dyspraxia), intestinal gas (flatulence), parasitic worm infections, and skin disorders. It is also used to increase urine flow (as a diuretic), disinfect the urine, and as an appetite stimulant.

Some people apply thyme directly to the skin for hoarseness (laryngitis), swollen tonsils (tonsillitis), sore mouth, and bad breath. Thyme oil is used as a germ-killer in mouthwashes and liniments. It is also applied to the scalp to treat baldness and to the ears to fight bacterial and fungal infections. Thymol, one of the chemicals in thyme, is used with another chemical, chlorhexidine, as a dental varnish to prevent tooth decay.

Possibly Effective For

1. Bronchitis: Some research suggests that taking thyme by mouth, in combination with various other herbs, improves symptoms of bronchitis such as coughing, fever, and increased production of sputum in adults, children, and teenagers.

2. Cough: Some research suggests that taking thyme by mouth, alone or in combination with various other herbs, reduces coughing in people with bronchitis, upper respiratory tract infections, or common colds.

Insufficient Evidence To Rate Effectiveness For

- Agitation
- Hair loss (alopecia areata)
- Movement disorders (dyspraxia)
- Colic.
- Ear infections.
- Swelling (inflammation) of the tonsils.
- Preventing bedwetting.
- Sore throat.
- Bad breath.
- Swelling (inflammation) of the lungs and mouth.

How Does Thyme Work?

Thyme contains chemicals that might help bacterial and fungal infections and minor irritations. It also might relieve smooth muscle spasms, such as coughing.

Are There Safety Concerns?

Thyme is likely safe when consumed in normal food amounts. Thyme is possibly safe when taken as medicine for short periods. It can cause digestive system upset. Thyme oil is possibly safe when applied to the skin. In some people, applying the oil to the skin can irritate. But there isn't enough information to know whether thyme oil is safe to take by mouth in medicinal doses.

Special Precautions & Warnings:

- Children
- Allergy to oregano and similar plants
- Bleeding disorders
- Hormone-sensitive conditions such as breast cancer, uterine cancer, ovarian cancer, endometriosis, or uterine fibroids
- Surgery

12. Allspice

Allspice is a plant. The unripe berries and leaves of the plant are used to make medicine. Allspice is used for indigestion (dyspepsia), intestinal gas, abdominal pain, heavy menstrual periods, vomiting, diarrhea, fever, colds, high blood pressure, diabetes, and obesity. It is also used for emptying the bowels. Some people apply allspice directly to the affected area for muscle pain and toothache or put it on the skin to kill germs. Some dentists use eugenol, a chemical contained in allspice, to kill germs on teeth and gums.

Insufficient Evidence To Rate Effectiveness For

- Intestinal gas
- Indigestion
- Vomiting
- Diarrhea
- Fever & Flu
- Colds
- Heavy menstrual bleeding
- Emptying the bowels

How Does Allspice Work?

Allspice contains a chemical called eugenol, which might explain some of its traditional uses for toothache, muscle pain, and as a germ-killer.

Are There Safety Concerns?

Allspice is safe for most adults when used as a spice. However, there is not enough information available to know if allspice is safe in medicinal amounts. When applied directly to the skin, allspice can cause allergic skin reactions in sensitive people.

Special Precautions & Warnings

1. Pregnancy And Breastfeeding: Allspice is safe for pregnant and breastfeeding women in food amounts. But larger medicinal amounts should be avoided until more is known.

2. Surgery: Allspice can slow blood clotting. There is some concern that it might increase the chance of bleeding during and after surgery. Stop using allspice at least 2 weeks before a scheduled surgery.

Are There Any Interactions With Medications?

1. Medications That Slow Blood Clotting (Anticoagulant / Antiplatelet Drugs) Interaction Rating: Moderate Be cautious with this combination. Talk with your health provider.

2. Allspice Might Slow Blood Clotting: Taking allspice along with medications that also slow clotting might increase the chances of bruising and bleeding.

3. Allspice Contains Eugenol: Eugenol is the part of allspice that might slow blood clotting. Eugenol is very fragrant and gives allspice and cloves their distinctive smell.

Some medications that slow blood clotting include aspirin, clopidogrel (Plavix), diclofenac (Voltaren, Cataflam, others), ibuprofen (Advil, Motrin, others), and others.

Dosing Considerations For Herbs Of Wealth And Power

The appropriate dose of those herbs of wealth and power listed above should be appropriately followed depending on several factors such as the user's age, health, and several other conditions. At this time there is not enough scientific information to determine an appropriate range of doses for thyme. Keep in mind that natural products are not always necessarily safe and dosages can be important. Be sure to follow relevant directions on product labels and consult your pharmacist or physician or other healthcare professional before using.

CHAPTER 2: HERBS FOR HEALING

1. Anise

Anise is an herb. The seed and oil are used to make medicine. Less commonly, the root and leaf are used to make medicine as well. Do not confuse anise with other herbs called star anise or fennel. These are sometimes called anise. Anise is most commonly used for indigestion (dyspepsia) and a long-term disorder of the large intestines that causes stomach pain (irritable bowel syndrome or IBS). It is also used for many other conditions, but there is no good scientific evidence to support most of these uses.

In foods, anise is used as a flavoring agent. It has a sweet, aromatic taste that resembles the taste of black licorice. It is commonly used in alcohols and liqueurs, such as anisette and ouzo. Anise is also used in dairy products, gelatins, meats, candies, and breath fresheners. In manufacturing, anise is often used as a fragrance in soap, creams, perfumes, and sachets.

How Does It Work?

There are chemicals in anise that may have estrogen-like effects. Chemicals in anise may also act as insecticides and decrease swelling or inflammation.

Uses & Effectiveness?

Possibly Effective For

Indigestion (Dyspepsia): Some research shows that taking anise powder daily for 4 weeks reduces stomach discomfort, bloating, and pain following a meal in people who have indigestion after eating.

A Long-Term Disorder Of The Large Intestines That Causes Stomach Pain (Irritable Bowel Syndrome Or IBS): Some research shows that taking a capsule containing anise oil daily reduces pain and bloating in people with IBS.

Insufficient Evidence For

- Asthma
- Depression
- Diabetes
- Lice
- Symptoms of menopause
- Migraine
- Premenstrual syndrome (PMS)

- Cough
- Increasing breast milk
- Increasing sex drive
- Itchy skin infection caused by mites (scabies)
- Scaly, itchy skin (psoriasis)
- Spasms
- Starting menstrual periods

Side Effects

When Taken By Mouth: Anise is likely safe for most adults when taken in amounts typically found in foods. Anise powder and oil are possibly safe when taken as medicine for up to 4 weeks.

Special Precautions And Warnings

- Pregnancy and breast-feeding
- Children
- Allergies
- Diabetes

Hormone-sensitive condition such as breast cancer, uterine cancer, ovarian cancer, endometriosis, or uterine fibroids

Surgery

2. Arnica

Arnica is an herb that grows mainly in Siberia and central Europe, as well as temperate climates in North America. The flowers of the plant are used in medicine. Arnica is most commonly used for pain caused by osteoarthritis, sore throat, surgery, and other conditions. Arnica is also used for bleeding, bruising, swelling after surgery, and other conditions, but there is no good scientific evidence to support these uses. Arnica can also be unsafe when taken by mouth.

In foods, arnica is a flavor ingredient in beverages, frozen dairy desserts, candy, baked goods, gelatins, and puddings. In manufacturing, arnica is used in hair tonics and anti-dandruff preparations. The oil is used in perfumes and cosmetics.

How Does It Work?

The active chemicals in arnica may reduce swelling, decrease pain, and act as antibiotics.

Uses & Effectiveness?

Possibly Effective For

Osteoarthritis

Early research shows that using an arnica gel product (A. Vogel Arnica Gel, Bioforce AG) twice daily for 3 weeks reduces pain and stiffness and improves function in people with osteoarthritis in the hand or knee. Other research shows that using the same gel works as well as the painkiller ibuprofen in reducing pain and improving function in the hands.

Possibly Ineffective For

Reducing pain, swelling, and complications of wisdom tooth removal. In most research, taking arnica by mouth does not seem to reduce pain, swelling, or complications after wisdom tooth removal. One early study suggests that taking six doses of homeopathic arnica 30C might reduce pain, but not bleeding.

Insufficient Evidence For

- Bleeding
- Stroke
- Acne
- Chapped lips
- Insect bites
- Painful, swollen veins near the surface of the skin
- Sore throats

Side Effects

Arnica is possibly safe when taken by mouth in the amounts commonly found in food or when applied to unbroken skin short-term. Amounts that are larger than the amount found in food are likely unsafe when taken by mouth. Arnica is considered poisonous and has caused death. When taken by mouth it can also irritate the mouth and throat, stomach pain, vomiting, diarrhea, skin rashes, shortness of breath, a fast heartbeat, an increase in blood pressure, heart damage, organ failure, increased bleeding, coma, and death. Arnica is often listed as an ingredient in homeopathic products; however, these products are usually so dilute that they contain little or no detectable amount of arnica.

Special Precautions And Warnings

Pregnancy and breast-feeding

Allergy to ragweed and related plants: Arnica may cause an allergic reaction in people who are sensitive to the Asteraceae/Compositae family. Members of this family include ragweed, chrysanthemums, marigolds, daisies, and many others. If you have allergies, be sure to check with your healthcare provider before applying them to your skin. Do not take arnica by mouth.

- Broken skin
- Fast heart rate
- High blood pressure
- Surgery

3. Boldo

Boldo is a tree that grows in the Andes mountains in South America. Interestingly, fossilized boldo leaves dating from over thirteen thousand years ago have been found in Chile. These fossils have imprints of human teeth, suggesting that boldo has a long history of dietary or medicinal use. Boldo is used for mild gastrointestinal (GI) spasms, gallstones, achy joints (rheumatism), bladder infections, liver disease, and gonorrhea. It is also to increase urine flow to rid the body of excess fluids, reduce anxiety, increase bile flow, and kill bacteria.

Insufficient Evidence To Rate Effectiveness For

- Gallstones
- Achy joints (rheumatism)
- Bladder infections
- Liver disease
- Anxiety
- Gonorrhea
- Fluid retention
- Constipation or flushing out of the bowels
- Mild stomach or intestinal spasms

How Does Boldo Work?

Boldo contains chemicals that might increase urine output, fight bacterial growth in the urine, and stimulate the stomach.

Are There Safety Concerns?

Boldo might be UNSAFE when used for medicinal purposes. Poisoning by ascaridole, a chemical that occurs naturally in boldo, has occurred in people taking boldo. Boldo might cause liver damage when taken by mouth. If you take boldo, use only ascaridole-free preparations. When applied to the skin, boldo can irritate.

Special Precautions & Warnings

Pregnancy and breast-feeding

Bile duct blockage: Boldo seems to be able to increase the flow of bile, a fluid produced by the liver and stored in the gallbladder. Bile passes through small channels (ducts) in the intestine where it plays an important role in digesting fats. These ducts can become blocked. There is a concern that the extra bile flow caused by boldo might be harmful in people with blocked bile ducts.

Liver disease

Surgery

4. Bacopa

Brahmi is a plant that has been used in traditional Indian medicine (Ayurveda). Be careful not to confuse Brahmi (Bacopa monnieri) with Gotu kola and other natural medicines that are also sometimes called Brahmi. Brahmi is used for Alzheimer's disease, improving memory, anxiety, attention deficit-hyperactivity disorder (ADHD), allergic conditions, irritable bowel syndrome, and as a general tonic to fight stress. People also take Brahmi to treat backache, hoarseness, mental illness, epilepsy, joint pain, and sexual performance problems in both men and women. It is also sometimes used as a "water pill."

Possibly Effective For

Improving memory. Some research shows that taking specific Bacopa extracts (KeenMind; BacoMind) improves some measure of memory in otherwise healthy older adults. Also, taking Bacopa extract seems to improve some measures of memory and hand-eye coordination in children aged 6-8 years.

Possibly Ineffective For

Irritable bowel syndrome (IBS). Bacopa appears to be no more effective than a sugar pill in keeping IBS symptoms from returning after remission.

Insufficient Evidence To Rate Effectiveness For

Anxiety: Early research suggests that taking 30 mL of Bacopa syrup daily for 4 weeks reduces symptoms of anxiety, including nervousness, racing heart, trouble sleeping, headaches, tiredness, difficulty concentrating, and stomach discomfort.

Epilepsy (seizures): Early research suggests that taking Bacopa extract for 5 months prevents seizures in some people with epilepsy.

- Asthma
- Backache
- Hoarseness
- Mental illness
- Joint pain (rheumatism)
- Sexual problems
- Fluid retention

How Does Bacopa Work?

Brahmi might increase certain brain chemicals that are involved in thinking, learning, and memory. Some research suggests that it might also protect brain cells from chemicals involved in Alzheimer's disease.

Are There Safety Concerns?

Bacopa extract is POSSIBLY SAFE for adults when taken by mouth appropriately and short-term, up to 12 weeks. Common side effects include increased bowel movements, stomach cramps, nausea, dry mouth, and fatigue.

Special Precautions & Warnings

Pregnancy And Breastfeeding: There is not enough reliable information about the safety of taking Bacopa if you are pregnant or breastfeeding. Stay on the safe side and avoid use.

Slow Heart Rate (Bradycardia): Bacopa might slow down the heartbeat. This could be a problem in people who already have a slow heart rate.

Gastrointestinal tract blockage

Ulcers

Lung conditions

Thyroid disorders

Urinary tract obstruction

Dosing Considerations For Bacopa.

The following doses have been studied in scientific research:

By Mouth:

For Improving Memory And Thinking: A dosage of 300 mg Brahmi extract per day for 12 weeks.

5. Cannabis

Cannabis, (genus Cannabis), a genus of medicinal, recreational, and fiber plants belonging to the family Cannabaceae. By some classifications, the genus Cannabis comprises a single species, hemp (Cannabis sativa), a stout, aromatic, erect annual herb that originated in Central Asia and is now cultivated worldwide.

What Is Cannabis?

Cannabis is a plant. People use dried leaves, seed oil, and other parts of the cannabis plant for recreational and medicinal purposes. It can have a pleasurable effect and may soothe the symptoms of various conditions, such as chronic pain.

Ways Of Using It Include:

- Smoking or vaping it
- Brewing it as a tea
- Consuming it in the form of edibles, such as brownies or candies
- Eating it raw
- Applying it as a topical treatment
- Taking it as capsules or supplements

Some of the ingredients in cannabis are psychoactive (mind-altering), but others are not. The potency and balance of the ingredients vary, depending on how the manufacturer grows and processes the plant.

What Are CBD And THC?

Cannabis contains at least 120Trusted Source active ingredients, or cannabinoids. The most abundant ones are cannabidiol (CBD) and delta-9-tetrahydrocannabinol (THC). Some cannabinoids can have euphoric or psychoactive effects. THC produces both effects. CBD is present in various forms, including:

- Oils for applying to the skin

- Capsules, to take as a supplement
- Gummy candies

So far, most studies have focused on CBD and THC, but scientists are looking into the effects of other cannabinoids, too.

Medical Uses

According to the National Academies of Sciences, Engineering, and Medicine, there is conclusive evidence that cannabis or cannabinoids can help manage:

Chronic pain in adults

Nausea and vomiting resulting from chemotherapy treatment

Some symptoms of multiple sclerosis (ms)

There is moderate evidence that it can help with sleep problems relating to sleep apnea, fibromyalgia, chronic pain, and MS. Other conditions that it may be helpful for include:

- Low appetite
- Tourette's syndrome
- Anxiety, in some individuals

Effects

There are different ways of using cannabis, and the method can determine the effects of the drug.

1. Smoking Or Inhaling: A sense of elation can start within minutes and peak after 10–30 minutes. The feeling will typically wear off after about 2 hours.

2. Ingesting: If a person consumes products containing cannabis by mouth, they will usually feel the effects within 1 hour, and the sensations will peak after 2.5–3.5 hours. One study suggests that the type of edible affects the time it takes to feel the effect, with hard candies kicking in quicker.

3. Topical: Transdermal patches allow the ingredients to enter the body over a prolonged period. This steady infusion can benefit people who are using cannabis to treat pain and inflammation.

How Do Cannabinoids Work?

The human body naturally produces some cannabinoids through the endocannabinoid system. They act in a similar way to neurotransmitters, sending messages throughout the nervous system. These neurotransmitters affect brain areas that play a role in memory, thinking, concentration, movement, coordination, sensory and time perception, and pleasure. The receptors that respond to these cannabinoids also react to THC and other cannabinoids. In this way, cannabinoids from an outside source can change and disrupt normal brain function.

- THC appears to affect areas of the brain that control:
- Memory and attention
- Balance, posture, and coordination
- Reaction time

Due to these effects, a person should not drive a car, operate heavy machinery, or engage in risky physical activities after using cannabis. THC stimulates specific cannabinoid receptors that increase the release of dopamine. Dopamine is a neurotransmitter that relates to feelings of pleasure. THC can also affect sensory perception. Colors may seem brighter, music more vivid, and emotions more profound.

What Does A Person Feel?

When people use cannabis, they may notice the following effects:

- A feeling of elation or euphoria, known as a high Relaxation
- Changes in perception, for example, of color, time, and space
- An increase in appetite
- Feeling more talkative
- Risks

Using cannabis can also entail some risks. These include:

- Impairment of judgment
- Immune response
- Gum disease
- Memory loss
- Testicular cancer
- Cannabis Withdrawal

Quitting cannabis, after becoming dependent, is not life-threatening, but it can be uncomfortable.

Symptoms May Include:

- Irritability
- Mood changes
- Insomnia
- Cravings
- Restlessness
- Decreased appetite
- General discomfort

Symptoms tend to peak within the first week after stopping and last up to 2 weeks. Experts do not know exactly how frequent and long-term cannabis use affects a person's health. Both the short- and long-term effects may vary among individuals.

Takeaway

Cannabis contains chemicals that can have various effects on the human body. It is a popular recreational drug with some medicinal uses. Anyone who is considering using cannabis for any purpose should first check that it is legal to use in their state. They should also consider its possible effects on their mental and physical health. A doctor can be a good person to ask for advice.

Dosing Considerations For Herbs Of Healing.

The appropriate dose of herbs of healing for use as treatment depends on several factors such as the user's age, health, and several other conditions. At this time there is not enough scientific information to determine an appropriate range of doses for boldo. Keep in mind that natural products are not always necessarily safe and dosages can be important. Be sure to follow relevant directions on product labels and consult your pharmacist or physician or other healthcare professional before using.

CHAPTER 3: HERBS OF PROTECTION, GOODLUCK, AND FERTILITY

1. Belladonna

Description

Belladonna, more commonly known as deadly night-shade, Atropa belladonna, devil's cherries, devil's herb, divide, dwale, Mayberry, great morel, naughty man's cherries, and poison black cherry, is a perennial herb that has been valued for its medicinal properties for over five centuries. Belladonna is a member of the Solanaceae (nightshade) family and can be identified by its bell-shaped, purple flowers and cherry-sized green berries that mature to a dark purple or black color. The tall, branching plant can grow to a height of at least 5 ft (1.5 m), and is native to Europe, North Africa, and Asia and cultivated in North America and the United Kingdom. Belladonna has also been introduced to several places, including the United States and Ireland, and now grows wild.

Belladonna leaves are large (up to 10 in [25.4 cm] in length) and grow in pairs on either side of the plant stem. Near the flowers or blossoms, one of each leaf pair is noticeably smaller in size. Both the leaves and roots have a sharp, unpleasant odor and bitter taste. As the name deadly nightshade suggests, the herb is highly toxic if taken even when taken in extremely low concentrations.

General Use

Belladonna has a long history of medicinal applications in healthcare. Belladonna alkaloids are anticholinergic, which means that it works by blocking the certain nerve impulses involved in the parasympathetic nervous system, which regulates certain involuntary bodily functions or reflexes, including pupil dilation, heart rate, secretion of glands and organs, and the constriction of the bronchioles in the lungs and the alimentary canal (digestive tract).

Belladonna relaxes the smooth muscles of the internal organs and inhibits or dries up secretions (e.g., perspiration, mucous, breast milk, and saliva). Belladonna alkaloids, the active ingredients of the plant, include atropine and scopolamine. These alkaloids are extracted from the leaves and roots of the plant and administered either alone or in combination with other herbal remedies or prescription medications.

Belladonna alkaloids are used to treat a variety of symptoms and conditions, including:

Gastrointestinal Disorders: Because the alkaloids relax the smooth muscles of the gastrointestinal tract and reduce stomach acid secretions, it is useful in treating colitis, diverticulitis, irritable bowel syndrome, colic, diarrhea, and peptic ulcer.

Asthma: By relaxing the bronchioles, belladonna alleviates the wheezing symptoms of an asthma attack.

Excessive Sweating: Belladonna slows gland and organ secretion, which makes it useful in controlling conditions that cause excessive sweating.

Nighttime Incontinence: Belladonna acts as a diuretic and can help treat excessive nighttime urination and incontinence.

Headaches And Migraines: The pain-relieving properties of atropine, a belladonna alkaloid, are useful in treating headaches.

Muscle Pains And Spasms: Belladonna is frequently prescribed to ease severe menstrual cramps.

Motion Sickness: Scopolamine, an alkaloid of belladonna, helps treat motion sickness and vertigo.

Parkinson's Disease: Belladonna can alleviate the excessive sweating and salivation associated with the disease, as well as controlling tremors and muscle rigidity.

Biliary Colic: Muscle spasm, or colic, of the gallbladder and liver, can be relieved through the muscle-relaxing properties of belladonna.

Homeopathic Use

Belladonna is a frequently prescribed homeopathic remedy used to treat illnesses that manifest symptoms similar to those that belladonna poisoning triggers (i.e., high fever, nausea, delirium, muscle spasms, flushed skin, dilated pupils). These include the common cold, otitis media (earache), fever, arthritis, menstrual cramps, diverticulitis, muscle pain, sunstroke, toothache and teething, conjunctivitis, headaches, sore throat, and boils, and abscesses. As with all homeopathic remedies, the prescription of belladonna depends on the individual's overall symptom picture, mood, and temperament. When used as a homeopathic remedy, belladonna is administered in a highly diluted form to trigger the body's natural healing response without the risk of belladonna poisoning or death.

Preparations

Belladonna leaf is harvested between May and July and dried at temperatures no warmer than 140°F (60° C). The roots of Atropa belladonna plants that have reached two to four-year-old maturity are also harvested for herbal preparations in early fall between mid-October and mid-November. The roots are then cleaned and dried at temperatures no warmer than 122°F (50°C). After drying, the leaves and roots are crushed for use in several forms, including decoctions, tinctures, infusions, plasters, pills, suppositories, liquid solutions or suspensions, and powders. They can be used both alone and in combination with other herbs and medications.

It is extremely dangerous to self-prescribe belladonna, and it should always be taken under the direction of a doctor or other qualified healthcare professional. The frequency and quantity of dosage will depend on both the patient and the illness the herb is prescribed for, but the doses are always extremely small. For example, the Physicians Desk Reference (PDR) for Herbal Medicines recommends an average single dose of 0.05-0.10 g. Each patient's illness is different and some patients experience toxicity at unusually low doses.

For homeopathic remedies, the plant is broken apart and juice is extracted through a pressing process. The extract is then mixed with a water/alcohol solution by a ratio of either 1:10 or 1:100, and this process is repeated up to 30 times to form an extremely diluted dose of the extract. Homeopathic belladonna remedy is generally added to pellets of sugar for easier administration. The dilution and dosage frequency depends on the symptoms being treated, but homeopathic remedies are typically administered only until the patient starts to show signs of improvement so that the body's natural healing response can take over.

Belladonna is available by prescription both alone (in high concentration strength) and in combination with other drugs. Currently, available prescription combinations include belladonna with opium (for uterine pain), kaolin and pectin (for diarrhea), pheno-barbital (for menopausal symptoms and migraine prophylactic), other barbiturates (for insomnia and cramping and muscle spasms in the digestive tract), or belladonna and opium suppositories (for severe intestinal cramping).

Belladonna preparations should be stored in air-tight containers away from direct light. Under these conditions, most preparations will remain potent for up to three years.

Precautions

Ingestion of high concentrations of atropine, a potent alkaloid found in belladonna, can cause severe illness and death. Atropine is fatal in doses as small as 100 mg, which equals 5-50 g of belladonna herb, depending on the potency of the particular plant. For children, a fatal dose is even significantly less. For this reason, belladonna should never be used unless prescribed by a trained practitioner.

Individuals suffering from kidney disease, intestinal blockage, glaucoma, enlarged prostate, urinary blockage, severe ulcerative colitis, or myasthenia gravis are advised not to take belladonna, as are those patients with a known allergy to belladonna. Patients with any chronic health conditions should never take belladonna without a doctor's prescription.

Pregnant or breastfeeding women should avoid all but homeopathic belladonna unless prescribed by a doctor. Because of the sedative qualities of belladonna, individuals taking the herb should use caution when driving or operating machinery. Alcohol and other central nervous systems (CNS) depressants should also be avoided, as they may increase drowsiness and dizziness in the patient taking belladonna.

If individuals taking homeopathic dilutions of belladonna experience worsening of their symptoms (known as a homeopathic aggravation), they should contact their healthcare professional. A homeopathic aggravation can be an early indication that a remedy is working properly, but it can also be a sign that a different remedy is called for.

Side Effects

Toxic signs of belladonna include dry mouth, drowsiness, dizziness, constipation, and nausea. Some side effects, including pupil dilation, blurred vision, fever (due to the inability to perspire), inability to urinate, arrhythmia, and excessive dry mouth and eyes, can also be early indications of belladonna overdose. Individuals experiencing these side effects should inform their health care practitioner immediately.

Belladonna overdose is also indicated by a burning throat, delirium, restlessness and mania, hallucinations, difficulty breathing, and flushed skin that is hot and dry. Without proper treatment, constriction of the airway can cause suffocation. If any of these symptoms occur, individuals should seek emergency medical attention immediately.

Treatment of belladonna overdose is typically gastric lavage, which involves inserting a tube down the patient's throat and washing out the stomach with a solution of activated charcoal or tannic acid to neutralize the atropine. Oxygen may also be required until breathing is stabilized, and barbiturates may be administered to counteract mania and/or excitation.

Interactions

Certain medications may increase the effects of belladonna. These include central nervous system (CNS) depressants, monoamine oxidase (MAO) inhibitors, tricyclic antidepressants, quinidine, amantadine, antihistamines, and other anticholinergics. Other medications, including anticoagulants (blood thinners) and corticotropin (ACTH), become less effective when used with belladonna, while some drugs, such as diarrhea medicines containing kaolin and attapulgite, may decrease the therapeutic response to belladonna when they are taken with the herb. If you are taking these or any other medications or herbal remedies, let your healthcare professional know.

Individuals considering treatment with homeopathic dilutions of belladonna should consult their healthcare professional about possible interactions with certain foods, beverages, prescription medications, aromatic compounds, and other environmental elements that could counteract the efficacy of belladonna treatment.

2. Cactus

The cactus family or Cactaceae is made up of about 2,000 species of perennial plants with succulent stems, most of which are well-armed with sharp spines. The natural distribution of most cacti is American, ranging from southern British Columbia and southern Ontario in Canada, through much of the United States, to the tip of southern South America. One genus, Rhipsalis, occurs in Africa, Madagascar, and India, and is probably native there. Cacti usually inhabit deserts and other dry, open places. The major use of cacti by humans is as attractive, ornamental plants in gardens, or as indoor house plants. A few species produce edible fruits, and one yields peyote, a hallucinogenic drug.

Cacti are xerophytic plants, meaning they are physiologically and morphologically adapted to coping with the extreme water deficiencies of dry habitats, such as deserts. The xerophytic adaptations of cacti include:

Their succulent, water-retaining stems.

A thick, waxy cuticle and few or no leaves to greatly reduce the losses of water through transpiration.

Stems that are photosynthetic, so leaves are not required to execute this function.

Stems that are cylindrical or spherical, which reduces the surface to volume ratio, and helps to preserve moisture

Tolerance of high tissue temperatures

Protection of the biomass and moisture reserves from herbivores by an armament of stout spines

A physiological tolerance of long periods of drought, and

A periodic pattern of growth, productivity, and flowering, which takes advantage of the availability of moisture during the brief, rainy season, while the plant remains dormant at drier times of the year.

Cacti have a so-called crassulacean-acid metabolism, in which atmospheric carbon dioxide is only taken up during the night when the stomates are open. The carbon dioxide is fixed into four-carbon, organic acids, and can later be released within the plant, to be fixed into sugars by photosynthesis when the sun is shining during the daylight hours. Because this system allows stomates to be kept tightly closed during the day, crassulacean-acid metabolism is an efficient way of conserving water in dry environments.

Some plant species of dry habitats that are not related to cacti are nevertheless remarkably similar in appearance (at least, apart from their flowers and fruits, which are always distinctive among plant families). This is the result of convergent evolution, the similar evolutionary development of unrelated species or families that are subjected to comparable types of environmental selective pressures. Some species of spurges (family Euphorbiaceae) that grow in dry habitats are commonly thought by non-botanists to be cacti, even though they are quite unrelated.

Importance Of Cacti

Many species of cacti are highly prized by horticulturalists as botanical oddities and ornamental plants. These may be cultivated for their beautiful flowers, the aesthetics of their stems and spines, or merely because the plants have a strange-looking appearance. In addition, many people like to grow cacti because they are relatively easy to maintain, it does not matter much if you forget to water your cacti for a few days, or even a few weeks or more. Over-watering is usually the greatest risk to most cacti that are kept as house plants, because too much moisture will pre-dispose these drought-adapted plants to developing fungal and bacterial diseases, such as soft rot.

Virtually any of the native species of cacti of North America may be used in horticulture, as are many of the species of Central and South America. The genera Mammillaria and Opuntia are most commonly grown, but virtually any species may be found in cultivation around or in homes and greenhouses. One of the most common and familiar species is the Christmas cactus (Zygocactus elegans), a flat-stemmed, red-, pink-, or white-flowered species that is grown as a garden and house plant. This species blooms during the winter, and florists often induce this plant to bloom around Christmas-time when it is commonly sold as a living ornament to brighten homes during that festive season.

Many species of cacti can be rather easily transplanted from natural habitats into the vicinities of homes and businesses, where they may be used as central components of low-maintenance gardens in places where rainfall is sparse, and the development of grassy lawns would require excessive use of scarce and expensive water. Wild cacti are also collected to grow in or around the home and to develop private collections of these interesting plants.

The most commonly edible cactus fruit is that of Opuntia species, especially O. ficus-indica. The fruits of prickly pears, sometimes known as apples or tunas, can be eaten directly or used to make jelly. Prickly-pear fruits are considered to be a delicacy around Christmas time in some regions. Peyote or mescal buttons (Lophophora williamsii) is a cactus containing several alkaloids in its tissues that are used as a hallucinogen and folk medicine. Peyote is important in the culture of some tribes of native Amerindians in the southwestern United States and Mexico, especially in the vicinity of the Rio Grande River. These aboriginal peoples use peyote to induce religious experiences and revelations. Peyote is also commonly used as a recreational drug by many people, and by several religious cults. Some species of spiny cacti, such as Opuntia, are used as living fences, for example, to keep livestock out.

Key Terms

Berry: A soft, multi-seeded fruit, developed from a single, compound ovary.

Cuticle: A waxy, superficial layer that covers the foliage of vascular plants, and the stems of cacti.

Monoecious: This is a plant breeding system in which male and female reproductive structures are present on the same plant, and in the case of cacti, in the same flowers.

Perfect: In the botanical sense, this refers to flowers that are bisexual, containing both male and female reproductive parts.

Stomate: These are microscopic pores in the leaf or stem cuticle, bordered by guard cells that control the opening or closing of the pore.

Succulent: Having thick, fleshy leaves or stems that conserve moisture.

Xerophyte: A plant adapted to dry or drought-prone habitats of gardens. The long, sharp spines of other cacti were used as needles in some of the earliest types of phonographs. The "wood" of the saguaro cactus has long been used by Amerindian peoples and is still utilized to make crafts and novelty furniture.

3. Fennel

Description

Fennel (Foeniculum vulgare), also known as F. officinale, is a member of the Umbelliferae (Apiaceae) or carrot family, along with dill (Anethum graveolens), caraway (Carum carvi), and anise (Pimpinella anisum). Fennel has a thick, spindle-shaped taproot that produces a pithy, smooth, or finely-fluted round stem that may reach 6 ft (1.8 m) in height. The finely divided leaves, with numerous thread-like segments, grow from a sheath surrounding the stalk at the base of the leaf stem. The delicate, blue-green filiform leaf segments have a pungent scent, somewhat similar to licorice, and an anise-like flavor. This characteristic is due to the presence of the phytochemical anethole, also a primary constituent of anise oil. Fennel's tiny yellow flowers form in large, compound umbels. The blossoms are frequently visited by bees, wasps, and other insects, and fennel leaf is a favorite food of the swallowtail-butterfly.

Fennel was introduced to North America by Spanish missionaries for cultivation in their medicinal gardens. Fennel escaped cultivation from the mission gardens and is now known in California as wild anise. English settlers brought the herb with them to the New England colonies where it became part of their kitchen gardens. In Puritan folk medicine fennel was taken as a digestive aid. The herb is still found growing on the sites of these early English settlements. This attractive, aromatic, and sun-loving herb thrives on roadsides, embankments, sea cliffs, and in dry, stony fields.

General Use

The seeds, leaves, and roots of fennel are safe and edible. The essential oil, extracted from the seeds, is toxic even in small amounts. Fennel has been widely used in culinary and medicinal preparations for centuries. The herb acts as a carminative and was traditionally employed as a digestive aid and remedy for flatulence. An infusion or decoction of the dried seeds is anti-spasmodic and will ease stomach pains and speed up the digestion of fatty foods. Fennel is a proven remedy for colic in infants and is safe when administered as a mild infusion of the leaf and seed. It is also used for coughs and colds. Fennel exerts a calming influence on the bronchial tissues. The seeds contain large amounts of phytochemical alpha-pinene, which acts as an expectorant and helps to loosen phlegm in the lungs. An eyewash, prepared from a decoction of the crushed seeds, is said to improve eyesight and reduce irritation and eye strain. Fennel has a long history of use as a galactagogue. The seed, when boiled in barley water, acts to increase the flow of breast milk in nursing mothers. A poultice of the herb may be helpful to relieve swelling of the breasts during lactation. A leaf and seed tea has been used to expel hookworm and kill intestinal bacteria. Fennel has also been used to promote appetite. The entire herb is used in culinary dishes, and the fleshy sheaths surrounding the base of the leaf stems are a staple in Italian cuisine. The foliage, known as fennel weed, is used to flavor eggs, fish, stews, and vegetables. The root is sometimes grated fresh and added to salads. The licorice-flavored seeds are traditionally served after meals in India to cleanse the breath.

Preparations

Harvest fennel leaf from time to time throughout the growing season. Use the fresh leaf when possible as the herb may lose much of the flavor when dried. The leaves may also be frozen for later use. Harvest the seeds in autumn. Seeds are fully ripe just as the color fades and the seed-bearing umbels turn from yellow-green to a light brown. Cut the brown umbels from the stalk and place them in a paper bag to dry in a warm room. Shake the dried seeds from the number and store them in tightly sealed, clearly labeled, dark-glass containers. Harvest the root late in the fall at the same time the stems are harvested as a vegetable. The root is generally less medicinally potent than the seeds.

Seed Infusion: Crush 1 tsp–1 tbsp of the dried seed, add to 1 cup of unchlorinated water, fresh milk, or barley water, in a non-metallic pot. Bring to a boil; then steep, covered, for about 10 minutes. A standard dosage of the tea is two to three cups per day.

Root Decoction: Add one ounce of the clean, thinly sliced dry root, or 2 oz of the thinly-sliced fresh root, to 1 pt of unchlorinated water in a non-metallic pot. Bring to a boil and simmer for about 10 minutes. Strain and cover. A decoction may be refrigerated for up to two days and retain its healing qualities.

Tincture: Combine half a cup of dried fennel seeds with 1 pt of brandy or vodka in a glass container. Seal the container with an airtight lid. Leave to macerate in a darkened place for two weeks. Shake daily. Strain the mixture through a cheesecloth or muslin bag and pour it into a dark bottle for storage for up to two years. Dosage is 2–4 ml of the tincture two times a day.

Precautions

Pregnant women should not use the herb, seeds, tincture, or essential oil of fennel in medicinal remedies. Small amounts used as a culinary spice are considered safe. In large doses, fennel acts as a uterine stimulant. The essential oil of fennel is toxic in doses as small as 5 ml and may cause skin irritation, vomiting, seizure, and respiratory problems. The volatile oil should not be ingested. The herb and seed oil may cause contact dermatitis in sensitive individuals.

4. Vitex

Vitex (Vitex agnus-castus) is a plant used in herbal medicine. Also known as chaste tree or chasteberry, it's often taken as a remedy for women's health problems. Vitex supplements typically contain extracts of the fruit and/or seed of the plant. Vitex may influence hormone levels in several ways. For example, it's said to promote the release of luteinizing hormone and, in turn, increase levels of progesterone (a hormone known to play a key role in regulating the menstrual cycle). Vitex is also thought to affect levels of prolactin, which is involved in stimulating breast development and milk production in women.

Health Benefits

Vitex has a long history of use as a folk remedy for a range of female conditions, such as post-partum hemorrhage, and to help with the "passing of afterbirth." The name "chaste tree" comes from the belief in folk medicine that it could suppress libido. In alternative medicine, vitex is frequently used in the treatment of the following issues:

- Premenstrual syndrome (PMS)
- Acne
- Fibrocystic breast disease
- Infertility in women
- Heavy menstrual periods
- Menopausal symptoms
- Benign prostatic hyperplasia
- Migraines
- Joint conditions
- Possible Side Effects

Vitex may trigger several side effects including; bleeding between menstrual periods, dry mouth, hair loss, headache, itching, mild digestive upset, nausea, rapid heartbeat, and skin rash. Use of vitex should be avoided by pregnant or nursing women. In addition, people with hormone-sensitive conditions (such as endometriosis, uterine fibroids, and cancers of the breast, ovaries, or prostate) shouldn't take vitex. Because vitex may influence levels of the neurotransmitter dopamine, individuals with Parkinson's disease, schizophrenia, or any other condition in which dopamine levels are affected should avoid vitex (unless under the supervision of a qualified health professional). In addition, there's some concern that vitex may decrease the effectiveness of oral contraceptives or hormone replacement therapy.

Dosage And Preparation

There is not enough scientific evidence to establish a recommended dose of vitex or chaste berry. Different doses have been studied in research studies investigating the herb's effect on various conditions. The right dose for you may depend on various factors including your age, medical conditions, and the specific formulation (extract) used. Speak to your healthcare provider to get personalized advice.

5. Maca Root

Maca (Lepidium meyenii) is the root of a vegetable native to the Andes region of Peru. Known as "Peruvian ginseng" (even though it doesn't belong to the same botanical family as ginseng), maca is consumed as a food and is said to boost energy and libido. Typically added to smoothies, juice, and shakes, the ground root powder can also be used as an ingredient in such foods as coffee, chocolate, or oils. In Peru, whole maca root is often added to soup and oatmeal, roasted and consumed as a vegetable, or made into a fermented beverage known as "maca chica."

Uses

Proponents claim that maca may benefit conditions such as erectile dysfunction, low libido, depression, hair loss, and hot flashes, and other symptoms associated with menopause. As a cruciferous vegetable (like cabbage, broccoli, arugula, Brussels sprouts, and kale), maca contains glucosinolates, plant compounds that are being studied for their role in cancer prevention. In Peruvian folk medicine, maca is sometimes used to raise energy levels.

Health Benefits

- Sexual Function and Libido
- Antidepressant-Induced Sexual Dysfunction
- Fertility
- Depression

Possible Side Effects

Little is known about the safety and side effects of the short-term or long-term use of maca. Since it is a natural food, it is generally believed to be safe in large doses. Maca's effect on hormone levels is poorly understood. For instance, some studies have found no effect on sex hormones, while animal studies have reported elevated levels of luteinizing hormone, progesterone, and testosterone. If you have a hormone-sensitive condition, such as endometriosis, uterine fibroids, or breast, uterine, or ovarian cancer, you shouldn't take maca without consulting your doctor. Excessive or regular intake of raw maca may interfere with thyroid function. As with other supplements, maca hasn't been tested for safety in pregnant women, nursing mothers, children, and those with medical conditions or those who are taking medications.

Dosage And Preparation

Maca is sold as a powder, in capsules, as gelatin, and as a tincture. It is also sometimes added to foods, its nutty, earthy flavor pairs well with cinnamon. There is no standard recommended daily allowance for maca root. Alternative medicine practitioners recommend starting with 3 grams (1 Tbs. powder) and working your way up to 9 grams a day.

6. Tribulus

The puncture vine is the green climbing plant known as Tribulus, the abbreviated form of its botanical name, Tribulus Terrestris, a leafy green climbing plant that grows in various parts of the United States, as well as in warm weather climates such as those of India and Sri Lanka. The Tribulus is regarded as a noxious weed for agricultural purposes in most U.S. states.

Tribulus, or its regional variations, has been held in high regard in the ancient medical practices of India (where the herb is known as Gokshura in the Ayurveda holistic medical teachings) and the traditional Chinese medicines for many centuries. In both cultures, Tribulus leaves were valued for their use in herbal formulations and tonics to elevate mood, as well as to ease the discomfort caused to the digestive and urinary tracts by conditions such as colic. Tribulus was also believed to act as a remedy for male impotence in both cultures, as well as working as an agent to alleviate the symptoms of menopause in women.

It is the connection believed to exist between the ingestion of Tribulus and the increase in male sexual potency that has fueled a more recent interest in Tribulus as a weight training supplement. The active chemical ingredient contained in the leaf of the Tribulus plant is steroidal saponins, also known as furostanol. There has been significant analysis of this chemical concerning its impact, if any, on increased levels of testosterone within the body. Testosterone, the male sex hormone, is a key regulator of many important functions within the body, including the formation, development, and maintenance of muscle mass. Taken as a freestanding supplement to build greater strength, testosterone is a banned performance-enhancing substance in almost all international athletic competitions. Testosterone, when ingested as a training supplement, is classed as an illegal anabolic steroid by the World Anti-Doping Agency (WADA), given its muscle-building properties.

Tribulus and its active ingredient furostanol are not anabolic substances, as Tribulus itself does not directly affect the growth of human muscle. The Tribulus research has been focused on the relationship between Tribulus ingestion and its impact on the chemical that occurs naturally in the human body, the luteinizing hormone (LH). LH plays an important role in the regulation and maintenance of testosterone levels in the body, which provided the theoretical basis for the proposition that a positive impact by Tribulus on LH might itself increase levels of testosterone production. There has not been any conclusive scientific research to support the proposition that Tribulus consumption will definitively increase testosterone production within the body. The chief difficulty with any determination that Tribulus consumption raises testosterone levels is connected to the fact that all exercise will temporarily increase the production of testosterone. It is therefore difficult to scientifically differentiate between the purported effect of Tribulus and the known effect of the exercise.

Persons engaged in strength training who use Tribulus are now more likely to stack Tribulus with a mineral supplement known by the acronym ZMA, a compound that is commercially available in several formulations. The most popular ZMA mixture is generally constituted with zinc, magnesium, and vitamin B-6; zinc is a component of over 3,000 different proteins within the body, and magnesium is essential to both nervous system function and bone formation. The popularity of this

Tribulus stack is rooted in word-of-mouth endorsements from users than it is supported by hard science. Few side effects have been identified from the use of the combination of Tribulus and ZMA.

7. Red Raspberry

Red raspberry is a plant that is the source of a widely eaten, tasty, sweet berry. Red raspberry fruit and leaf have also been used as medicine for centuries. Some people take red raspberry leaf by mouth for easing labor and delivery, for gastrointestinal (GI) disorders including diarrhea; for infection of the airways including flu, and heart problems. Red raspberry leaf is used in a gargle for sore throat and applied to the skin for rashes. In foods, red raspberry fruit is eaten and processed into jams and other foods. Red raspberry leaf in small quantities is a source of natural flavoring in Europe.

How Does It Work?

The chemicals in red raspberry might have antioxidant effects and help relax blood vessels. They might also cause muscles to contract or relax, depending on the dose and the muscle involved. This is the theory behind red raspberry's use in easing labor and delivery.

Uses & Effectiveness?

Possibly Ineffective For

Labor Pain: Taking red raspberry leaf does not reduce the length of labor or decrease the need for pain-relieving medication around the time of delivery.

Insufficient Evidence For

- Abnormally heavy bleeding during menstrual periods (menorrhagia)
- Aging skin
- Diabetes
- Diarrhea
- Flu (influenza)
- Gastrointestinal disorders
- Heart disease
- Heart failure and fluid build-up in the body (congestive heart failure or CHF)
- High blood pressure
- Infection of the airways
- Menstrual cramps (dysmenorrhea)
- Morning sickness
- Preventing miscarriage
- Skin rash
- Sore throat (pharyngitis)
- Vitamin deficiencies
- Side Effects

When Taken By Mouth: Red raspberry fruit is likely safe for most people when eaten in food amounts. It is possibly safe when taken in larger amounts as medicine. No side effects from taking red raspberry fruit have been reported. But a full evaluation of the safety of red raspberry has not been conducted.

Special Precautions And Warnings

1. Pregnancy And Breastfeeding: It's likely safe to eat red raspberry fruit in food amounts during pregnancy. red raspberry leaf is possibly safe for use by mouth in medicinal amounts during late pregnancy, but only under the direct supervision of a healthcare provider. Red raspberry leaf is used by nurse-midwives to ease delivery. But don't take it on your own. It is likely unsafe to take red raspberry leaf as medicine throughout pregnancy without the direct supervision of a healthcare provider. The concern is that red raspberry might act like the hormone estrogen. This might harm the pregnancy.

2. Diabetes: Red raspberry leaf might lower blood sugar levels in people with diabetes. Watch for signs of low blood sugar (hypoglycemia) and monitor your blood sugar carefully if you have diabetes and use red raspberry leaf.

3. Hormone-Sensitive Conditions Such As Breast Cancer, Uterine Cancer, Ovarian Cancer, Endometriosis, Or Uterine Fibroids: Red raspberry might act like estrogen. If you have any condition that might be made worse by exposure to estrogen, don't use red raspberry.

8. Dang Gui

Dang Gui is one of the most commonly used herbs in the Chinese herbal system. It is primarily known as a "women's herb," though many men consume it as well. Most famously and importantly, it is known as a superior blood tonic, and that is one reason women use so much of it. It is also used conjunctively as a "blood vitalizer," meaning that it supports healthy blood circulation, especially in the abdomen and pelvic basin. Men and women benefit from superior circulation. Dang Gui is very widely used to help establish, support and maintain healthy menstrual balance in women. It also has analgesic and mild sedative (calming, relaxing) actions.

As always, quality matters a great deal when selecting Dang Gui. This herb comes in a very wide range of qualities from Asia. It is one of the herbs that people choose very carefully and for which they develop a "connoisseur" state of mind. Ron Teeguarden has been sourcing Dang Gui for over three decades. Dragon Herbs Dang Gui is grown in a specific region of northwestern China, from a valley known for centuries as a premier Di Tao (authentic and superior grade) source. Our Dang Gui is always made from fresh roots with rich, sweet aromatic volatile oils and a perfect balance of constituents. Dang Gui has a very characteristic fragrance that is very evident in Dragon Herbs Dang Gui extract due to the presence of n-butylidene phthalide and ligustilide in the volatile oil.

9. Mints

Mint is an aromatic herb produced by various species of the mint plant (Mentha). Native to the eastern Mediterranean, mint gets its name from a mythic nymph named Minthe (Minto). Jealous Persephone turned her into a lowly mint plant after she had an affair with Pluto, the god of the underworld. The mint plant is common and a favorite of many gardeners, so it's easy to grow your own. As an herb, it is gluten-free and suitable for vegan, vegetarian, and paleo diets.

Varieties

Spearmint and curly mint are the varieties most often grown to use as herb in cooking and beverages. Peppermint is a little too strong to use fresh for most culinary purposes. Instead, it is grown and processed into peppermint oil, which is then used as a flavoring, and it can be further refined into a menthol. You can find other varieties of mint that have interesting flavors and aromas. Apple mint has an apple scent; orange mint has a citrus flavor; chocolate mint has a bit of chocolate taste.

Recipes

Mint traditionally complements lamb and poultry. It is widely used in Middle Eastern and Greek dishes, including salads, side dishes, and sauces. Fresh mint is a favorite for herbal tea.

- Lamb burgers with mint
- Fresh mint tea
- Mint sauce for lamb

Uses

In the home, mint has long been used as an aromatic. As a strewing herb, it was scattered around the house as a deodorizer. Today, it is commonly used in sachets and potpourris. Some soap makers add small amounts of dried mint to their soaps, while peppermint oil is sometimes used in aromatherapy to improve alertness.

Storage

Store fresh mint in the refrigerator or place the stems in a container of water and cover the leaves loosely with a plastic bag. Dried mint should be stored in a cool, dark place in a sealed jar.

Health Benefits

Modern medical research has focused on peppermint oil, which is now often sold as a dietary supplement capsule, medicinal tea, or topical preparation. In combination with caraway oil, it may help indigestion. Topical peppermint oil has some limited evidence of being helpful for tension headaches. There isn't enough evidence to show peppermint oil or peppermint leaf is useful for any other condition. The usual doses of peppermint oil capsules should be safe, but they can be toxic in excessive doses. Peppermint oil should not be applied to children or infants as it can cause serious respiratory side effects. It can also result in rashes and skin irritation for adults as well.

10. Chamomile

Chamomile (or camomile) is a flowering herb. It looks like a tiny daisy, with a yellow central disc surrounded by delicate white petals. Chamomile is more fragrant than similar flowers, giving off a gentle floral, almost apple-like aroma that is very relaxing. For this reason, and due to its many reported health benefits, chamomile is popular in herbal teas and aromatherapy.

What Is Chamomile Tea?

A member of the Asteraceae family, chamomile is closely related to echinacea, sunflowers, marigolds, and other daisy-like flowers. The name comes from the Greek word chamaimēlon, meaning "ground apple." The flowering herb has been used as a medicinal tonic and topical remedy for thousands of years. Though its use likely predates the period, it is known to have been drunk by Ancient Egyptians. Chamomile was also used as both a beverage and incense by the Romans.

There are two main types of chamomile: Anthemis nobilis (Roman chamomile) and Matricaria chamomilla (German or wild chamomile). The Roman variety was named by a botanist in the 19th century who found it growing near the Colosseum in Rome. German chamomile tends to have a more robust, almost pungent scent, while Roman chamomile is sweeter and fruitier.

The chamomile plant's flowers and buds are harvested for tea as the flowers open. It continually blooms for a few months, depending on the climate in which it's grown. Egypt and Eastern Europe lead chamomile cultivation, though it's grown worldwide, and German chamomile often grows wild. After harvest, the flowers are dried to prolong the shelf life. When this occurs, the white petals turn a pale yellow and may fall off the yellow head, which is its most recognizable form.

3 Health Benefits Of Chamomile

Although chamomile is a flavorful and aromatic herb, it is often sought out specifically for its health benefits. It has longstanding medicinal and spiritual uses. Chamomile has been used for centuries to treat a variety of health conditions. While it is widely used today in alternative and natural medicine, researchers continue to study chamomile's potential. It may help relieve colic, anxiety disorders, irritable bowel syndrome (IBS), and canker sores. Some preparations may help with inflammation and improve the quality of life for cancer patients, as well. Studies also suggest that it may be helpful for people with diabetes, cardiovascular conditions, and osteoarthritis.

1. Stress Relief: As a stress reliever and to help with insomnia, chamomile is one of the best herbs you can choose. The tea can be very calming, acting as a natural sedative. This effect can be enhanced by combining chamomile with other soothing herbs, such as lavender and rosemary, whether in tea or aromatherapy applications such as massage oils, herbal baths, or sleep pillows.

2. Anti-Inflammatory: In various preparations, including tea, chamomile is touted for its anti-inflammatory properties. It may reduce symptoms associated with muscle spasms and pain, menstrual cramps and disorders, and gastrointestinal disorders. It may also have some effect on lowering blood sugar levels for people with diabetes. Topical preparations may reduce inflammation of the skin, such as dark circles under the eye, eczema, sunburns, and rashes.

3. Immune Boost: Though studies into the matter continue, there is evidence that chamomile may help boost the immune system. The tea is also a popular option for relieving some symptoms of the common cold, including a sore throat. The effect seems to be minimal and may be linked more to its calming properties.

General Use

The aromatic flower heads and herbs (leaves) of both Roman and German chamomile are used medicinally. They are highly scented with volatile, aromatic oil, including the heat-sensitive Azulene, which is the blue chamomile essential oil. The phytochemical constituents in chamomile also include flavonoids, coumarins, plant acids, fatty acids, cyanogenic glycosides, choline, tannin, and salicylate derivatives. This bittersweet herb acts medicinally as a tonic, anodyne, antispasmodic, anti-inflammatory, antibacterial, anti-allergenic, and sedative. Traditionally, a mild infusion of the herb has been safely used to calm restless children, and to ease colic and teething pain in babies. It is also effective in relieving acid indigestion and abdominal pain. Its carminative properties relieve intestinal gas, and it helps in cases of diarrhea, constipation, and peptic ulcers. The herbal tea can ease symptoms of colds and flu by relieving headaches and reducing fever. The infusion is also helpful to treat toothache, arthritis, gout, and premenstrual tension. It may also be used in douche preparations or sitz baths. As an external wash in strong infusion, or decoction, or as part of a hot compress, the herb can soothe burns and scalds, skin rashes, and sores. Chamomile can be used in a douche, as a gargle for mouth ulcers, as soothing eyewashes for conjunctivitis, and as a hair rinse to brighten the hair. Chamomile blossoms may also be used as an herbal aromatic treatment, providing a tonic lift with its pleasing scent.

Preparations

Chamomile is most often prepared as an infusion of the blossoms of German chamomile, and less commonly of Roman chamomile. Traditionally the tiny blossoms are picked on midsummers' eve. The best time to harvest is on a sunny day when the mass of blossoms is at its fullness in the morning. Harvesting chamomile blossoms can be painstaking work, requiring a gardener's best patience. Pinch off the flower head, leaving the stem. Fresh or dried blossoms may be used in herbal preparations.

Blossoms to be dried for storage should be spread singly on a screen or mat and placed in a well-ventilated place, out of the direct sun, with a temperature close to 95°F (35°C). The rapid drying will preserve much of the volatile oil and other medicinal properties. A few blossoms go a long way with this pleasant and safe herbal ally. Store dried blossoms in tightly sealed, glass containers, away from light. They will maintain potency for about one year. Chamomile is prolific, and the plant blossoms frequently throughout the summer. Sometimes two or three harvests can be made in one season.

Chamomile tea may be made from an infusion of blossoms prepared as a tisane, for a single, soothing cup, or in a larger quantity for use throughout the day. Chamomile combines well with mints, such as lemon balm (Melissa officinalis) or spearmint (Mentha spica-ta), combined in equal quantity. For a tisane, use 1 tsp of dried blossoms, or 1.5 tsp of freshly picked flowers in a warm cup. Heat water to the boiling point and pour over the blossoms in a glass container. Cover, and infuse for 3–5 minutes. Let strain. Be careful not to overstep chamomile, lest it loses its delicate flavor to a bitter edge. The standard dose is up to three cups per day. The prepared tea will keep for a day or two in the refrigerator.

To prepare a chamomile decoction, which is a stronger preparation, let the plant parts steep in a covered nonmetallic pot for at least ten minutes. The decoction may be used as a skin wash, hair rinse, mouth wash, or to bathe wounds. An extract of the essential oil can be prepared by placing 2 oz (57 g) of fresh blossoms into a glass container and covering the plant with 0.5–1 pt (0.24–0.47 l) of olive oil. Place the mixture on a sunny window sill for about one week. Strain and store in a dark container with a tight-fitting lid. The oil remains potent for up to one year. It is best when applied warm.

Precautions

Chamomile has been used over the centuries and is generally considered a safe and gentle herbal remedy that may be used daily as a calming tea. Persons who may be allergic to such pollen-bearing plants as chamomile would be wise to experiment with this herbal remedy with some caution.

Side Effects

Despite its many health benefits, chamomile isn't for everyone. It is not recommended for women who are breastfeeding or pregnant. There are also interactions between chamomile and some drugs, which should be taken into consideration and discussed with your doctor. Chamomile can cause allergic reactions in people with hay fever and some types of flower allergies. If you are allergic to ragweed, chrysanthemums, or other plants in the Asteraceae family, it's best to avoid chamomile. The moderate internal use of chamomile preparations has no known side effects; however, some herbalists warn that the herb, when taken internally in excessive doses, can induce vomiting and produce vertigo (dizziness).

Interactions

There are no contraindications for using this gentle, healing herb. Chamomile does combine well with other herbs that enhance its pleasant and medicinal qualities.

11. European Five-Finger Grass

European five-finger grass is an herb. The dried plant is used to make medicine. People take European five-finger grass for diarrhea and fever. European five-finger grass is sometimes applied directly to the affected area for swollen mouth and gums, toothache, and heartburn. It is also used to treat open wounds by helping to dry out the tissue. Don't confuse European five-finger grass (Potentilla reptans) with dwarf cinquefoil (Potentilla Canadensis).

Insufficient Evidence to Rate Effectiveness For

- Diarrhea
- Fever
- Swollen mouth and gums, when applied directly to the affected area
- Toothache, when applied directly to the affected area
- Heartburn, when applied directly to the affected area
- Wounds, when applied directly to the affected area

How Does European Five-Finger Grass Work?

European five-finger grass contains chemicals called tannins that might help reduce skin inflammation and have a drying (astringent) effect on the tissues.

Are There Safety Concerns?

There isn't enough information available to know if European five-finger grass is safe or what the possible side effects might be.

Special Precautions & Warnings

Pregnancy and breastfeeding: Not enough is known about the use of European five-finger grass during pregnancy and breastfeeding. Stay on the safe side and avoid use.

Dosing Considerations For Herbs Of Protection, Goodluck, And Fertility.

The appropriate dose for herbs of protection, good luck, and fertility depends on several factors such as the user's age, health, and several other conditions. Keep in mind that natural products are not always necessarily safe and dosages can be important. Be sure to follow relevant directions on product labels and consult your pharmacist or physician or other healthcare professional before using.

CHAPTER 4: HERBS FOR LOVE AND BEAUTY

1. Coriander

The word coriander refers to a plant, Coriandrum sativum, of which both the leaves and the seeds are used in the culinary arts. When the coriander leaves are used, they are considered an herb. Coriander leaves, also known as cilantro, have a bright, almost citrus-like flavor. Coriander leaves are used in all sorts of cuisines, from Latin American to Asian. In Mexico and the United States, fresh coriander leaves are frequently used as a garnish for salsas and spicy soups. Coriander seed, which is the dried fruit of the coriander plant, is used as a spice. Typically used ground, coriander seed has a spicy, citrus flavor. Coriander seed is used extensively in Indian, Middle Eastern, and Asian cuisines. Whole coriander seed is sometimes used in pickling and bringing.

Also Known As:

- Cilantro
- Chinese parsley

2. Ginseng

Ginseng refers to two closely related herbs of the genus Panax. Asian ginseng (P. ginseng) and American ginseng (P. quinquefolius) have traditionally been used for healing. Asian ginseng is also known as Korean red ginseng, Chinese ginseng, Japanese ginseng, ginseng radix, Sinjin, sang, and ren shen. American ginseng is also known as Canadian ginseng, North American ginseng, Ontario ginseng, Wisconsin ginseng, red berry, sang, and ren shen. Siberian ginseng (Eleutherococcus senticosus) is a plant with different properties that belong to a completely different genus. Ginseng in this entry refers only to Asian and American ginseng of the genus Panax.

Purpose

Ginseng has been used for about 2,000 years in Traditional Chinese Medicine (TCM) to boost energy, hasten recovery from illness or injury, reduce stress, improve mental and physical performance (including sexual performance), and treat several dozen different infections, gastrointestinal disorders, circulatory problems, and conditions as diverse as burns, cancers, diabetes, migraine headaches, and weight loss. The genus name Panax means "heal all," and ginseng is considered by herbalists to be an almost universal remedy. Most of these traditional uses of ginseng have not yet been substantiated by conventional medicine, however encouraging results from some well-designed, controlled human studies strongly suggest that ginseng may improve mental performance and have other health benefits.

Health Claims

Dozens of health claims are made for ginseng, many based on traditional or folk use of the herb. These claims are difficult to substantiate in ways that satisfy conventional medicine for several reasons including:

The amount and strength of ginseng in dietary supplements is not standardized and a wide range of doses are used in different studies

Ginseng is often one of several herbs contained in herbal remedies, making it difficult to tell if the effects are due to ginseng or another herb

Many studies done on ginseng are poorly designed so that it is impossible to show a direct link between cause and effect, or they poorly reported, making analysis of the results difficult

Many rigorous and well-designed human studies have a small sample size

Key Terms

Alternative Medicine: A system of healing that rejects conventional, pharmaceutical-based medicine and replaces it with the use of dietary supplements and therapies such as herbs, vitamins, minerals, massage, and cleansing diets. Alternative medicine includes well-established treatment systems such as homeopathy, Traditional Chinese Medicine, and Ayurvedic medicine, as well as more recent, fad-driven treatments.

Alzheimer's Disease: An incurable disease of older individuals that results in the destruction of nerve cells in the brain and causes gradual loss of mental and physical functions.

Conventional Medicine: Mainstream or Western pharmaceutical-based medicine practiced by medical doctors, doctors of osteopathy, and other licensed health care professionals.

Dietary Supplement: A product, such as a vitamin, mineral, herb, amino acid, or enzyme, that is intended to be consumed in addition to an individual's diet with the expectation that it will improve health.

Traditional Chinese Medicine (TCM): An ancient system of medicine based on maintaining a balance in vital energy or qi that controls emotions, spiritual, and physical well-being. Diseases and disorders result from imbalances in qi, and treatments such as massage, exercise, acupuncture, nutritional and herbal therapy are designed to restore balance and harmony to the body.

Some health claims for ginseng appear more promising than others. There is good evidence that ginseng can cause short-term improvement in mental performance in both healthy young adults and elderly ill adults. Not enough information is available to determine if long-term gains also occur, but the results have been promising enough that ginseng is being studied in patients with Alzheimer's disease and other dementias. Along with improved mental performance, some studies have shown that ginseng improves the sense of well-being and quality of life. Results of these studies are mixed, with some finding improvements and others finding no change. The situation is complicated by the fact that different studies define and measure "well-being" and "quality of life" in different ways. In general, people with the worst quality of life report the most improvement.

Many claims are made that ginseng boosts the immune system, thus helping to prevent disease and promote more rapid recovery from illness and injury. There is good evidence that ginseng lowers blood sugar in people with type 2 (non-insulin-dependent) diabetes. The effect of ginseng on blood sugar in people with type 1 (insulin-dependent) diabetes has not been studied enough to produce any definite findings.

Studies of the effect of ginseng on the circulatory system are mixed. Some studies find that ginseng lowers blood pressure and in combination with other herbs prevents coronary artery disease and possibly congestive heart failure. Other studies find no effect, or that the effect is apparent only at very high, and possibly unsafe, doses. The effect of ginseng on the circulatory system continues to be investigated.

Many other health claims are made for herbal mixtures that contain ginseng. These claims are extremely difficult to evaluate because of the number of variables, including the strength of the mixture, the effects of the different herbs, and potential interactions among other herbs. Until much more is known about the chemical properties and active ingredients of common medicinal herbs, it is almost impossible to evaluate these mixtures in a way that satisfies the demands of conventional medicine.

Precautions

Ginseng is generally safe and causes few side effects when taken at recommended doses. The generally recommended dose is 100–200 mg of standardized ginseng extract containing 4% ginsenosides once or twice daily. The safety of ginseng in children and pregnant and breastfeeding women has not been studied. Pregnant and breastfeeding women should be aware that some tinctures of ginseng contain high levels of alcohol. Some herbalists recommend that individuals take ginseng for 2–3 weeks and then take a break of 1–2 weeks before beginning the herb again.

Independent laboratory analyses have repeatedly found that many products labeled as ginseng contain little or none of the herb. True ginseng is expensive, and unscrupulous manufacturers often substitute low-cost herbs for ginseng. Another problem is that some ginseng products are contaminated with pesticides and other chemicals that can cause serious side effects.

Interactions

Ginseng appears to interact with blood-thinning and anti-coagulant medicines such as warfarin (Coumadin), clopidogrel (Plavix), aspirin, and nonsteroidal anti-inflammatory drugs (e.g. Advil, Motrin). Individuals taking these drugs should not begin taking ginseng without consulting their health care provider.

Because ginseng lowers blood sugar levels, individuals who are taking insulin or other medications that also lower blood sugar, and those with type 2 diabetes, should be monitored for low blood sugar if they begin taking ginseng. Adjustments are needed in their other medications.

Ginseng may also interact with monoamine-oxi-dase (MAO) inhibitors used to treat certain kinds of depression and mental illness. Examples of MAOs include isocarboxazid (Marplan), phenelzine (Nardil), and tranylcypromine (Parnate). Individuals taking MAOs with ginseng may develop headaches, tremors, increased anxiety, restlessness, sleeplessness, and mania.

Preliminary evidence suggests that ginseng may interact with certain blood pressure and heart medications. The herb may also interfere with the way the liver processes other drugs and herbs.

Before beginning to take a supplement containing ginseng, individuals should review their current medications with their health care provider to determine any possible interactions.

Complications

Serious side effects of ginseng are rare. The most common side effects are increased restlessness, insomnia, nausea, diarrhea, and rash. Allergic reactions are possible but uncommon. Some of the more serious side effects reported are thought to be the result of contamiNation with pesticides, heavy metals, or other chemicals rather than a side effect caused by ginseng.

Parental Concerns

Parents should be aware that the safe dose of many herbal supplements has not been established for children. Accidental overdose may occur if children are given adult herbal supplements.

3. Juniper

Juniper (Juniperus communis) is an evergreen shrub found on mountains and heaths throughout Europe, Southwest Asia, and North America. The tree grows to a height of 6-25 ft (2-8 m) and has stiff, pointed needles that grow to 0.4 in (1 cm) long. The female bear's cones produce small round bluish-black berries, which take three years to fully mature.

Juniper belongs to the pine family (Cupressaceae). Juniper has diuretic, antiseptic, stomachic, antimicrobial, anti-inflammatory, and antirheumatic properties. The tree's therapeutic properties stem from a volatile oil found in the berries. This oil contains terpenes, flavonoid glycosides, tannins, sugar, tar, and resin. Terpinene-4-of (a diuretic compound of the oil) stimulates the kidneys, increasing their filtration rate. The flavonoid amentoflavone exhibits antiviral properties. Test tube studies show that another constituent of juniper, desoxypodophyllotoxins, may act to inhibit the herpes simplex virus. The resins and tars contained in the oil benefit such skin conditions as psoriasis.

Juniper has also been used as a traditional remedy for cancer, arthritis, gas, indigestion, warts, bronchitis, tuberculosis, gallstones, colic, heart failure, intestinal disease, gout, and back pain. The berries were often eaten to relieve rheumatism or to freshen bad breath. When treating patients, doctors often chewed juniper berries to prevent infection.

General Use

Modern herbalists prescribe juniper to treat bladder infections, kidney disease, chronic arthritis, gout, rheumatic conditions, fluid retention, cystitis, skin conditions, inflammation, digestive problems, menstrual irregularities, and high blood pressure. The German Commission E has approved juniper berries for use in treating heartburn and dyspepsia (indigestion), belching, and other digestive disturbances.

Juniper Is A Powerful Diuretic: The volatile oil contained in juniper is composed of compounds that stimulate the kidneys to remove fluid and bacterial waste products from the body. This diuretic action is useful in such conditions as congestive heart failure, urinary infections, and kidney disease.

The oil also has antiseptic properties, which makes it a useful disinfectant treatment for urinary and bladder infections. The German Commission E reported that juniper caused an increase in urine flow and smooth muscle contractions. Juniper may be combined with other herbs such as uva ursi, parsley, cleavers, or buchu to treat bladder infections. Juniper may help treat bladder infections more effectively when combined with other herbs.

Juniper's anti-inflammatory properties help to relieve the inflammation, stiffness, and pain that are present in conditions like arthritis, rheumatism, and gout. The berries can be made into an ointment and rubbed on the affected joints and muscles.

The tree needles may be crushed and added to a bath to ease aching muscles. Some people may find relief from the nerve, muscle, joint, and tendon pains of gout and rheumatoid arthritis by applying a compress made from an infusion of juniper berries. Juniper is also warming to the digestive system and increases the production of stomach acid, stimulates the appetite, settles the stomach, and relieves gas.

Preparations

The ripe, berries and needles from the tree are used in herbal medicine. Juniper is available in bulk form as whole berries, or as a supplement in the form of capsules or tinctures.

The recommended tincture dosage is 10-20 drops four times daily.

Teas are often taken to relieve digestive problems. To make a tea, 1 cup of boiling water is poured over 1 tablespoon of juniper berries. The mixture is covered and steeped for 10-20 minutes. One cup can be drunk two times daily. The tea should not be used for longer than two weeks at a time. A clean cloth may be soaked in the cooled mixture to create a compress.

Precautions

Juniper should be used only for short periods. High doses or prolonged use of juniper may irritate the kidneys and urinary tract, causing damage. People with kidney problems should not use this herb. Juniper stimulates contractions of the womb. Pregnant women should not use juniper. Breast-feeding women also should not use juniper. Juniper may increase blood sugar levels in diabetics. Therefore, diabetics should consult with their doctor before using juniper. When taking juniper for a bladder infection, consumers should see their doctor if the infection is still present after several days of use, or if lower back pain, fever, or chills develop.

Side Effects

External application of juniper oil may cause a skin rash.

People with allergies may experience allergy symptoms such as nasal congestion.

Symptoms of juniper overdose include diarrhea, purplish urine, blood in the urine, kidney pain, intestinal pain, elevated blood pressure, and a quickened heartbeat. If these effects occur, consumers should stop taking juniper and call their doctor immediately.

Interactions

Consumers should use juniper cautiously with other diuretic drugs or substances because excessive fluid loss may occur.

3. Lavender

Lavender is a hardy perennial in the Lamiaceae, or mint, family. The herb is a Mediterranean native. Many species of Lavendula vary somewhat in appearance and aromatic quality. English lavender, L. Angustifolia, also known as true lavender, is commercially valuable in the perfume industry and is a mainstay of English country gardens. French lavender, L.stoechas, is the species most probably used in Roman times as a scenting agent in washing water. The species L. Officinalis is the official species used in medicinal preparations, though all lavenders have medicinal properties in varying degrees.

General Use

Lavender is best known and loved for its fragrance. The herb has been used since ancient times in perfumery. As an aromatic plant, lavender lifts the spirits and chases melancholy. Taking just a few whiffs of this sweet-smelling herb is said to dispel dizziness. Traditionally, women in labor clutched sprigs of lavender to bring added courage and strength to the task of childbearing. A decoction of the flower may be used as a feminine douche for leucorrhoea.

The dried blossoms, sewn into sachets, may be used to repel moths and to scent clothing or may be lit like incense to scent a room. Because of its fumigant properties, the herb was hung in the home to repel flies and mosquitoes, and strewn about to sanitize the floors. The lavender essential oil was a component of smelling salts in Victorian times.

The essential oil of certain lavender species has a sedative, antispasmodic, and tranquilizing effect. Lavender has been long valued as a headache remedy. It can be taken in a mild infusion, or can be rubbed on the temples, or sniffed like smelling salts to provide relief from headaches caused by stress. Lavender oil is antiseptic and has been used as a topical disinfectant for wounds. In high doses, it can kill many common bacteria such as typhoid, diphtheria, streptococcus, and pneumococcus, according to some research. The essential oil has also been used as a folk treatment for the bite of some venomous snakes. When used in hydrotherapy as part of an aromatic, Epsom salt bath, the essential oils of some species will soothe tired nerves and relieve the pain of neuralgia. They are also used topically on burns and have been shown to speed healing. It is also a fine addition to a foot bath for sore feet. Lavender essence makes a pleasant massage oil for kneading sore muscles and joints. Acting internally, lavender's chemical properties increase the flow of bile into the intestines, relieving indigestion. Its carminative properties help expel intestinal gas. Lavender is an adjuvant and may be used in combination with other herbs to make a tonic cordial to strengthen the nervous system.

Preparations

The medicinal properties of lavender are extracted primarily from the oil glands in the leaf and blossom. The plant contains volatile oil, tannins, coumarins, flavonoids, and triterpenoids as active chemical components. These phytochemicals are the plant constituents responsible for the medicinal properties. Lavender's volatile oil is best when extracted from flowers picked before they reach maximum bloom and following a long period of hot and dry temperatures. The flower spikes dry quickly when spread on a mat in an airy place away from direct sun.

Distilled Oil: The essential oil of lavender is extracted by steam distillation. Just a few drops of this essential oil are effective for topical applications. Commercial distillations of this essential oil are readily available.

Lavender Tea: An infusion of the fresh or dried flowers and leaf can be made by pouring a pint of boiling water over one ounce of the dry leaf and flower, or two ounces of fresh herb, in a non-metallic pot. It can be steeped (covered) for about ten minutes, strained, and sweetened to taste. It should be drunk while still warm. Lavender tea may be taken throughout the day, a mouthful at a time, or warm, by the cup, up to three cups per day. Lavender works well in combination with other medicinal herbs in infusion.

Lavender Oil Extract: In a glass container, one ounce of freshly harvested lavender flowers can be combined with 1-1/2 pints of olive oil, sufficient to cover the herb. It should be placed on a sunny windowsill for about three days and shaken daily. After three days, the mixture should be strained through muslin or cheesecloth. The lavender extract can be safely used internally to treat migraines and nervous indigestion. A few drops on a sugar cube can speed headache relief. Externally, a small amount of lavender oil, rubbed on sore joints, can relieve rheumatism. The essential oil 297 twill297 been used to minimize scar tissue when applied to burned skin.

Lavender Sachet: Dried lavender blossoms and leaves can be sewn into a small cloth bag to scent linens and deter insects. The bag may be placed beneath the pillow as aromatherapy.

Lavender Vinegar: Fresh leaves and blossoms may be steeped in white vinegar for seven days, then strained and stored in a tightly capped bottle.

Precautions

Lavender has a long history of use as an essential oil and as a mildly sedative tea. When taken in moderation the tea is safe. It is important to note that, as with all essential oils, high or chronic doses of lavender essential oil are toxic to the kidney and liver. Infants even more easily overdose than adults.

Side Effects

No known side effects.

Interactions

As an adjuvant, lavender can enhance the helpful properties of other herbs when used in combination. Lemon balm (Melissa officinalis) leaves can be combined with lavender as a headache infusion. For cramping, an infusion of lavender and valerian (Valeriana officinalis) makes a soothing tea. Lavender's pleasant scent works well to cover disagreeable odors of other herbs in medicinal combinations. A tonic cordial can be made by combining fresh rosemary (Rosmarinus officinalis) leaves, cinnamon, nutmeg, and sandalwood with the lavender blossoms and steeping the mixture in brandy for about a week.

4. Patchouli Oil

The warm, spicy, musky, and sensuous scent of Patchouli Essential Oil is commonly associated with the hippy generation and referred to as "the scent of the sixties." This oil is derived from the leaves of the highly-valued Patchouli plant, which belongs to a family of other well-known aromatic plants, including Lavender, Mint, and Sage. Patchouli is native to and extensively cultivated in tropical regions such as Brazil, Hawaii, and Asian regions like China, India, Malaysia, and Indonesia. In Asian countries, it was traditionally used in folk medicine to treat hair problems like dandruff and oily scalp, as well as skin irritations like dryness, acne, and eczema.

There are 3 species of Patchouli, which are called Pogostemon Cablin, Pogostemon Heyneanus, and Pogostemon Hortensis. Of these, the Cabin species is the most popular and is the one cultivated for its essential oil, as its therapeutic properties lend it a relative superiority over other species. Patchouli Essential Oil is presently used for various purposes including perfumery, aromatherapy, cosmetic products, home cleaning products, and clothing detergents. Through any of these methods, the calming scent of the essential oil relieves anxiety, stress, and depression, making it effective for achieving relaxation, especially in meditation.

Benefits Of Patchouli Oil

Patchouli Essential Oil's active chemical components contribute to the therapeutic benefits that give it the reputation of being a grounding, soothing, and peace-inducing oil. These constituents make it ideal for use in cosmetics, aromatherapy, massage, and home cleaning products to purify the air as well as surfaces. These healing benefits can be attributed to the oil's anti-inflammatory, antidepressant, antiphlogistic, antiseptic, aphrodisiac, astringent, cicatrisant, cytophylactic, deodorant, diuretic, febrifuge, fungicide, sedative, and tonic qualities, among other valuable properties.

The main constituents of Patchouli Essential Oil are: Patchoulol, α-Patchoulene, β-Patchoulene, α-Bulnesene, α-Guaiene, Caryophyllene, Norpatchoulenol, Seychellene, and Pogostol.

Patchoulol is known to exhibit the following activity:

- Grounding
- Balancing
- Mood-harmonizing
- α-Bulnesene is known to exhibit the following activity:
- Anti-inflammatory

α-Guaiene is known to exhibit the following activity:

- An earthy, spicy fragrance
- Caryophyllene is known to exhibit the following activity:
- Anti-inflammatory
- Anti-bacterial
- Neuro-protective
- Anti-depressant
- Anti-oxidant
- Analgesic
- Anxiolytic

Used topically after dilution in a carrier oil or a skin care product, Patchouli Essential Oil can deodorize body odors, soothe inflammation, fight water retention, break up cellulite, relieve constipation, promote weight loss, facilitate the faster healing of wounds by stimulating the growth of new skin, moisturize rough and chapped skin, and reduce the appearance of blemishes, cuts, bruises, and scars. It is known to fight infections that contribute to fevers, thereby reducing body temperatures. It can also relieve discomfort associated with digestive issues. By boosting circulation and thus increasing oxygen to the organs and cells, it helps the body retain a healthy-looking, youthful appearance. Patchouli Oil's astringent properties help prevent the early onset of sagging skin and hair loss. This tonic oil improves metabolic functions by toning and strengthening the liver, stomach, and intestines and regulating proper excretion, which leads to an immune system boost that protects against infection and encourages alertness.

Used in aromatherapy, it is known to eliminate unpleasant odors in the environment and to balance emotions. The sedative scent stimulates the release of pleasure hormones, namely serotonin, and dopamine, thereby improving negative moods and enhancing the feeling of relaxation. It is believed to work as an aphrodisiac by stimulating sensual energy and boosting the libido. When diffused at night, Patchouli Essential Oil can encourage restful sleep, which can, in turn, improve mood, cognitive function, and metabolism.

Cosmetic: Antifungal, Anti-inflammatory, Antiseptic, Astringent, Deodorant, Fungicide, Tonic, Cytophylactic.

Odorous: Anti-depressant, Anti-inflammatory, Aphrodisiac, Deodorant, Sedative, Anti-phlogistic, Febrifuge, Insecticide.

Medicinal: Anti-fungal, Anti-inflammatory, Anti-depressant, Anti-septic, Astringent, Anti-phlogistic, Cicatrisant, Cytophylactic, Diuretic, Fungicide, Febrifuge, Sedative, Tonic.

Uses Of Patchouli Oil

The uses for Patchouli Essential Oil are abundant, ranging from medicinal and odorous to cosmetic. Its many forms include oils, gels, lotions, soaps, shampoos, and sprays, to name a few suggestions for homemade products.

When diluted and used topically in cosmetic products, Patchouli Essential Oil provides skin with many benefits such as a complexion that looks vibrant and feels healthy and smooth. It is used to slow the look of aging by tightening and toning the skin, thereby reducing the appearance of wrinkles and blemishes. 1-2 drops of the oil can be mixed into a skin care product of personal preference and used to moisturize problem skin that is blemished or wrinkled. Used as a massage balm, 1-2 drops of Patchouli Essential Oil can be diluted with a carrier oil such as Fractionated Coconut Oil before being applied to the body. It is beneficial for all skin types and can also be massaged into the face to relieve dryness or to balance oily and acne-prone skin. For the faster healing of scars, wounds, or blemishes caused by measles, pox, or acne, 5 drops of Patchouli Oil can be added to a face wash or a face cream to minimize the appearance of unwanted marks. This oil is also known to strengthen hair and it can be applied to the scalp by diluting 5 drops in a hair conditioner.

Used in aromatherapy, the mood-enhancing fragrance of Patchouli Essential Oil is inhaled and scent receptors in the brain's emotional powerhouse process the smell as grounding and emotionally balancing, allowing the brain and body to relax with the calming down of emotions. Similarly, 1-2 drops smoothed onto a pillow may reduce insomnia and promote the faster onset of deeper sleep by reducing anxiety and improving sleep quality. Diffusing 3-4 drops of this anti-inflammatory oil can also reduce fevers and colds by eliminating infectious bacteria, thus reducing body temperature and the pain commonly associated with illness. When diluted and applied topically to the hands, neck, stomach, or temples, Patchouli Essential Oil can offer a cooling sensation that will also reduce feverish body temperatures. When diffused during spiritual practices, it can be used on its own or in blends during prayer and meditation to enhance concentration and to feel a stronger mystical connection.

Patchouli Essential Oil acts as a natural perfume and an air freshener that creates a relaxing atmosphere, especially for the bedroom. Its antiseptic and anti-fungal properties make it beneficial for use in natural cleaning products. A spray cleaner can be made by blending 10 drops of Patchouli Essential Oil with 10 drops of Orange Essential Oil and diluting the blend in a 16 oz. (470 ml) bottle of warm water. This can be used to clean any surfaces including counters, walls, and floors.

5. Yarrow

Yarrow (Achillea millefolium) is an aromatic member of the Asteraceae (Compositae) family. This perennial European native with lovely, fern-like foliage is also named milfoil, or thousand leaves, because of its finely divided leaves. There are many species and subspecies of yarrow, including a similar native American variety known as A. Millefolium var. Granulosa.

Yarrow is naturalized throughout North America and can be found growing wild in meadows, fields, and along roadsides. Introduced to North America by early colonists, yarrow soon became a valued remedy used by many tribes of indigenous people. American Shakers gathered yarrow for use in numerous medicinal preparations. The plant was listed in the official U.S. Pharmacopoeia from the mid-to-late nineteenth century.

Yarrow's hardy rhizome, or underground stem, develops from underground runners as the extensive root system spreads. The lacy, finely-divided leaves are multi-pinnate, and grow alternately, clasping at the base along the simple, erect, and angular stem. The feather-like leaves may reach 6 in (15.2 cm) in length. The mound near the ground in early growth; then the slightly hairy stems reach upwards to 3 ft (0.91 m) in height during flowering. The tiny blossoms may be rose or lilac-colored, or a creamy white; they flower from June until October. Yarrow blossoms grow in flat-topped composite clusters at the top of the stems.

The herb was also believed to be useful in love charms and conjuring. One folk name for yarrow is devil's nettle. Other names include bloodwort, carpenter's weed, sanguinary, staunched, dog daisy, old man's pepper, field hops, nosebleed, knight's milfoil, soldier's woundwort, and military herb. Yarrow accompanied soldiers into battle and was relied upon for its hemostatic action to treat wounds. This use may have been the source of yarrow's generic name, taken from the legend of Achilles.

General Use

Scientists have identified over one hundred active chemical compounds in yarrow, including the intensely blue-colored azulene derivatives found in the essential oil of yarrow and at least two species of chamomile (Chamaemelum Nobile (L.) and Matricaria recutita).

Other chemical constituents in yarrow include lactones, flavonoids, tannins, coumarins, saponins, sterols, sugars, bitter glycoalkaloids, and amino acids. The aerial parts of yarrow, particularly the wild white-flowered variety, are most often used in medicinal remedies.

External Uses

Yarrow is well known for its wound-healing capabilities, particularly in staunching the flow of blood. The herb is considered vulnerable and hemostatic with antiseptic and antibacterial properties. The astringent action of the leaf, when inserted into a nostril, may stop a nosebleed. An infusion of the leaf, stems, and flowers will speed the healing of rashes, hemorrhoids, and skin ulcers. Dried and powdered yarrow sprinkled on cuts and abrasions may also facilitate healing. Native Americans used yarrow in poultice form to treat skin problems. Infusions of yarrow have been used as a hair rinse in attempts to prevent baldness.

Internal Uses

In folk medicine, freshly gathered yarrow root mashed in whiskey was used as a primitive anesthetic. Yarrow has also been used to stop internal bleeding, and as a bitter digestive tonic. Its emmenagogic action promotes the flow of bile. Yarrow tea taken warm acts as a diaphoretic, or medication given to induce sweating. It is particularly beneficial in the treatment of fever, colds, and influenza, as well as the early stages of measles and chickenpox. The essential oil, extracted by steam distillation of the flowers, is dark blue and has anti-inflammatory, anti-allergenic, and antispasmodic properties. Fresh yarrow leaf chewed slowly is said to relieve toothache. The herb has also been used to induce nosebleeds in an attempt to relieve migraine headaches. Yarrow appears to be beneficial in reducing high blood pressure. Flavonoids in the herb act to dilate the peripheral arteries and help to clear blood clots.

Preparations

Yarrow should be harvested while the herb is in flower, on a dry day after the morning dew has evaporated. The leaves, stems, and blossoms are all used medicinally. The leaves should be cut from the stems and spread out on a paper-lined tray to dry in a bright, airy room, out of direct sunlight. Blossoms may be left on the stems and hung in small bunches upside-down in a very warm room. Dried flowers should be stored separately, and dry stems cut into small segments before storage in an airtight, dark glass container, clearly labeled to indicate the contents and the date and place of harvest.

Leaf Infusion: Place 2 oz of fresh yarrow leaf, less if dried, in a warmed glass container. Bring 2.5 cups of fresh, nonchlorinated water to the boiling point and add it to the yarrow. Cover. Steep the tea for 10 to 15 minutes, then strain. Drink warm or cold throughout the day, up to three cups per day. The prepared tea can be stored for about two days in the refrigerator.

Tincture: Combine 4 oz of fresh yarrow leaf and stalks cut fine (or 2 oz dry powdered herb) with 1 pint of brandy, gin, or vodka in a glass container. The alcohol should be enough to cover the plant parts and have a 50/50 ratio of alcohol to water. Cover and store the mixture away from the light for about two weeks, shaking several times each day. Strain and store in a tightly capped clearly labeled dark glass bottle. A standard dose is 10 to 15 drops of the tincture in water, up to three times a day.

Precautions

Yarrow may have a cumulative medicinal effect on the system. Patients should avoid the frequent use of yarrow in large doses for long periods. Yarrow is a uterine stimulant; pregnant or lactating women should therefore not use the herb internally.

Side Effects

People with allergies to ragweed, another member of the Asteraceae family of plants, may also want to avoid taking yarrow internally. In some cases, yarrow may cause skin rashes or photosensitivity after ingestion.

Interactions

No interactions between yarrow and standard pharmaceutical preparations have been reported.

6. Vanilla

Vanilla is the fruit of an orchid plant, which grows in the form of a dark brown bean pod that is long and skinny. Vanilla orchids are grown in tropic climates, including Mexico, Tahiti, Reunion, Mauritius, Comoro, Indonesia, Uganda, and Tongo. Three-fourths of the world's supply comes from Madagascar. Vanilla is enjoyed throughout the world. The beans are used to add real vanilla flavor to sauce, frosting, syrup, ice cream, beverages, and a variety of desserts.

What Is A Vanilla Bean?

There are over 110 varieties of vanilla orchids. Only one, Vanilla planifolia, produces the fruit responsible for 99 percent of commercial vanilla. Another genus, the Vanilla tahitensis is grown in Tahiti. Its fruit has a more pronounced aroma, but debatably less flavor. To produce the fruit, the orchid flowers are hand-pollinated at a specific time of the day when the flowers are open during a short flowering period. The fruit is not permitted to fully ripen since this will cause the beans to split and lose their commercial value. Hand-harvesting occurs four to six months after the fruit appears on the vines. Once harvested, the green beans go through a treatment process that lasts another six months.

Some areas produce beans with higher vanillin content, which is responsible for the flavor and aroma. The resulting dark brown vanilla bean is usually 7 to 9 inches long, weighs about 5 grams, and yields about ½ teaspoon of seeds.

Vanilla Bean Uses

Most often, vanilla beans are processed into vanilla extract, a common ingredient in baked goods and other food recipes. Pure vanilla extract is made from real vanilla beans and imitation vanilla extract uses artificial vanillin flavoring. Whole vanilla beans or their seeds are used in recipes, just not as frequently because of the higher cost. The tiny seeds add texture and the bean has an intense flavor, plus they can add to the beauty of a light-colored dessert. Vanilla beans are simple to prepare. They're also often used whole to infuse the natural flavor into sugar, syrups, and beverages, including liquors.

How To Cook With Vanilla Bean

Preparing a vanilla bean is easy. For most recipes, use a sharp knife to slice the bean in half lengthwise while leaving the underside intact. Then scrape the seeds out and incorporate them into the recipe's other ingredients. The outer pod can be used to infuse the vanilla flavor into milk, cream, or sugar—a good use for dried-out and old vanilla beans, too. For whole bean recipes, generally cut off the ends then chop up the remainder (save the ends for vanilla infusions as well).

You can also use whole beans to make your vanilla extract. It's an easy infusion but takes about two months for the flavor to develop. Another option is to use them to make vanilla bean paste. It's a faster process but does require more work. This can be used as a replacement for either vanilla bean or vanilla extract in many recipes. It also retains the little black flecks that make vanilla bean recipes beautiful. If the beans dry out, they can be rehydrated. Soak them in milk or warm water for several hours.

What Does It Taste Like?

Vanilla beans have the most intense vanilla flavor and aroma that you will find. Generally, vanilla can be described as a sweet, rich, and warm woody or smoky flavor.

Vanilla Bean Substitute

The easiest substitute for whole vanilla beans is pure vanilla extract. The flavor intensity of a bean is much higher than the extract. The general rule is that 1 inch of vanilla bean is equal to 1 teaspoon of pure vanilla extract. That means one tablespoon will replace one whole bean; for extra flavor, increase it to two tablespoons. Generally, when a recipe calls for vanilla extract, it's measured in teaspoons, though. Adding tablespoons can negatively affect the consistency of your food, so you'll need to cut back on another liquid by a tablespoon or two. You would need even more imitation vanilla extract to match the flavor of a whole bean. Vanilla bean paste is another substitute, though it's not as common as the extract. Again, use 1 tablespoon of the paste to replace 1 whole vanilla bean. Since there's not as much moisture in the paste, you may not have to adjust the recipe's liquids.

Storage

To maintain the freshness of vanilla beans, store them in an airtight container, removing as much air as possible. Keep it in a cool, dry, and dark place. Refrigerating vanilla beans may cause mold growth and speed up drying. Open the container for about 15 minutes every few weeks to air out the beans. It's best to use beans within six months as they will dry out over time, even under the best conditions. They can be stored for eight to 12 months, and sometimes up to two years.

Commercial vanilla bean paste can have a shelf life of up to three years; homemade versions are typically good for one year. It should also be stored in an airtight container (typically a glass jar) at room temperature.

Nutrition and Benefits

The vanilla bean has trace amounts of calcium, iron, magnesium, manganese, potassium, and zinc.

1. However, the amount added to recipes likely isn't going to affect your daily nutrition significantly. It is better nutritionally than artificially flavored vanilla products, though. A real benefit of using the bean may be in the mood-enhancing aroma and taste.

2. The happy, relaxed feeling you get when burning a vanilla-scented candle can be found in naturally flavored food as well.

8. Aloe

Appearance

Aloe vera, a member of the lily family, is a spiky, succulent, perennial plant. It is indigenous to eastern and southern Africa, but has been spread throughout many of the warmer regions of the world, and is also popularly grown indoors. There are about 300 identified species, but Aloe vera ("true aloe") is the most popular for medical applications. It has also been known as Aloe Vulgaris ("common aloe") and Aloe barbadensis. The plant has yellow flowers and triangular, fleshy leaves with serrated edges that arise from a central base and may grow to nearly 2 ft (0.6 m) long. Each leaf is composed of three layers. A clear gel, that is the part of the plant used for topical application is contained within the cells of the generous inner portion. Anthraquinones, which exert a marked laxative effect, are contained in the bitter yellow sap of the middle leaf layer. The fibrous outer part of the leaf serves a protective function.

General Use

Few botanicals are as well known or as highly thought of as the Aloe vera plant. Throughout recorded history, it has been used to keep skin beautiful and restore it to health. A frequent moisturizing ingredient in cosmetics and hair care products, it also promotes the healing of burns and superficial wounds, but should not be used on deep or surgical wounds of punctures. Topical application has been successful in the treatment of sunburn, frostbite, radiation injuries, some types of dermatitis, psoriasis, cuts, insect stings, poison ivy, ulcerations, abrasions, and other dermatologic problems. Healing is promoted by the anti-inflammatory components, including several glycoproteins and salicylates, and substances that stimulate the growth of skin and connective tissue. Aloe vera contains several vitamins and minerals that are necessary for healing, including vitamin C, vitamin E, and zinc. It also exerts antifungal and antibacterial effects and thus helps to prevent wound infections. One study showed it to have a little more activity than the antiseptic silver sulfadiazine against several common bacteria that can infect the skin. It has moisturizing and pain-relieving properties for skin lesions, in addition to healing effects.

Aloe vera gel products may also be used internally. They should not contain the laxative chemicals found in the latex layer. There is some evidence that Aloe vera juice has a beneficial effect on peptic ulcers, perhaps inhibiting the causative bacteria, Helicobacter pylori. It appears to have a soothing effect on the ulcer and interferes with the release of hydrochloric acid by the stomach. Colitis and other conditions of the intestinal tract may also respond favorably to the internal use of gel products. Aloe vera has been shown to exert a stabilizing effect on blood sugar in studies done on mice, indicating a possible place for it in the treatment of diabetes. One study suggested that giving Aloe vera extract orally to patients with asthma who are not dependent on steroids could improve symptoms. A health care provider should be consulted about these uses. Other suggested, but insufficiently proven, indications for oral Aloe vera gel include prevention of kidney stones and relief of arthritis pain.

Aloe vera products derived from the latex layer are taken orally for the laxative effect. They can cause painful contractions of the bowel if taken in high doses. Milder measures are recommended first. The concentration of the immune stimulant acemannan is variable in the natural plant, as well as gel and juice products, 304 twil is also available in a purified, standardized, pharmaceutical-grade form. An injectable type is used in veterinary medicine to treat fibrosarcoma and feline leukemia, a condition caused by a virus in the same family as AIDS.

Preparations

Commercial Products

Choosing effective Aloe vera products can be challenging. Once a leaf is cut, enzymes start to break down some of the long-chain sugars which make Aloe vera gel an effective healing product, so the plant needs to have been properly handled and stabilized. Ask for help in selecting a reputable company to buy from. When shopping for a product to use for topical healing, look for Aloe vera to be one of the first products listed to ensure that it is not too dilute to be efficacious. Commercial, stabilized gel products may not work as well as fresh gel, but cold processing is thought to best retain beneficial properties. The FDA does not regulate the labeling of Aloe vera products.

Aloe vera juice is most often the form of a gel that is used internally. At least half of the juice should be Aloe vera gel. If laxative properties are not desired, be sure that the juice does not contain latex. A product that is made from the whole leaf does not necessarily contain anthraquinones from the latex layer, as those are water-soluble and can be separated during processing. Capsules and tinctures of the gel are also available. Oral forms of the latex extract are generally capsules, as it is extremely bitter.

Growing Aloe At Home

For common topical use, keeping an Aloe vera plant at home is one of the easiest ways to get the freshest and most concentrated gel. It is easy to cultivate, requiring only good drainage, mild temperatures, and occasional watering. Bring the plant inside if outside temperatures are less than 40°F (4.4°C). It will tolerate either full or partial sunlight but will require more frequent watering in full sun. Water it only when the soil has become dry. To use the gel, break off a leaf and cut it lengthwise to expose the inner layer. Scoop the gel out and apply generously to the area needing treatment. Discard whatever gel is not used immediately, as 305 twill degenerate quickly. The inner portion of the leaf may also be applied directly to a skin injury and bound to it.

Precautions

Aloe vera gel is generally safe for topical use, but it is best to apply it to a small area first to test for possible allergic reactions. Stinging and generalized dermatitis may result in individuals who are sensitive to it. The vast majority of the warnings apply only to products containing anthraquinones, such as aloin and barbaloin (as well as numerous others), which are found in the latex layer of the plant. Aloe vera latex should not be used internally by women who are pregnant or lactating, or by children. This product can cause abortion or stimulate menstruation. It may pass into the milk of breastfeeding mothers. People who have abnormal kidney function, heart disease, or gastrointestinal diseases are best advised to avoid any product containing Aloe vera latex or anthraquinones. Prolonged, internal use in high doses may produce tolerance so that more is required to obtain the laxative effect. Be aware of the possibility that any Aloe vera product for internal use that is supposed to contain only the gel portion can become contaminated by the anthraquinones of the latex layer. For this reason, people who have a contraindication for using Aloe vera latex should use caution when taking an Aloe vera gel product internally.

Side Effects

Internal use of Aloe vera latex may turn the urine red, and may also cause abdominal pain or cramps when products containing anthraquinones are consumed.

Interactions

Chronic internal use of products containing Aloe vera latex may increase the likelihood of potassium loss when used concomitantly with diuretics or corticosteroids. It may compound the risk of toxicity when used with cardiac glycosides (both prescription and herbal types) and antiarrhythmic drugs. Absorption of other oral medications can be decreased. Aloe vera latex should not be used with other laxative herbs, which may also lead to excessive potassium loss.

Internal use of Aloe vera gel can cause changes in blood sugar, so diabetics should monitor blood glucose levels during use, particularly if insulin or other pharmaceuticals are being used to control hyperglycemia. Topical Aloe vera may enhance the effect of topical corticosteroids and allow a reduction in the amount of the steroid being used.

CHAPTER 5: HERBS FOR DIVINATION

7. Honeysuckle

Honeysuckle is a large, volubilate shrub of the genus Lonicera. There are over 300 species of honeysuckle in the Caprifoliaceae family, found from Asia to North America. The shrub reaches heights of 20–30 ft (6–9 m), with thin, hairy branches. It has ovoid leaves that range 1.2–3.2 in (3–8 cm) long by 0.6–1.6 in (1.5–4.0 cm) wide. The plant flowers in late spring or early summer, depending on the species. Japanese honeysuckle (Lonicera japonica) blooms in the spring from April to May, with fragrant white flowers touched with a shade of purple that fades to yellow as they mature. The species of honeysuckle that is found in North America, the United Kingdom, and western Asia, Lonicera caprifolium, flowers in June. Generally, honeysuckle flowers are 1.2–1.6 in (3–4) cm long, with an inner tube of approximately the same length. All varieties of honeysuckle are famous for this tube, which is extracted and sucked for its sweet nectar. The shrub also produces a blackberry.

General Use

Japanese honeysuckle (L. japonica, also called Japanese jin yin Hua, which means gold and silver flower) and common honeysuckle (L. caprifolium, also called Italian honeysuckle, Dutch honeysuckle, and woodbine) are both widely used for their medicinal qualities. Although the Chinese most commonly use the bud of the flower in their medical practice, in other countries it is mostly the flowers and leaves that are used for their healing properties. Japanese honeysuckle works well as a detoxifier and is best used for acute infections and inflammations. As an alternative, which cleanses and purifies the blood, and an antipyretic, which reduces fever with its cooling properties, Japanese honeysuckle is best used for such ailments as sore throats, swollen eyes, headaches, etc.

Acute Infections And Inflammations

Japanese honeysuckle is most useful in treating acute illnesses, infections, and inflammations. At the onset of a cold, honeysuckle should be taken in combination with chrysanthemum flowers. Several popular Chinese formulas, such as yin-chair and ganmaoling, contain this herbal combination. Because it is a natural antibiotic, honeysuckle can also be used to treat infections caused by staphylococcal or streptococcal bacteria. Honeysuckle should be used for acute conditions and is not meant to be used in the treatment of chronic illnesses.

Skin Infections

Honeysuckle works well against internal infections, and it can also be used externally for skin irritation and infections. Honeysuckle has been found useful in alleviating rashes ranging from skin diseases to poison oak. For these types of skin ailments, honeysuckle is best used as a poultice. For cuts and abrasions that may become infected, a honeysuckle infusion can be applied externally. It is in treating skin infections that the stems of honeysuckle are used.

Circulatory System

John Gerard, a master herbalist of the sixteenth century, said that honeysuckle's "floures, be steeped in oil, and set in the Sun, are good to anoint the body that is benumbed, and growne very cold." Indeed, L. caprifolium as a fixed oil is good for the circulatory system. When it is heated and smoothed onto the skin, it has been shown to have a vasodilatory effect, causing the blood to flow into the dermis, which is the thick layer of skin beneath the epidermis.

Asthma And Coughs

L. caprifolium can be used for asthma on account of its antispasmodic properties. An herbal infusion of the leaves is the best method for treating asthma. A decoction of honeysuckle flowers can be used for coughs.

Other Uses

The seeds of L. caprifolium can be used as a diuretic. L. villosa, also known as American honeysuckle, has been used as a kidney stimulant. L. japonica has been used to treat dysentery and diarrhea.

Preparations

Three teaspoons of the leaf infusion can be taken three times a day. For skin irritation, honeysuckle should be made into an infusion or poultice and applied externally to the skin. When honeysuckle is compounded in capsule form, 10–17 g can be taken daily.

Precautions

Although honeysuckle poultices are used for skin irritations, there have been cases of contact dermatitis reported from pulling up Japanese honeysuckle. A patient that had come into contact with L. japonica reported developing a line of itchy blisters. People often taste honeysuckle tubes for their nectar; however, several cases of plant poisoning have been reported in children. The symptoms include gastrointestinal discomfort and muscle cramps.

Side Effects

There are no known side effects from using honeysuckle.

Interactions

No known adverse drug interactions have been reported with honeysuckle.

8. Iris

Irises are plants in the family Iridaceae, which contains 1,500-1,800 species and 70-80 genera. The center of diversity of this family is in southern Africa, but species are found on all of the habitable continents. The largest groups in the family are the true irises (Iris spp.) with 200 species and gladiolus (Gladiolus spp.) with 150 species. Many species in the iris family have large, attractive flowers. The major economic importance of this family involves the cultivation of many species in horticulture. In France and Quebec, the iris is generically known as the fleur-de-lis, and it is an important cultural symbol.

Biology Of Irises

Most species in the iris family are perennial herbs. These plants die back to the ground surface at the end of the growing season and then redevelop new shoots from underground rhizomes, bulbs, or corms at the beginning of the next growing season. A few species are shrubs.

The leaves of iris species are typically long, narrow, and pointed at the tip with parallel veins and sheathing at the base of the plant or shoot. The large, colorful, showy flowers are erect on a shoot and contain both female (pistillate) and male (staminate) organs.

The floral parts are in threes: three petals, three sepals, three stamens, and a pistil composed of three fused units. The sepals are large and petal-like, and they enclose the petals which are erect and are fused into a tube-like structure in some species. The flowers may occur singly or in a few-flowered inflorescence, or cluster. The flowers produce nectar, are pleasantly scented, and are pollinated by flying insects or birds, although some species are wind-pollinated. The fruits make up a three-compartmented capsule containing numerous seeds. The leaves and the rhizomes of Iris species contain an irritating chemical that is poisonous if eaten.

Horticultural Irises

Many species and cultivars in the iris family are grown in gardens and greenhouses for their beautiful flowers. These plants are typically propagated by splitting their rhizomes, bulbs, or corms, and sometimes by seed.

Various species of iris are cultivated in gardens. These include the yellow-flowered water-flag (Iris pseudacorus and blue-flowered species such as the true fleur-de-lis (I. germanica), the Siberian iris (I. sibirica), the stinking iris (I. foetidissima), and the butterfly iris (I. ochroleuca). Some cultivated species of iris have become naturalized in parts of North America and can be found in wild habitats and old gardens near abandoned houses.

Many of the approximately 80 species of crocuses are grown in gardens. In places where there is a snowy winter, crocuses are often blooming very soon after the snow melts and air temperatures become mild. The most commonly cultivated species is the European spring crocus (Crocus Verna).

Another commonly cultivated group is the gladiolus, including Gladiolus Byzantines from southwestern Asia and many horticultural hybrids. The tiger flower (Tigridia pavonia) is native to Mexico and is sometimes cultivated in temperate gardens.

Key Terms

Bulb: An underground thickened stem with many fleshy leaves surrounding a bud and fibrous roots emerging from the bottom. New shoots develop from bulbs at the beginning of the growing season.

Corm: A thick broad vertically growing underground stem that is covered with papery leaves and from which new shoots develop at the beginning of the growing season.

Cultivar: A distinct variety of a plant that has been bred for particular, agricultural or culinary attributes. Cultivars are not sufficiently distinct in the genetic sense to be considered to be subspecies.

Inflorescence: A grouping or arrangement of florets or flowers into a composite structure.

Rhizome: This is a modified stem that grows horizontally in the soil and from which roots and upward-growing shoots develop at the stem nodes.

Stigma: The part of the female organs of a plant flower (the pistil) upon which pollen lands in the first stage of fertilization.

Style: A stalk that joins the pollen-receptive surface of the stigma, to the ovary of the female organ of a plant (i.e., the pistil). Fertilization occurs in the ovary, which is reached by the male gametes through the growth of an elongate pollen tube from the pollen grain.

9. Jasmine

Jasmine is a plant. The flower is used to make medicine. Jasmine has been used for liver disease (hepatitis), liver pain due to cirrhosis, and abdominal pain due to severe diarrhea (dysentery). It is also used to cause relaxation (as a sedative), to heighten sexual desire (as an aphrodisiac), and in cancer treatment. In foods, jasmine is used to flavor beverages, frozen dairy desserts, candy, baked goods, gelatins, and puddings. In manufacturing, jasmine is used to add fragrance to creams, lotions, and perfumes.

Insufficient Evidence To Rate Effectiveness For

- Mental alertness
- Liver problems such as hepatitis and cirrhosis
- Stomach pain due to severe diarrhea (dysentery)
- Increasing sexual desire (as an aphrodisiac)
- Cancer treatment
- To cause relaxation (as a sedative).

How Does Jasmine Work?

There isn't enough information to know how jasmine might work.

Are There Safety Concerns?

Jasmine is likely safe for most people in food amounts. It is not known if jasmine is safe when used as medicine. Jasmine may cause allergic reactions.

Special Precautions & Warnings:

Pregnancy And Breastfeeding: There is not enough reliable information about the safety of taking jasmine in medicinal amounts if you are pregnant or breastfeeding. Stick to food amounts.

10. Lemon Balm

Lemon balm is a citrus-scented, aromatic herb. It is a perennial member of the Lamiaceae (formerly Labiatae), or mint, family and has proven beneficial to the nervous system. This lovely Mediterranean native, dedicated to the goddess Diana, is bushy and bright. Greeks used lemon balm medicinally over 2,000 years ago. Honey bees swarm to the plant.

Lemon balm grows in bushy clumps to 2 ft (0.6 m) tall and branches to 18 in (45.7 cm). It thrives in full sun or partial shade in moist, fertile soil from the mountains to the sea. The heart-shaped, deeply-veined leaves exude a pleasant lemon scent when brushed against or crushed. They have scalloped edges and square stems. The tiny white or golden blossoms grow in the leaf axils and bloom from June through October. The plant is hardy, self-seeding, and spreads easily in the right soil conditions. The plant has a short rhizome, producing erect, downy stems. The essential oil content appears to be highest in the uppermost third of the plant.

General Use

Lemon balm is a soothing, sedative herb that can relieve tension and lift depression. An infusion of this citrus-scented herb will improve digestion, reduce fever, ease spasms, and enhance relaxation. The plant has anti-histaminic properties and helps with allergies. Lemon balm infusions, taken hot, will induce sweating. Lemon balm has been used for centuries to calm the mind, improve memory, and sharpen wit. A daily infusion of lemon balm is said to promote longevity. It is a helpful herb in cases of hyperthyroid activity, palpitations of the heart, and tension headache. It can relieve pre-menstrual tension and menstrual cramping. It helps promote good digestion, relieve flatulence, and colic, and can ease one into a restful sleep. Lemon balm has antiviral and antibacterial properties. Used externally as a skin wash, this gentle herb can ease the sting of insect bites, soothe cold sore eruptions (herpes simplex), and treat sores and wounds. Lemon balm's highly aromatic qualities make it a good insect repellent. It is also valued in aromatherapy to relax and soothe a troubled mind. Fresh leaves are often added to salads, or used with fish, mushroom, and cheese dishes. In France, the herb is used in making cordials and is called Tea de France.

Preparations

Lemon balm leaves and flowers are used in medicinal remedies. The herb is at its best when used fresh from the harvest. The leaves may be picked throughout the summer, but the flavor is at its prime just before flowering. When the plant is dried for storage, the volatile oils diminish, reducing the medicinal potency of the herb. Freezing the fresh harvest is a good way to preserve the leaves for later use.

To create a tea, place two ounces of fresh lemon balm leaves in a warmed glass container; bring 2.5 cups of fresh, nonchlorinated water to the boiling point; add it to the herbs; cover, and infuse the tea for about 10 minutes. Once strained, the tea can be consumed warm. The prepared tea will store for about two days in the refrigerator. Lemon balm infusion is a gentle and relaxing tea. It may be enjoyed by the cupful three times a day. Lemon balm combines well with the leaves of peppermint (Mentha piperita), and nettle (Urtica dioica), and the flowers of chamomile (Matricaria chamomilla).

Precautions

Lemon balm has been used safely for thousands of years. However, pregnant women and individuals with hypothyroidism should avoid use unless under consultation with a physician. Use caution when harvesting because of the likely presence of bees.

Side Effects

The sedative effect of lemon balm means that it can depress the central nervous system when given in high doses. In addition, it has been reported that persons with glaucoma should avoid using essential oil of lemon balm, as it can raise the pressure inside the eye.

Interactions

Lemon balm should be used in lower dosages when combined with other herbs, particularly such other sedative herbs as valerian. In addition, lemon balm should not be taken together with prescription sedatives or alcohol, as it can intensify their effects.

Lemon balm has been reported to interfere with the action of thyroid hormones. Persons taking any medication containing thyroid hormones should not take lemon balm. A physician should be consulted before taking lemon balm in conjunction with any other prescribed pharmaceuticals.

5. Mugwort

Mugwort (Artemisia vulgaris) also known as common artemisia, felon herb, St. John's herb, chrysanthemum weed, sailor's tobacco, and moxa is a perennial member of the Compositae family and a close relative of wormwood (Artemisia absinthium L.). Mugwort's generic name is from that of the Greek moon goddess Artemis, a patron of women. Mugwort has long been considered an herbal ally for women with particular benefits in regulating the menstrual cycle and easing the transition to menopause. The common name may be from the old English word naught meaning "moth," or mugwort, meaning "midgewort," referring to the plant's folk use to repel moths and other insects.

This tenacious herb has naturalized throughout North America and maybe found growing wild in rocky soils, along streams and embankments, and in rubble and other waste places, particularly in the eastern United States. In some areas, including North Carolina and Virginia, mugwort is characterized as a noxious, alien weed. Mugwort root is about 8 in (20 cm) long with many thin rootlets. It spreads from stout and persistent rhizomes.

General Use

Mugwort leaf and stem are used medicinally. Mugwort acts as a bitter digestive tonic, uterine stimulant, nervine, menstrual regulator, and antirheumatic. The volatile oil of mugwort includes thujone, linalool, borneol, pinene, and other constituents. The herb also contains hydroxy-coumarins, lipophilic flavonoids, vulgar, and triterpenes.

Mugwort acts as an emmenagogue, an agent that increases blood circulation to the pelvic area and uterus and stimulates menstruation. It is a useful remedy for painful and irregular menstruation. A compress of the herb has been used to help promote labor and assist with the expulsion of the afterbirth. A mild infusion of mugwort is useful as a digestive stimulant. It is helpful in cases of mild depression and nervous tension.

The herb also may stimulate the appetite. A weak infusion of mugwort has sedative properties that may quiet restlessness and anxiety. Its antispasmodic action may relieve persistent vomiting and has been used in the treatment of epilepsy. Mugwort added to bathwater is an aromatic and soothing treatment for the relief of aches in the muscles and joints. In a clinical trial, crushed fresh mugwort leaves applied to the skin were shown to be effective in eradicating warts. Taken as an infusion, mugwort helps rid the system of pinworm infestation. Dried mugwort leaf also acts as a natural tinder, useful in holding a smoldering fire. The dried herb has also been smoked as nicotine-free tobacco. A species of mugwort (A. douglasiana), common in the southwestern United States, was used by some western Native Americans as prevention for poison oak rash. The fresh mugwort leaf was rubbed over areas of exposed skin before walking into the poison oak habitat. The two plants often grow near one another.

In Chinese medicine mugwort, known as Ai ye or Hao-shu is highly valued as the herb used in moxibustion, a method of heating specific acupuncture points on the body to treat physical conditions. Mugwort is carefully harvested, dried, and aged, then it is shaped into a cigar-like roll. This "moxa" is burned close to the skin to heat the specific pressure points. It has been used in this way to alleviate rheumatic pains aggravated by cold and damp circumstances. Mugwort has also been used in various size cones that are placed on the skin directly or on top of an herb or some salt and burned. In Japan, some practitioners only use moxa for treatment.

In Chinese medicine, mugwort is ingested to stop excessive or inappropriate menstrual bleeding. Mugwort has also been used in Brazilian folk medicine as a remedy for stomach ulcers. Researchers have found that the plant contains antioxidants which help to explain its protective effects on gastric tissues.

More recently, mugwort has attracted attention as the source of a natural compound, artemisinin, which has been shown to have antimalarial properties. Artemisinin is a promising natural remedy for malaria because of its low toxicity and its effectiveness against drug-resistant mutations of the malaria parasite. In addition to its effectiveness in treating malaria, artemisinin is also being tested as a possible anticancer drug. A group of researchers in Mississippi has shown that artemisinin is toxic to several different types of human cancer cells.

Preparations

Mugwort is harvested just as the plant comes into flower before the blossoms are fully open. The leaves are removed from the stalks and dried on paper-lined trays in a light, airy room, away from direct sunlight. The flowerheads should be dried intact and the dried herb stored in clearly labeled tightly-sealed, dark glass containers.

For infusion, 1 oz of fresh mugwort leaf, less if dried, is placed in a warmed glass container. One pint of fresh, nonchlorinated boiling water is added to the herb. The mixture is covered to prevent the loss of volatile oils. The tea should be infused for five to 10 minutes. A mild infusion is best. After straining, it is recommended to drink two cups of mugwort tea per day. Use should be discontinued after six days.

Four ounces of finely-cut fresh or powdered dry herb can be combined with 1 pt of brandy, gin, or vodka, in a glass container. The alcohol should be enough to cover the plant parts and have a 50/50 ratio of alcohol to water. The mixture should be kept in a dark place for about two weeks, shaking several times each day. It can then be strained and stored in a tightly capped, dark glass bottle. Dosage recommendations vary, with some herbalists cautioning against ingestion of mugwort in medicinal preparations.

In traditional Chinese medicine, the herb is burned slightly in a pan before simmering with other herbs to stop menstrual bleeding.

Precautions

Mugwort should be avoided during pregnancy and lactation. The herb is a uterine stimulant. Women should avoid its use during lactation as the chemical constituent thujone may be passed to the baby through the mother's milk. Mugwort should no be ingested if uterine inflammation or pelvic infection is present.

Side Effects

High doses of mugwort may cause liver damage, nausea, and convulsions. Some people develop contact dermatitis, or allergic skin rash if they are in contact with mugwort and certain other spices. This food allergy has been called the mugwort-spice syndrome, or sometimes the mugwort-celery-spice syndrome. Other foods and spices that are part of this syndrome include carrots, paprika, curry, cumin, birch, and pepper. In addition, mugwort pollen has been reported to cause asthma in susceptible children.

Interactions

People who are allergic to mugwort are also highly likely to be allergic to chamomile and should not take preparations made from either herb.

6. St. John's Wort

St. John's wort is a perennial, yellow-flowering plant that grows in the wild throughout Europe and is now found also in North America. The plant tends to be in blossom in June, around the day considered to be the birthday of John the Baptist; hence its popular name. The plant's Latin name is Hypericum perforatum.

St. John's wort has been used as a popular herbal folk remedy for centuries. More recently, practitioners of conventional Western medicine have been exploring its utility for treating depression and anxiety.

Purpose

Writings since the Middle Ages have been described using St. John's wort as a treatment for inflammation, injuries, burns, muscle pain, anxiety, high blood pressure, stomach problems, fluid retention, insomnia, hemorrhoids, cancer, and depression. Research conducted over the last decade of the twentieth century in Europe studied the efficacy of St. John's wort for the treatment of depression and anxiety. Research protocols have been developed in the United States to study the same issues, to determine appropriate dosages, to develop standard formulations, and to define whether it can be used for all forms of depression or only for more mild forms of the condition. The leaves and flowers of St. John's wort are both used. St. John's wort is available as pills, capsules, extracts, dried herbs for tea, and oil infusions for skin applications.

Recommended Dosage

Because dosages of herbal preparations are not always standardized, it is important to discuss with a knowledgeable practitioner the most reliable form of St. John's wort. Recommendations call for 300-500 mg (of a standardized 0.3% hypericin extract) three times daily. It can take four to six weeks to notice the antidepressant effects of this preparation.

Alternatively, one to two teaspoons of dried St. John's wort can be put into a cup of boiling water and steeped for 10 minutes to make tea. The recommended dosage of tea is one to two cups daily. Again, four to six weeks may be necessary to notice the improvement in symptoms of depression.

Precautions

The following precautions should be considered and discussed with a knowledgeable practitioner before St. John's wort is taken:

Some people may become more sensitive to the sun.

Key Terms

Immunosuppressant: Medications that suppress or lower the body's immune system, primarily used to help the body accept a transplanted organ.

Monoamine Oxidase Inhibitors: A group of anti-depressant drugs that decrease the activity of monoamine oxidase, a neurotransmitter found in the brain that affects mood.

Reserpine: Medication to treat high blood pressure. Brand names include Serpalan, Novoreser-pine, and Reserfia.

Theophylline: A medication used to treat asthma. Sold under many brand names, including Aerolite Sr, Respbid, and Theolair.

Warfarin: A medication that helps to prevent the formation of clots in the blood vessels. Sold as Coumadin in the U.S.

Patients taking MAOIs must carefully avoid taking St. John's wort due to the serious adverse effects of combining the two. Because the effects of St. John's wort are still being studied, pregnant and breastfeeding women should avoid its use. Depression can be a serious, even life-threatening, condition; therefore, depressed patients using St. John's wort must be carefully monitored.

Side Effects

People taking St. John's wort may develop one or all of the following side effects:

Skin rash due to sun sensitivity, the most common side effect

Headache, dizziness, dry mouth, constipation

Abdominal pain, confusion, sleep problems, and high blood pressure are less frequently experienced

Interactions

Again, a knowledgeable professional should be consulted before St. John's wort is taken to determine the appropriateness of its use and avoid serious interactions. Interactions include:

Possible decrease in the effectiveness of reserpine, warfarin, theophylline, immunosuppressant medications such as cyclosporine, and antiviral drugs such as indinavir.

Dangerous interactions when used with other anti-depressant medicines (especially MAOIs), digoxin, and loperamide.

Interactions with oral birth control pills. St. John's wort may interfere with the effectiveness of birth control pills, increasing the risk of pregnancy; an alternative form of birth control should be considered while taking St. John's wort. In addition, women taking both birth control pills and St. John's wort may notice bleeding between menstrual periods.

7. Wormwood

Wormwood (Artemisia absinthium) is a perennial that is native to Europe and parts of Africa and Asia but now grows wild in the United States. It is extensively cultivated. Also called shrub wormwood, Artemisia absinthium is a member of the daisy or Asteraceae family. The species name, absinthium, means "without sweetness." Many species of the genus Artemisia have medicinal properties.

Wormwood grows alongside roads or paths. This shrubby plant is 1-3 ft (0.3-0.9 m) tall and has gray-green or white stems covered with fine hairs. The yellowish-green leaves are hairy and silky and have glands that contain resinous particles where the natural insecticide is stored. Wormwood releases an aromatic odor and has a spicy, bitter taste.

Wormwood is a strong bitter that affects the bitter-sensing taste buds on the tongue that sends signals to the brain to stimulate the entire digestive system (salivation, stomach acid production, intestinal tract movement, etc.). This bitter taste also stimulates the production of bile by the liver and the storage of bile in the gall bladder. The azulenes in wormwood have anti-inflammatory activity. The sesquiterpene lactones are insecticidal and have anti-tumor activity. The toxin thujone is a brain stimulant. Wormwood also has anti-inflammatory, antidepressant, carminative (relieves intestinal gas), tonic (restores tone to tissues), antibacterial, antifungal, antiamoebic, antifertility, hepatoprotective (prevents and cures liver damage), febrifugal (reduces fever), and vermifugal (expels intestinal worms) activities.

General Use

Wormwood has been used in European traditional medicine as a restorative of impaired cognitive functions (thinking, remembering, and perception). Wormwood is often used as a digestive stimulant. It helps treat indigestion, heartburn, irritable bowel syndrome, stomach pain, gas, and bloating. By increasing the production of stomach acids and bile, wormwood can be useful to persons with poor digestion. It helps persons recover after a long illness and improves the uptake of nutrients.

As the name suggests, wormwood is used to eliminate intestinal worms, especially pinworms and roundworms. It is also used as an insect repellent and insecticide. Wormwood is also helpful in treating gall bladder inflammation, hepatitis, jaundice, fever, infections, and mild depression. Wormwood may also protect the liver from harmful chemicals and stimulate menstruation or miscarriage. It has been used to treat the pains associated with childbirth, cancers, muscle aches, arthritic joints, sprains, dislocated joints, and broken bones.

Wormwood has a historical dark side: absinthe. This clear green alcoholic beverage, which contains essential oil of wormwood and other plant extracts, is highly toxic and presently banned in many countries. A favorite liqueur in nineteenth-century France, absinthe was addictive and associated with a collection of serious side effects known as absinthism (irreversible damage to the central nervous system). The toxic component of wormwood that causes absinthism is thujone. Wormwood may contain as much as 0.6% thujone. On the other hand, wormwood soaked in white wine is used to produce the liqueur called vermouth (derived from the German word for wormwood, Wermuth), which contains very little thujone.

Preparations

Wormwood is harvested immediately before or during flowering in the late summer. All the aerial portions (stem, leaves, and flowers) have medicinal uses. Wormwood is used either fresh or dried.

Wormwood may be taken as an infusion (a tea), as a tincture (an alcohol solution), or in pill form. Wormwood should be taken only under the supervision of a professional. It should be taken in small doses as directed, and for no longer than four to five weeks at a time. The infusion is prepared by steeping 0.5-2 tsp of wormwood in 1 cup of boiling-hot water for 10-15 minutes. The usual dosage is 3 cups daily, for a period not to exceed four weeks.

Wormwood tincture can be prepared by adding 1.5 cups of fresh, finely chopped wormwood or 8 tbsp of powdered wormwood to 2 cups of whiskey. The herb and alcohol mixture is shaken daily and allowed to steep for 11 days. The solids are strained out and the tincture is stored in a tightly capped bottle in a cool place. This tincture may be used externally (to relieve pain) or internally. Ten to twenty drops of tincture are added to water, which is taken 10–15 minutes before each meal. As with the infusion, wormwood tincture should not be taken for longer than four weeks.

Wormwood preparations are usually sipped because the strong bitter taste is an important component of its therapeutic effect on stomach ailments. The bitter taste of wormwood infusion or tincture may be masked with honey or molasses when the bitter action is not necessary, as in the treatment of worms, fever, or liver ailments.

Insect repellent can be made from wormwood by mixing thoroughly crushed fresh wormwood leaves with apple cider vinegar. This mixture is put into a small piece of gauze or cheesecloth. The ends are folded up and tied to make a little bag, and the bag is rubbed over the skin of humans or pets to repel mosquitoes, gnats, and horseflies.

Precautions

Excessive use of wormwood leads to toxic levels of thujone in the body. The long-term use of wormwood oil containing thujone, or alcoholic drinks containing thujone oil (e.g., absinthe) can be addictive and cause seizures, brain damage, temporary kidney failure, and possibly death. Using wormwood for longer than four weeks or at higher than recommended doses may lead to nausea, vomiting, restlessness, insomnia, vertigo, tremors, and seizures. Women who are pregnant or lactating (breastfeeding) should not use wormwood.

Side Effects

Significant side effects are not encountered when wormwood is taken in small doses for only two to four weeks. One report stated, however, that using as much as 1 mL of wormwood tincture three times a day for up to nine months caused no side effects.

Interactions

As of mid-2000, there are no identified interactions between wormwood and any other drug or herbal medicine.

CONCLUSION

This an excellent beginning to managing stress holistically. We encourage you to consider which of the practices mentioned above would be most beneficial and suggest creating a customized stress-management plan that is unique to your needs. We think you'll find the combination of lifestyle habits and herbal support to not only help you manage stress but also strengthen and improve your overall wellness. Generally considered safe and can provide a natural way for soothing acid reflux that works for some people. This approach doesn't work for everyone. We are all different. You may have to try different natural remedies to find one that works for you.

Consult your doctor before using supplements. With your doctor's help, you can come up with a treatment plan that's right for you. If you're pursuing an alternative route for healing, make sure your doctor is aware of the supplements you take or plan to take. Herbal supplements and other alternative forms of medicine can have negative health effects and can affect the absorption of medications.

Several other herbs have historically been used to lend support to healthy digestive function. These include:

- Chamomile
- Catnip
- Skullcap
- Lemon Balm
- Flax Seed
- Chia Seed
- Psyllium Seed
- Cascara Sagrada
- Senna Leaf
- Triphala
- Blackberry Root
- Boldo Leaf e.t.c.

Most herbalists will tell you that they became interested in herbs because they had some conditions that they wanted to find a better way to address. For me, it was more about learning to be in charge of my emotions. It's not that they were out of control, but I studied psychology in college, and this interest has never left me. Strong emotions can be uncomfortable and do considerable damage to various bodily systems. Herbs with nervine and adaptogenic actions have been shown to ease and support the body's response to stress. Nervines work to lessen overactive stress responses and help bring the mind and body back to a state of rest. They do this by shifting the nervous system from the active, sympathetic system to the parasympathetic system. All nervines are unique and work slightly differently from one another; some are uplifting, working to ease anxiety and boost mood, while others have more relaxing, sedative qualities. Many nervines work well in teas and tinctures to provide support. Many herbalists use adaptogens to boost immune function, increase stamina, improve stress response, and provide general support to the body as a whole. The benefits of these herbs are not always seen immediately. They usually work best when taken over some time. Many adaptogens work well in tinctures, teas, and rolled pills and can be added to daily food preparations, such as Adaptogenic Bliss Balls and Nourishing Herbal Broth.

Activating your metabolism will help you burn more fat and give you more energy throughout the day. This is something we all want and can get! It can start with this tea recipe using plant-based ingredients that are high in nutrients that naturally activate your metabolism.

To train your body to crave the right foods, we have to set the foundation for that every single day. This morning tea uses a splash of apple cider vinegar, fresh lemon juice, cayenne pepper, and cinnamon to wake up your metabolic system naturally. We've added some raw honey and ginger root to make it taste better and help your digestive system as well.

NATIVE AMERICAN ESSENTIAL OILS

A Complete Medical Handbook of Native American Essential Oils

Taahira Maskwa

INTRODUCTION

Essential oil is a highly volatile substance isolated by a physical process from an odoriferous plant of a single botanical species. The oil bears the plant's name from which it is derived, for example, rose oil or peppermint oil. Such oils were called essential because they were thought to represent the very essence of odor and flavor.

Distillation is the most common method for isolating essential oils, but other processes, including enfleurage (extraction using fat), maceration, solvent extraction, and mechanical pressing, are used for specific products. Younger plants produce more oil than older ones, but old plants are richer in more resinous and darker oils because of the continuing evaporation of the lighter fractions of the oil.

Out of many plant species, essential oils have been well characterized and identified from only a few thousand plants. The oils are stored as microdroplets in the glands of plants. After diffusing through the walls of the glands, the droplets spread over the plant's surface before evaporating and filling the air with perfume. The most odoriferous plants are found in the tropics, where solar energy is the greatest.

The function of the essential oil in a plant is not well understood. Odors of flowers probably aid in natural selection by acting as attractants for certain insects. Leaf oils, wood oils, and root oils may protect against plant parasites or depredations by animals. Oleoresinous exudations that appear when the trunk of a tree is injured prevent loss of sap and act as a protective seal against parasites and disease organisms. Few essential oils are involved in plant metabolism, and some investigators maintain that many of these materials are simply waste products of plant biosynthesis.

Commercially, essential oils are used in three primary ways: as odorants, they are used in cosmetics, perfumes, soaps, detergents, and miscellaneous industrial products ranging from animal feeds to insecticides to paints; as flavors, they are present in bakery goods, candies, confections, meat, pickles, soft drinks, and many other food products; and as pharmaceuticals, they appear in dental products and a wide, but diminishing, group of medicines.

The first records of essential oils come from ancient India, Persia, and Egypt. Greece and Rome conducted extensive trade in odoriferous oils and ointments with the countries of the Orient. These products were probably extracts prepared by placing flowers, roots, and leaves in fatty oils. In most ancient cultures, what used odorous plants or their resinous products directly. Only with the coming of the golden age of Arab culture was a technique developed to distill essential oils. The Arabs were the first to distill ethyl alcohol from fermented sugar, thus providing a new solvent for the extraction of essential oils in place of the fatty oils that had probably been used for several millennia.

The knowledge of distillation spread to Europe during the Middle Ages, and the isolation of essential oils by distillation was described during the 11th to 13th centuries. These distilled products became a specialty of medieval European pharmacies by about 1500, who had introduced the following products: oils of cedarwood, calamus, costus, rose, rosemary, spike, incense, turpentine, sage, cinnamon, benzoin, and myrrh. The Swiss physician and alchemist Paracelsus alchemical theories played a role in stimulating physicians and pharmacists to seek essential oils from aromatic leaves, woods, and roots.

Starting from the time of Marco Polo, the much-prized spices of India, China, and the Indies served as the impetus for European trade with the Orient. Naturally, such spices as cardamom, sage, cinnamon, and nutmeg were subjected to the pharmacists' stills by the middle of the 18th century in Europe, introducing about 100 essential oils.

However, there was little understanding of the nature of the products. As chemical knowledge expanded in the late 1800s and early 1900s, many well-known chemists took part in the chemical characterization of essential oils. Improvement in the understanding of essential oils led to a sharp expansion in production. The use of the volatile oils in medicine became entirely subordinate to uses in foodstuffs, beverages, and perfumes.

In the United States, what produced oils of turpentine and peppermint before 1800; within the next several decade's oils of four indigenous American plants became important commercially, namely, sassafras, wormwood, wintergreen, and sweet birch. Since 1800 many essential oils have been prepared, but only a few have attained commercial significance.

Methods Of ProductionThe first step in isolating essential oils is crushing or grinding the plant material to reduce the particle size and rupture some of the cell walls of oil-bearing glands. Steam distillation is the most common and essential production method, and extraction with cold fat (enfleurage) or hot fat (maceration) is chiefly of historical importance.

Three different methods of steam distillation are practiced. In the oldest and most straightforward method, a vessel containing water and the chopped or crushed plant material is heated by a direct flame. A water-cooled condenser recovers the water vapor and volatile oil.

This original method is being replaced by a process in which the plant material is suspended on a grid above the water level, and steam from a second vessel is introduced under the grid. The volatiles is condensed, and the oil is separated. In the third process, the ship containing the plant material on a grid is heated to prevent steam condensation, so that dry distillation is attained. In southern France, essential oils were extracted with cold fat long before introducing extraction with volatile solvents.

This process is applied to flowers that do not yield an appreciable quantity of oil by steam distillation or whose odor is changed by contact with boiling water and steam. In this process, flowers are spread over a highly purified mixture of tallow and lard and are left for a period varying from 24 hours to 72 hours. During this time, most of the flower oil is absorbed by the fat. The petals are then removed (effleurage), and the process is repeated until the fat is saturated with oil. The final product is called pomade (e.g., pomade de jasmine).

In most cases, it is possible to shorten the long enfleurage process by extracting the essential oils using molten fat for one to two hours at a temperature ranging from about 45° to 80° C (110° to 175° F). The fat is filtered after each immersion, and after 10 to 20 extraction cycles, the pomade is sold as such, or who may extract it with alcohol to yield the oil residue.

Since both enfleurage and maceration are rather expensive processes, some essential oil specialists have shifted almost entirely to using volatile solvents to recover crucial oils from plant materials that could not be processed by steam distillation. Petroleum naphthas, benzene, and alcohol are the primary solvents.

A procedure called expression is applied only to citrus oils. The outer colored peel is squeezed in presses, and the oil is decanted or centrifuged to separate water and cell debris. The method is used for sweet and bitter orange oil, lemon, lime, mandarin, tangerine, bergamot, and grapefruit. Much oil is produced as a by-product of the concentrated-citrus-juice industry.

EXPLANATION OF ESSENTIAL OIL

Essential Oils

Essential oils are produced in various parts of a plant, such as in the flower, seeds, bark, root, leaves, resin, or wood, and can be responsible for a plant's distinctive odor or fluent. Among the plants notable for their essential oils and used as a source of fragrances and flavorings are members of the following plant families.

- Carrot family (anise, dill, angelica)
- Ginger family (cardamom, ginger)
- Laurel family (cinnamon, camphor)
- The mint family (peppermint, rosemary, thyme)
- Myrtle family (clove, allspice)
- The orchid family (vanilla)
- Nutmeg family (nutmeg, mace)
- Pepper family (black pepper)

Oils derived from plants, namely vegetable oils, have been used for thousands of years. Plants have been a healthy alternative to animal-derived oils since their discovery, containing virtually no cholesterol. Most vegetable oils are pressed from seeds; however, oils are pressed from the fruit pulps in a few cases, such as olives and palm fruits. About 70% of the world's plant oil production comes from four plant species: soybeans, oil palm, rape, and sunflower. Of these, only sunflower (Helianthus annuus) can claim North America as its original home.

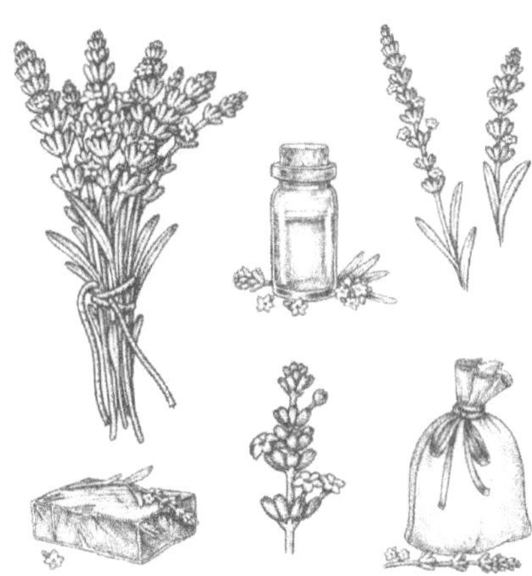

Evidence suggests that Native Americans in present-day Arizona and New Mexico cultivated the sunflower about 3,000 BC. Sunflower seeds were eaten and crushed for oil. Wild, weedy populations of this annual species still occur throughout Canada, the United States, and Mexico. Wild plants are branched, bearing numerous relatively small heads. Domesticated sunflowers usually have one central authority atop a single flowering stem.

Some archaeologists suggest that sunflower may have been domesticated before corn. The seed of the native perennial herb, arrowleaf balsamroot, Balsamorhiza sagittata, was a prized source of oil for many Native Americans. Arrowleaf balsamroot is a showy member of the sunflower family. "Balsamorhiza" refers to the balsam-like taste and smell of the resinous and woody root.

Native American Healing

Native American traditions focused on healing rather than curing. While physicians today look for ways to make symptoms disappear, ancient healing traditions of tribes like the Cherokee concentrate on creating a whole person and restoring harmony in the human body.

More focus has been given to the nature of holistic medicine as people look for natural ways to end dependency on harmful drugs and expensive treatments. The spiritual healing of herbs and essential oils has been studied for thousands of years, and there is still much to learn about the practice. However, one thing is certain. Holistic medicine and treatments provide relief and even empower those who use it properly.

Native American healers also combine medicine with healing ceremonies and prayers. A caring community envelopes a sick individual so that everyone can show their love and ask the Great Spirit for healing. This type of healing calls on the power of nature, human connections, and spirit.

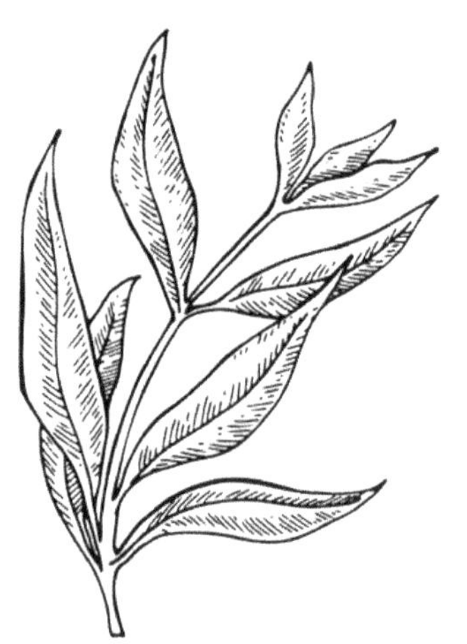

To heal means much more than taking away a symptom. It means improving a person's quality of life. With nature's gifts and caring communities, we can find a whole different way to look at the world of medicine and find better solutions for those experiencing pain and illness.

The meaning of the term medicine to an American Indian is quite different from that ordinarily held by modern societies. To most American Indians, medicine signifies various ideas and concepts rather than remedies and treatment alone. There is no separation between religion and medicine in tribal culture, and healing ceremonies are integral to the community experience.

To the American Indian, the natural or correct state of all things, including man, is harmony. Far from being dominant over nature, man is interdependent with other living beings and physical forces. All thinking is grounded in relationships. More emphasis is given to the connectedness of one thing to another than to the individual thing itself. To maintain a correct or natural relationship is to be in harmony. The universe is a complex matrix of interdependence. There is a proper set of connections for each being, a good existing in harmony with the universe.

George Bird Grinnell, who was intimately associated with northern Plains tribes, has written:

"All these things which we speak of as medicine the Indian calls mysterious, and when he calls them mysterious this only means that they are beyond his power to account for. He whom we call a medicine man may be called a doctor, a healer of diseases; or if he is a worker of magic, he is a mystery man. All Indian languages have words which are the equivalent of our word medicine, sometimes with curative properties; but the Indian's translation of "medicine," used in the sense of magical or supernatural, would be mysterious, inexplicable, unaccountable."

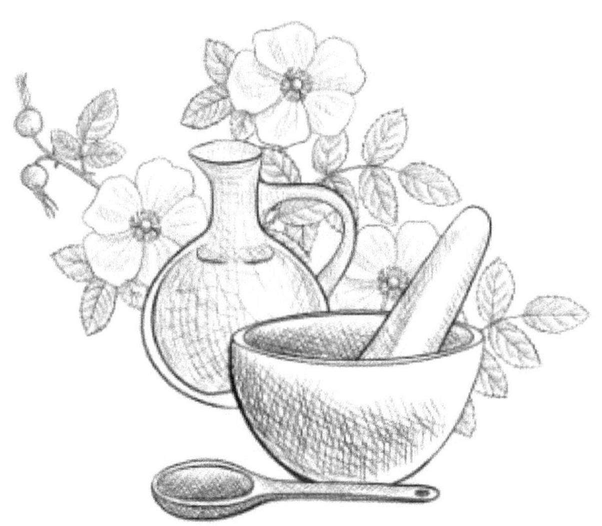

Tribal cultures interpret disease and human suffering as disharmony. An individual suffers because, in some way, they have fallen out of harmony. The person who does not feel well has become out of phase with the correct relationships.

Their medical theory arises from the reasoning that the medicine man can control the forces of nature and hence make disease yield to his personal effects. Consequentially, curative agents are medicine, but only one type of medicine, and then only when associated with prescribed rites. The medicine man is entrusted with ceremonies connected with birth and death, magical ceremonies, and the perpetuation of tribal lore. He is not only the primitive doctor but also the diviner, the rainmaker, the soothsayer, the prophet, the priest, and the chief. Some of the better-known American Indian leaders were medicine men: Sitting Bull, Geronimo, and Cochise.

Recent years have shown a surge of interest in the therapies of traditional cultures, in patients' use of alternative medicine, and the desire for mind-body therapies and spiritual treatment and behavioral medicine treatments for chronic medical illness. Some hospitals have included traditional Native American healers as part of their staff. Harvard University has created a Center to study alternative medicine.

Essential oils have enhanced lives for thousands of years, offering various benefits from cosmetic and dietary purposes to spiritual and religious use. Extracted through careful steam distillation, resin tapping, and cold pressing, the purest essential oils are far more powerful than the botanicals from which they come.

The term "essential oil" is a contraction of the original "quintessential oil." This stems from the Aristotelian idea that matter is composed of four elements: fire, air, earth, and water. The fifth element, or quintessence, was then considered to be spirit or life force. Distillation and evaporation were thought to be processes of removing the energy from the plant, and this is also reflected in our language since the term "spirits" is used to describe distilled alcoholic beverages such as brandy, whiskey, and eau de vie. The last of these again shows the reference to removing the life force from the plant. Nowadays, of course, we know that, far from being spirit, essential oils are physical and composed of complex mixtures of chemicals.

Native Americans stressed the development of the inner life, which was seen reflected in the outer world. The events of the external world spoke to internal processes for the person. A fire is burning on the mountain. The person is in agony. An awareness comes, which dissipates hell. Rain comes to quench the fire. The events are seen as related. The fire and the rain were messages about the internal processes of the person. Such ideas are more consistent with a dynamic energy systems (DES) approach. Systems interact in complex ways, communicating and creating shared memory through their common effects upon each other during that communication. While preposterous to the conventional psychotherapist that a human being can express agony to nature, modern DES theory parallels the traditional belief that the mountain could have responded with fire and then the sky with rain, both in response to the human and now also the burning mountain.

Native healing of externally caused injuries, in which the origin of the ailment is pronounced, is usually rational and often practical. Fractures, dislocations, snake and insect bites, skin irritation, and bruises in such a category. Minor internal illnesses, such as colds, headaches, and digestive disorders, are treated with herbal remedies. In cases of persistent internal disease where the cause is not apparent, the usual Indian custom is to attribute the illness to some supernatural agency.

If ordinary medicine did not soon bring relief, they would resort to shamanistic methods, such as incantations, charms, prayers, dances, rattles shaking, and drums beating. The supernatural causes of disease among American Indians societies included sorcery, taboo violation, disease-object intrusion, spirit intrusion, and soul loss, an additional disease cause prevalent among Iroquoian tribes, his unfulfilled dreams or desires. In certain tribes and areas, some of these causes are more important than others.

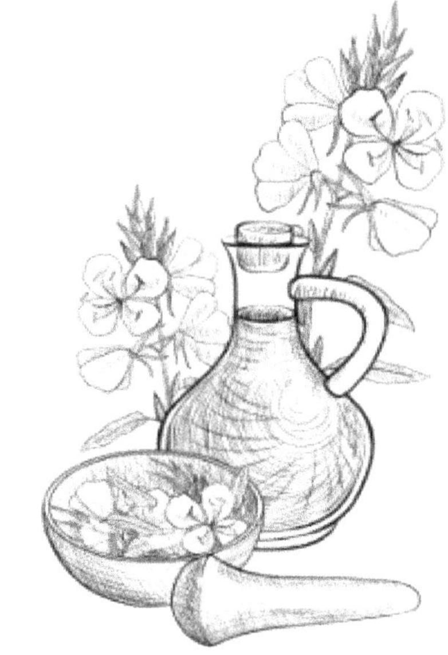

Of the supernatural causes of disease, the most important are the spirits of the animals, who thus gain revenge for slights and abuses. Disrespect toward the fire, such as urinating on the ashes, or spitting on it, will bring disaster. Insults to nature bring about a specific penalty. Human ghosts who naturally feel lonesome for their friends and relatives cause disease to provide friendly company. In contrast, an animal ghost will cause trouble if respect has not been shown to its body after being killed. A powerful disease-bringer is the magic used by witches to cause sickness. Other disease causes are dreams, omens, neglected taboos, and the evil influence attributed to a woman during her catamenial period.

The practice of the medicine man relates to the plant world in several ways. Some tribes believe that spirits inspire the healer to know which curative plants to use; others that a plant is protected by the heart" that has endowed it with medicinal properties. Offerings are often left to these spirits when the drug plant is picked. Healing is indicated by the soul's return or the medicine man claiming to produce the 'extracted object'. Massage and ritual 'sweat baths' are also used in the healing process. North American Indians used catnip tea for colic in babies.

As mentioned previously, the word "Medicine" has a different meaning for Native Americans. It encompasses well-being and spiritual health as well as physical health. A pipe ceremony is a ritual that Hopi Native Americans employ to pray to the Great Spirit. Great Spicomprisesd of the mother (the earth), the father (the heavens and celestial body), and the grandmothers and grandfathers. Grandmothers and grandfathers may be likened to angels. In the Hopi tradition, they are beings that have been in the universe since time began, and they are thought to carry specific medicines. That is, they each have different strengths or aptitudes, which the Hopi may call upon in other circumstances.

WHAT ARE ESSENTIAL OILS?

Essential oils are plant extracts. They're made by steaming or pressing various plant parts (flowers, bark, leaves, or fruit) to capture the compounds that produce fragrance. It can take several pounds of a plant to make a single bottle of essential oil. In addition to creating a scent, essential oils perform other functions in plants, too. Essential oil is a natural product extracted from a single plant species. Not all plants produce essential oils, and in the plants that do, what may find the essential oil in the roots, stems, leaves, flowers, or fruits.

Essential oils are highly concentrated plant extracts distilled into oil. Popular in complementary and alternative medicine, these oils, derived from flowers, leaves, roots, and other parts of plants, have been used for medicinal purposes in some cultures for centuries.

Continuing scientific research has found that certain essential oils have health benefits; in fact, many modern medications are derived from essential oils. However, while some fats are beneficial in small doses, others can be dangerous.

Popular Types

There are more than 90 essential oils, each with its unique smell and potential health benefits. Here's a list of 10 popular essential oils and the health claims associated with them:

- Peppermint: Used to boost energy and aid digestion
- Lavender: Used to relieve stress
- Sandalwood: Used to calm nerves and help with focus
- Bergamot: Used to reduce stress and improve skin conditions like eczema
- Rose: Used to improve mood and reduce anxiety
- Chamomile: Used to improve mood and relaxation
- Ylang-Ylang: Used to treat headaches, nausea, and skin conditions
- Tea Tree: Used to fight infections and boost immunity
- Jasmine: Used to help with depression, childbirth, and libido
- Lemon: Used to aid digestion, mood, headaches, and more

What Are Essential Oils Good For?

Although people claim essential oils are natural remedies for several ailments, there's not enough research to determine their effectiveness in human health. Some studies indicate a benefit to using essential oils, while others show no improvement in symptoms. Clinical trials have looked at whether essential oils can alleviate conditions such as:

- Anxiety
- Depression
- Nausea
- Insomnia
- Low appetite
- Dry mouth

How Can You Use Essential Oils Safely?

The quality of essential oils on the market varies greatly, from pure to those diluted with less expensive ingredients. And because there's no regulation, the label may not even list everything that's in the bottle you're buying. That's why who should not ingest essential oils.

Johns Hopkins also advises against using essential oil diffusers, small household appliances that create scented vapor. Diffusion in a public area or household with multiple members can affect people differently. For example, peppermint is often recommended for headaches. But if you use it around a child who's less than 30 months old, the child can become agitated.

It could have a negative effect. Additionally, someone with a fast heartbeat can react adversely to peppermint. The safest ways to use essential oils include:

- **Aromatherapy Accessories:** Necklaces, bracelets, and keychains made with absorbent materials you apply essential oils to and sniff throughout the day.
- **Body Oil:** A mixture of essential oils with a carrier oil such as olive, jojoba, or coconut oil that can massage into the skin. Because essential oils are concentrated, they can irritate. Avoid using them full-strength on the skin.
- **Aroma Stick:** An essential oil inhaler, these portable plastic sticks have an absorbent wick that soaks up the essential oil. They come with a cover to keep the scent under wraps until you're ready.

Allergic Reactions To Essential Oils

A small number of people may experience irritation or allergic reactions to certain essential oils. You're more likely to have a lousy reply if you have atopic dermatitis or a history of reactions to topical products. Although you can experience a response to any essential oil, some are more likely to be problematic, including:

- Oregano oil
- Cinnamon bark oil
- Jasmine oil
- Lemongrass oil
- Ylang-ylang oil
- Chamomile oil
- Bergamot oil

Because pure essential oils are potent, diluting them in carrier oil is the best way to avoid a bad reaction when applying directly to the skin. If you get a red, itchy rash or hives after using essential oils, see a doctor. You may be having an allergic reaction.

Which Essential Oils Are Best?

There are dozens of essential oils, all with different fragrances and chemical makeups. Which essential oils are best depends on what symptoms you're looking to ease or fragrances you prefer. Some of the most popular essential oils include:

- **Lavender Oil:** Many people find the lavender scent relaxing. It's often used to help relieve stress and anxiety and promote good sleep.
- **Tea Tree Oil:** Also called melaleuca, Australia's aboriginal people used this essential oil for wound healing. Today, it's commonly used for acne, athlete's foot, and insect bites.

- **Peppermint Oil:** There's some evidence peppermint essential oil helps relieve irritable bowel syndrome (IBS) symptoms when taken in an enteric-coated capsule (from a trusted health supplement provider). It may also relieve tension headaches when applied topically.
- **Lemon Oil:** Many people find the citrusy scent of lemon oil a mood booster. It's also often used in homemade cleaning products.

How To Find Quality Essential Oils

The most important thing to consider when shopping for essential oils is product quality. But figuring out which oils are the best is challenging since no government agency in the US provides a grading system or certification for essential oils. A big problem? Many companies claim their essential oils are "therapeutic grade," but that's just a marketing term. Unfortunately, there are many products you might find online or in stores that aren't harvested correctly or may have something in them that isn't listed on the label.

Here Are Some Tips To Help You Shop For Pure Essential Oils:

- **Look At The Label:** It should include the Latin name of the plant, information on purity or other ingredients added to it, and the country in which the plant was grown.
- **Evaluate The Company:** Purchase products from a well-known and reputable aromatherapy company that's been around for several years.
- **Choose Dark-Colored Glass Containers:** Pure essential oils are highly concentrated. They can dissolve plastic bottles over time, tainting the oil. Most companies package crucial oils in small brown or blue glass bottles to protect the quality.
- **Avoid "Fragrance Oils":** Fragrance or perfume oils are made from essential oils combined with chemicals or entirely from chemicals. They're not suitable for aromatherapy, instead, look for bottles that contain a single essential oil in its purest form (100% essential oil with no other fillers).
- **Compare Prices:** Essential oils range in price, depending on how involved harvesting and production are. There should be a wide variety of costs within a line. Rose absolute or sandalwood oils will be more expensive, while sweet orange oil will be less expensive. If you find a rock-bottom price for an expensive essential oil, it probably isn't pure.

How To Choose The Right Essential Oils

Many companies claim that their oils are "pure" or "medical grade." However, these terms aren't universally defined and therefore hold little weight. Given that they're products of an unregulated industry, the quality and composition of essential oils can vary greatly. Keep the following tips in mind to choose only high-quality oils:

- **Purity:** Find an oil that contains only aromatic plant compounds, without additives or synthetic oils. Pure oils usually list the plant's botanical name (such as Lavandula officinalis) rather than terms like "essential oil of lavender."
- **Quality:** True essential oils are the ones that have been changed the least by the extraction process. Choose a chemical-free essential oil that has been extracted through distillation or mechanical cold pressing.
- **Reputation:** Purchase a brand with a reputation for producing high-quality products.

Uses

Essential oils are often used to ease stress, boost mood, relieve pain from headaches and migraines, get a better night's sleep, quell nausea, and even repel insects. Most essential oils have antiseptic properties as well.

The beneficial compounds in oils often are delivered in three ways inhalation, topical application to the skin, and oral ingestion.

Inhalation: Essential oils typically are extracted using steam distillation, which involves applying steam to a plant until only oil remains. Essential oils contain volatile compounds, which make up the solid characteristic scent and their therapeutic effects. When inhaled, molecules in essential oils are believed to influence the nervous system and the limbic area of the brain and hormones, brain chemicals, and metabolism.

Topical: Essential oils sometimes are applied directly to the skin to treat pain in a specific body part to relieve backache, for example, or to ease sore muscles, or to relieve sinus pain, and who may use some topically for their antiseptic and anti-inflammatory properties, such as for acne or fungal infections.

However, many essential oils can be irritating and so should not be applied full-strength to the skin but instead diluted in a carrier oil (such as almond, apricot kernel, or avocado oil) first.

Essential Oils That Irritate Skin

These should never be applied directly to the skin unless properly diluted:

- Bay
- Cinnamon
- Clove
- Citronella
- Lemongrass
- Oregano
- Thyme

Always test essential oils on a small patch of skin before applying to a larger area. Essential oils are sometimes added to soap, lotion, shampoo, bath salts, and other products and used during massage and spa treatments.

Ingestion

who can use some essential oils in cooking or even be swallowed in small doses as medication, but should do this with great caution. While many are safe in small amounts, others are inherently poisonous and should never be ingested.

The potential risk of ingesting essential oils is heightened by the fact the FDA does not regulate them FDA, and there are no universal standards for ensuring the quality of the oil.

Essential oils should only be ingested with the guidance of a qualified important oil therapist and dosed and diluted appropriately for safety. Because essential oils are fat-soluble, it's necessary to eat some sort of dietary fat simultaneously they're taken.

Health Benefits

who can use essential oils to treat many physical and emotional health issues? At the molecular level, these oils contain beneficial compounds like antioxidants, terpenes, and esters that may help to boost wellness.

Although the body of research showing potential health benefits of essential oils is growing, many studies are limited to testing on animals and cell cultures. Large-scale human clinical trials looking at the effects of individual oils on specific health conditions are lacking. It evaluated the general health effects of supplements, herbs, and essential oils and found oils are as practical as other supplements in improving health.

In particular, study participants reported improved immunity, reduced pain and anxiety, and enhanced energy and mental clarity. Laboratory tests also found enhanced blood markers associated with cholesterol, diabetes, and heart disease.

Common Oils

There are dozens of essential oils, each with a unique scent and potential healing properties.

- Basil: Distilled from the popular cooking herb, basil oil is believed to ease coughs and congestion, enhance mood, improve digestion, increase alertness, and soothe muscle aches.
- Bergamot: This citrus oil gives Earl Grey tea its distinctive flavor and is used to relieve anxiety. Bergamot also is being studied for its potential to lower cholesterol.
- Calendula: A relative of the marigold, calendula may soothe rashes, wounds, yeast infections, and other skin irritations.
- Carrot seed: Used in cosmetics, this oil has antibacterial and anti-inflammatory properties.
- Cedarwood: Cedarwood oil may also ease stress and improve sleep when used to treat hair loss.
- Cinnamon: Research suggests the oil in this popular spice may improve circulation, relieve stress, ease pain, fight off infections, and improve digestion.
- Citronella: A natural insect repellant, citronella also may relieve stress and fatigue.
- Clove: Spicy clove oil can be used to treat toothaches and other types of pain.
- Eucalyptus: The active ingredient in VapoRub, eucalyptus is commonly used to treat colds, congestion, and coughs and is being studied for antibacterial benefits.
- Frankincense: This Biblical oil can help treat dry skin and reduce the appearance of wrinkles, age spots, scars, and stretch marks. It is also being investigated as an anti-cancer agent.
- Geranium: Commonly used in skincare, research shows this floral oil has antimicrobial properties.
- Grapefruit: This citrus oil is said to relieve hangovers and jet lag and reduce stress, stimulate circulation, increase energy, enhance mood, and improve digestion.
- Helichrysum: This oil has a medicinal scent and is often used to reduce inflammation, promote healing of wounds and burns, stimulate digestion, boost the immune system, and soothe the body and mind.
- Jasmine: A sweet-smelling floral oil, jasmine is touted as a stress-reliever with the potential to help treat dry skin and signs of aging, inflammation, and psoriasis.
- Lavender: One of the most widely used essential oils, lavender is used to relax and relieve insomnia.
- Lemon: Said to boost mood and energy, this citrus oil relieves anxiety and may help promote weight loss.
- Lemongrass: Used for stress relief and to help boost immunity, studies suggest this oil can treat dandruff and fungal infections and ease anxiety, headaches, and upset stomach.

- Myrrh: Myrrh is believed to ease coughs and colds, soothe digestive discomfort, and boost immunity.
- Neem: Neem is used to treat nail fungus and acne. It also is an effective insect repellent.
- Neroli: This sweet oil is used to relieve anxiety and may lower blood pressure.
- Orange: The bright citrus scent of orange can boost energy and improve mood. There's also research to suggest it can ease anxiety.
- Patchouli: This musky scent, popular in incense, has been found to improve sleep in studies.
- Peppermint: This popular oil is used for headaches, pain, and stomach issues like irritable bowel syndrome.
- Rose: One of the more expensive essential oils, this highly prized soothing floral scent may ease stress and menstrual cramps.
- Rosemary: Distilled from the cooking herb, rosemary essential oil is believed to enhance mental focus and is being studied to prevent dementia.
- Sandalwood: Popular in meditation centers and spas, this fragrant, earthy scent is thought to relieve anxiety and improve sleep.
- Tea Tree: Essential oil is said to have antimicrobial, antiseptic, and disinfectant qualities. It is commonly used in shampoos and skin care products to treat acne, burns, and bites. It features in mouth rinses, but it should never be swallowed, as it is toxic.
- Thyme: Essential oil is said to help reduce fatigue, nervousness, and stress.
- Yarrow: Essential oil is used to treat cold and flu symptoms and help reduce joint inflammation.
- Ylang ylang: Used to relieve pain, reduce inflammation, improve mood, and enhance libido.

Possible Side Effects

When used as directed, essential oils have few side effects or risks, although the way a given oil is used has a great deal of bearing on its safety.

Inhaling the scent of essential oils is the safest way to use them. The potential side effects of breathing in essential oil are minor and, depending on the oil, include headache, nausea, burning of eyes and throat, cough, or shortness of breath. These side effects typically resolve when the scent is no longer detectable.

Topical application of essential oils is generally safe. However, certain oils can cause a reaction that may include contact dermatitis, burns, and skin irritation. A patch test should always be done when using a new essential oil to see if you're sensitive to it.

Certain oils increase photosensitivity and may increase the risk of sunburn, especially citrus oils, such as lemon, lime, grapefruit, bergamot, and tangerine. It's advisable to stay out of the sun for 24 hours after applying any of these oils to your skin.

Ingesting essential oils is not always safe and depends on the oil. Many essential oils are FDA-approved as ingredients in food and fragrances and are labeled generally regarded as safe (GRAS). However, some oils can be toxic and only be ingested under medical supervision. Use caution when ingesting essential oils, and do not swallow large amounts.

Do not use essential oils near your eyes, genitals, or mucous membranes. If you get an oil in your eyes or mucous membrane, you can dilute it with a carrier oil.

Like any health supplement, essential oils may interact with prescription medications when taken internally. Check with your doctor or pharmacist before combining any essential oil with drugs.

ESSENTIAL OILS: BENEFITS, RISKS, AND SAFE STORAGE

Essential oils are highly-concentrated liquids made from plants. Examples include eucalyptus oil, clove oil, camphor, citronella, and tea tree oil. These products contain many active chemicals and have strong fragrances. This makes them popular ingredients in soaps, massage oils, perfumes, bath oils and salts, home fragrance diffusers, and potpourri. Essential oils smell great, reduce stress, treat fungal infections, and help you sleep. They are concentrated extractions from plants. Distillation turns the "essence" of a plant into a liquefied form for many medicinal and recreational uses.

There's a wide variety of essential oils available. Some are valued for their pleasing aroma. Others claim to have powerful healing properties. But their potency can have side effects you must be aware of.

Benefits & Risks Of Essential Oils

Proponents of aromatherapy and herbal remedies claim that some essential oils are therapeutic in treating specific health concerns. People may not realize, however, that some can also be very toxic. Upon contact with the skin or eyes, essential oils may irritate such as redness and burning, remarkably if undiluted. However, the real danger comes from swallowing them.

Children are attracted to sweet, citrusy, or minty fragrances and may mistake the products for familiar treats. Essential oils contain highly concentrated active chemicals, so it doesn't take a lot to cause health effects. These effects vary from oil to oil but may include nausea and vomiting, drowsiness, confusion, difficulty walking, restlessness, seizures, coma, or liver failure.

Children have died from drinking as little as one teaspoon of eucalyptus oil, camphor, or wintergreen oil. If you plan to use them in your home, treat them the same way you would treat medicines, cleaning products, or other household chemicals: Keep them stored up high, out of sight and reach of children.

Other Essential Oil Safety Tips

- Keep essential oils in their original containers. Transferring them to another container could lead to confusion.
- Only buy products in child-resistant containers, if possible.
- Always dilute essential oils if you plan to use them topically.
- Certain essential oils are flammable, so keep them away from flame sources.
- Many are unsafe to swallow. Consult an expert before ingesting them in any form.
- If you are pregnant or nursing, talk to your health care provider before using essential oils.

How Do You Use Essential Oils?

I will advises that the safest ways to use oils are to dilute them for topical use or diffuse them for direct inhalation. Essential oils should always be applied with a barrier substance (like oil, lotion, or aloe jelly) when using topically. It is even more critical to the first mix the oils with a barrier substance if used in a bath, as oil and water don't mix.

It also dispels the notion that applying essential oils to the bottom of the feet is the best way to absorb the properties. It says using oils to the tops of feet, arms, wrists, neck, and behind the ear generally produce better and more consistent results for most people. For those inhaling essential oils, I recommends using a waterless or water-based diffuser. Waterless diffusers are great for those with respiratory issues or immunocompromised states, as the deletion of water reduces the risk of waterborne bacteria being distributed.

HOW TO MAKE ESSENTIAL OILS

There are three methods to get essential oils. These are extraction, distillation, and expression. The distillation process is the most complicated. It requires specialized equipment and careful monitoring. As for the expression method, the product is not usually classified as an essential oil. This leaves us with the extraction method. In this tutorial, we will try rose essential oil-making, so let's get started!

What You'll Need:

- Flowers or plant parts to extract (in this case rose petals)
- 120-proof vodka
- Clear quart glass jar with a lid
- Small dark-colored bottle
- Porcelain-coated strainer
- Small glass bowl
- Tight-weave cheesecloth
- A spoon and medicine dropper

Step 1: Prepare Your Choice of Plant

You can use any kind of plant, from herbs, scented flowers to fruits. It all depends on the plant essence you want to be extracted. In this tutorial, we will be using roses. The more homegrown roses you have, the better.

You'll need pounds and pounds of plant material to make a small amount of essence. Prepare the roses by using a dehydrator to evaporate their natural water content. The roses will be ready when they start to wilt.

Step 2: Prepare The Jar

Prepare jars and fill them with rose petals. Pour vodka into the jar until the petals are submerged. Place the pot in a dark corner of the kitchen cupboard to sit undisturbed at room temperature.

Take the jar out three times a day and give it a good shake for several minutes. Repeat daily until you see the roses losing color, which could take up to a week.

Step 3: Straining Vodka Solution

Wearing protective gloves, take out the jar and prepare to strain. Strain out the plant material from the vodka by using a porcelain-coated strainer. Be careful not to spill any amount of liquid.

Shake the roses into the cheesecloth and squeeze it out by hand to get every last bit of vodka out. By this time, the vodka will smell terrible but don't worry, that's normal.

Step 4: Repeat Soaking Process

Repeat the rose soaking method several times with a new batch of rose petals using the same vodka. Make sure not to waste vodka when straining.

If needed, you can add a little more vodka to make sure the rose petals are submerged. The more you do this, you will be able to extract more of the essential oils.

Step 5: Storing Vodka Solution

Once you're done with the rose soaking, strain as usual. But this time, return the vodka into the quart glass and seal it. Put it in the dark corner of the cupboard again, leaving it undisturbed for a day or two. By this time, you will see some separation starting to occur. The vodka will separate from the essential oils and other plant matter.

Step 6: Freeze Solution

Place the jar in the freezer. This is the cool part–vodka does not freeze. So, only the essential oils and other plant materials will solidify.

Step 7: Strain Solution

Now, you will have to move fast with extra caution before the essential oil melts. You will need a piece of cheesecloth laid inside a glass bowl. Use another piece of cheesecloth secured around a clear canning jar, so it dips inside the neck. You will also need another small glass bowl and a small dark bottle which will hold the essential oil. Have a spoon and dropper ready as well.

Step 8: Harvest Essential Oils

Remove the jar from the freezer. Skim the gunky plant material off the vodka and place it on the cheesecloth laid inside the bowl. Pour the vodka into the other glass jar with the loose cheesecloth.

Move quickly to pick out any frozen bits using a dropper and place them inside the small dark bottle. The frozen bits are the essential oils.

What You Need To Know When Making Essential Oils

Essential oils are not oils that contain fatty acids. Instead, they are the concentrated plant essence. What is good in a plant reflects in its essential oil so that you can use it for personal care, disinfection, or healing.

Essential oil examples are peppermint, tea tree, and roses. They are known for their antibacterial, antifungal, and antiviral properties.

Essential oils are distinct from fragrance oils. They only mimic the scents of plants and do not have the important oil benefits.

Essential oils are hard to find in localities, which is why they are expensive. This is a good reason why it's good to learn the art of making essential oils from dried herbs yourself.

Mood-Boosting Essential Oils

There are many benefits of essential oils, and some essential oils are known to boost mood and increase serotonin levels in the body. Here are some mood-boosting essential oils:

- Mandarin Essential Oil
- Lime Essential Oil
- Sweet Orange Essential Oil
- Bitter Orange Essential Oil
- Bergamot Essential Oil
- Grapefruit Essential Oil
- Peppermint Essential Oil
- Spearmint Essential Oil
- Lavender Essential Oil
- Chamomile Essential Oil
- Tangerine Essential Oil

5 Ways To Use Essential Oils

There are different ways to use essential oils, and you can blend them as well! Here are five ways you can use your essential oils to boost your mood:

Diffuser Blend: Add two drops of desired essential oils with the required amount of water (depending on your diffuser) and enjoy!

Roller Blend: Add two drops of desired essential oils to a roller bottle and fill the rest of the bottle with jojoba oil or coconut oil. You can use this blend on your arms, legs, chest.

Massage Oil Blend: Blend 2 drops of desired essential oils into a 1oz, but then fill the rest of the bottle with almond and oil, then massages it onto your skin.

Bath Salt Blend: Add 3-5 drops of desired essential oils to castile soap and add it to your bathwater.

Room Spray Blend: Add two drops of desired essential oil into a 1oz spray bottle and fill the rest with distilled water

Reminder: Do not apply undiluted essential oils directly to your skin. Essential oils need to be diluted in a carrier oil before being used.

Dos And Don'ts of Essential Oils

1. DO Try It If You're Anxious: Simple smells such as lavender, chamomile, and rosewater may help keep you calm. You can breathe in or rub diluted versions of these oils on your skin. Scientists think they work by sending chemical messages to parts of the brain that affect mood and emotion. Although these scents alone won't take all your stress away, the aroma may help you relax.

DON'T Just Rub Them Anywhere: Oils that are fine on your arms and legs may not be safe to put inside your mouth, nose, eyes, or private parts. Lemongrass, peppermint, and cinnamon bark are some examples.

2. DO Check The Quality: Look for a trusted producer that makes pure oils without anything added. You're more likely to have an allergic reaction to oils that have other ingredients. Not all extras are nasty. Some added vegetable oil may be standard for sure more expensive essential oils.

DON'T Trust Buzzwords: Just because it's from a plant doesn't mean it's safe to rub on your skin, or breathe, or eat, even if it's "pure." Natural substances can be irritating, toxic, or cause allergic reactions. Like anything else you put on your skin, it's best to test a little bit on a small area and see how your skin responds.

3. DO Toss Out Older Oils: In general, don't keep them for more than three years. Older oils are more likely to be spoiled because of exposure to oxygen. They may not work as well and could irritate your skin or cause an allergic reaction. If you see a significant change in how an oil looks, feels or smells, you should throw it out because it has probably spoiled.

DON'T Put Edible Oils On Your Skin: Cumin oil, which is safe to use in your food, can cause blisters if you put it on your skin. Citrus oils that are safe in your food may be harmful to your skin, especially if you go out into the sun. And the opposite is true, too. Eucalyptus or sage oil may soothe you if you rub it on your skin or breathe it in. But swallowing them could cause a severe complication, like a seizure.

4. DO Tell Your Doctor: Your doctor can ensure it's safe for you and rule out any side effects, like affecting your prescriptions. For example, peppermint and eucalyptus oils may change how your body absorbs the cancer drug 5-fluorouracil from the skin. Or an allergic reaction may cause rashes, hives, or breathing problems.

DO Dilute Them: Undiluted oils are too strong to use straight. You'll need to dilute them, usually with vegetable oils or creams or bath gels, to a solution that only has a little bit 1% to 5% of the essential oil. Exactly how much can vary? The higher the percentage, the more likely you will react, so mixing them correctly is necessary.

5. DON'T Use On Damaged Skin: Injured or inflamed skin will absorb more oil and may cause unwanted skin reactions. Undiluted oils, which you shouldn't use at all, can be downright dangerous on damaged skin.

DO Consider Age: Young children and the elderly may be more sensitive to essential oils. So you may need to dilute them more. And you should avoid some oils, like birch and wintergreen. In even small amounts, those may cause severe problems in kids six or younger because they contain a chemical called methyl salicylate. Don't use essential oils on a baby unless your pediatrician says it's OK.

6. DON'T Forget To Store Them Safely: They can be very concentrated and may cause serious health problems, mainly if used at the wrong dose or in the wrong way. Just like anything else that little hands shouldn't reach, don't make your essential oils too handy. If you have young children, keep all essential oils locked away out of their sight and reach.

DO Stop Use If Your Skin Reacts: Your skin might love essential oils. But if it doesn't and you notice a rash, little bumps, boils, or just itchy skin, take a break. More of the same oil can make it worse. Whether you mixed it yourself or it's an ingredient in a ready-made cream,or oil, gently wash it off with water.

7. DO Choose Your Therapist Carefully: If you look for a professional aromatherapist, do your homework. By law, they don't have to have training or a license. But you can check to see if you went to a school certified by professional organizations like National Association for Holistic Aromatherapy.

DON'T Overdo It: More of a good thing is not always good. Even when diluted, the essential oil can cause a bad reaction if you use too much or use it too often. That's true even if you're not allergic or unusually sensitive to them.

8. DO Take Care If Pregnant: Some essential massage oils may make their way into the placenta, an organ in your uterus that grows along with your baby and helps to nourish it. It's not clear if this causes any problems unless you take toxic amounts, but to be safe, it's best to avoid certain oils if you're pregnant. Those include wormwood, rue, oakmoss, Lavandula stoechas, camphor, parsley seed, sage, and hyssop. Ask your doctor if you're unsure.

DON'T Be Afraid To Try Them: Used the right way, they can help you feel better with few side effects. For example, you may feel less nauseated from chemotherapy cancer treatment if you breathe in ginger vapors. You may be able to fight specific bacterial or fungal infections, including the dangerous MRSA bacteria, with tea tree oil.

ESSENTIAL OIL RECIPES CURE FOR AILMENTS

1. The Perfect Blend Of Essential Oils For Endometriosis

Prep Time: 5 Minutes

Total Time: 5 Minutes

Ingredients

- 4 ounces organic jojoba oil (see notes)
- 25 drops lavender
- 15 drops rosemary oil
- 5 drops peppermint oil

Instructions

- Combine the jojoba oil with lavender, rosemary, and peppermint oil.
- Then pour the blend into an amber jar (of any kind) for storage.

2. Aphrodisiac Essential Oil Recipe

Prep Time: 10 minutes

Ingredients

- 15 drops Ylang Ylang Essential Oil
- 15 drops Cardamon essential oil
- 10 drops vanilla essential oil
- Organic jojoba oil
- One blob Peru Balsam essential oil OPTIONAL
- 10ml 1 glass roll-on

Instructions

- Add the essential oil drops to a roll-on glass bottle.
- Fill up the 10 ml glass bottle with jojoba oil.
- Shake well!
- You can use this aphrodisiac perfume right away. However, it's best to allow 24h to let the essential oil blend well together. Enjoy!

3. Essential Oil Poison Ivy

Total Time: 2 minutes

Ingredients

- 2-ounce glass bottle
- 1 ½ tablespoon Aloe vera gel
- ½ tablespoon witch hazel
- 5 drops peppermint essential oil
- Five drops of geranium essential oil
- Five drops of rosemary essential oil

Instructions

- Pour the aloe vera gel and witch hazel into the bottle with a small funnel.
- Add the essential oil blend and shake well.

4. Thieves Essential Oil Blend Recipe

Prep Time: 5 minutes

Total Time: 5 minutes

Ingredients

- 2 tbsp clove essential oil
- 2 tbsp lemon essential oil
- 2 tbsp eucalyptus essential oil
- 2 tbsp rosemary essential oil
- 2.5 tbsp cinnamon bark oil

Instructions

- Gather all five essential oils and a 15 ml glass bottle, tinted blue or brown. Tinted glass bottles help reflect the sun's rays and protect the essential oil blend.
- Add all five ingredients to the bottle.
- Shake vigorously to blend the oils well. You can store the bottle in a cool, dark, and dry place.

5. Wellness Thieves Oil Tea

Cook Time: 2 min

Total Time: 2 minutes

Ingredients

- 1 cup hot water
- One drop of thieves young living essential oil
- Two drops of lemon young living essential oil
- One drop frankincense young living essential oil
- 1–2 teaspoons raw honey
- Optional: a slice of fresh lemon

Instructions

- Heat water up in the microwave for 2 minutes.
- Remove. Add essential oils and honey to the hot water. Stir and drink.

CONCLUSION

Essential oils are used every day to treat a variety of physical and emotional ailments. Some essential oils have been shown to have medicinal properties but should be used with caution. Ingesting essential oils should only be done under the supervision of a healthcare practitioner. Essential oils are the liquid extracts of potentially beneficial plants. People are beginning to use essential oils widely for various common conditions, and some research shows they may help relieve symptoms in some cases. Essential oils are generally safe when a person uses them correctly. Always dilute essential oils before applying them to the skin and never ingest them.

Essential oils have a variety of health benefits, from skincare to stress relief. The most common way to use essential oils is to inhale them, either directly out of the bottle or using a diffuser or humidifier. You can also dilute essential oils with a carrier oil and apply it now to your skin. Or you can get creative and add the mixture to a body wash, shampoo, or bath. Remember always to use caution with essential oils, especially when you first start trying them. Keep your eye out for any adverse reactions, and be mindful of potency.

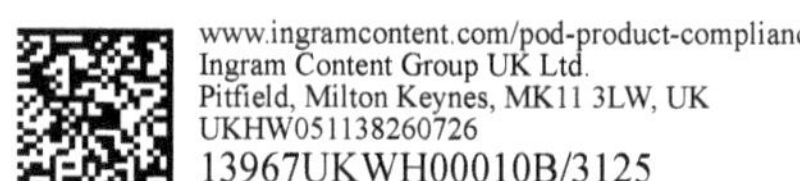

www.ingramcontent.com/pod-product-compliance
Ingram Content Group UK Ltd.
Pitfield, Milton Keynes, MK11 3LW, UK
UKHW051138260726
13967UKWH00010B/3125

9 781801 886130